W9-BZD-870

TOTAL HEALTH = WHOLENESS

A BODY, MIND, AND SPIRIT MANUAL

Dr. Keith Nemec

www.totalhealthinstitute.com

Total Health = Wholeness

A Body, Mind, & Spirit Manual

Copyright © 2000 by Total Health Institute

All Rights Reserved

For information about permission
to reproduce selections from this book,
write to Total Heath Institute
23 W 525 St. Charles Rd.
Wheaton, IL 60188

ISBN: 0-9700435-0-3

For information on how individual consumers can place orders,
or for orders of **10 or more** copies for special markets or premium use,
please call Total Health Institute at (630) 871-0000
or visit www.totalhealthinstitute.com

Published by Total Health Institute
by arrangement with Hosanna Publications, Inc.

Printed in the United States of America

CONTENTS

Forward	iv
Introduction	vi
1. Health, Wellness, and Wholeness	8
2. Disease	28
3. My Health: Where Did I Lose It?	50
4. The Interrelation of Total Health	70
5. Wholeness Assessment	79
6. You Are What You Eat	93
7. Water And Air	105
8. Toxicity - The Modern Day Cause of Disease	115
9. Spiritual Health	120
10. Mental Health	147
11. Nutritional Health	166
12. Digestive Health	209
13. Assimilative Health	232
14. Eliminative Health	247
15. Circulative Health	265
16. Immune Health	275
17. Oxidative Health	285
18. Organ/Gland Health	294
19. Light and Energy	302
20. Recommendations for Wholeness	308
Appendix I: Total Health Checklist	318
Appendix II: Total Health Institute's Products	320
Endnotes	331

FORWARD

This book was written out of an extension of a relationship between myself and the Living God. For me, the discovery of the Living God came when I entered into a deep, intimate, and personal relationship with Jesus Christ. He so changed my life forever that I realized that God is love, and His love is able to meet needs and change hearts and lives today. This book is not intended to offend anyone of any religious or non-religious belief. The Living God loves everyone of every race, creed, color, and belief. If you seek Him, you will find Him when you seek Him with all your heart. No matter what your beliefs are there are spiritual, mental, and emotional concepts that can give you a greater revelation in your own spiritual, mental, emotional journey. The physical health topics covered will be life changing for your body if you adopt them into your lifestyle. One last comment: The man or woman who has an open mind and heart and seeks revelation will find it, and sometimes in the most unlikely places.

This book is dedicated to Jesus Christ and my wife, Laurie, because they are the two most important individuals in my life. They are both responsible for me beginning this journey into wholeness and writing this book. Let me briefly share our story. After our second child, John Paul, was born, Laurie's health seemed to be declining. One day, while playing tennis, she became extremely weak and fatigued. This was very unusual for Laurie, a former professional ballerina, whose schedule was extremely demanding and who was never affected by all the long hours of intense physical activity. This fatigue was unlike any she had experienced since her teens, when she had developed mononucleosis. What we did not know was that this was just the tip of an iceberg of ill health. Over the course of the next 19 months her health continued to decline, and she experienced pain in many areas of her body, immune system suppression, and progressively debilitating fatigue. We went from doctor to doctor in search of a cure but found none. Finally, my beautiful, vibrant ballerina became unable to get out of bed except to care for the most basic necessities. I had to hire help to care for my two boys when we realized this condition was not going away. In the course of her being practically bedridden, my wife and I sought the Lord for answers. As the months went by, my wife became desperate due to her inability to care for her family and herself. Her reason for living was fading, and suicidal thoughts started to enter her mind. In a final through the Bible, as she had done so many times before, looking up all the scriptures where Jesus healed the sick. She asked, "If you did it then, why won't you do it now?" And as she sank into her bed, a still, quiet voice spoke inside her and said, "Believe in my Word and you will be healed." She then received a vision of herself in the wide open ocean; there in front of her was a life preserver, and it was the Word of God. Encouraged by these words from the Lord, my wife began her first steps of faith out of her sick bed, to which she never would return. As the months went by, she progressively began to get stronger, and again the Lord spoke to her heart and told her to change her diet.

This led to much research and eventually her recovery. Not only was she healed, or made whole, so was our oldest son, Joseph, who had struggled with many health problems from the time he was born. In this trial of life, Jesus showed my family and me what health really is, and that this precious gift should be cherished and always held in high regard.

Through this suffering, we were finally able to rejoice and praise the Lord, for His love endures forever. Although the Lord did not put us into this trial, He gloriously delivered us out of it. The benefit is not only for us, but for all those to whom we can teach the steps to total health = wholeness.

Dr. Keith J. Nemec

INTRODUCTION

In the first part of this book I will be dividing physical health into five categories: genetic, structural, chemical, eliminative, and physical. To these I will add mental health and spiritual health to build a foundation of wholeness. Therefore I named this book *Total Health = Wholeness*.

In the second part of the book I will further break down the categories of total health into ten. They are organ/gland(structural), oxidative, immune, circulative, eliminative, assimilative, digestive, nutritional, mental, and spiritual health. The reason for expanding the number of categories is to move beyond the basic concepts of the physical aspects of health to greater detail regarding all the ways you can improve your life, living and walking in total health = wholeness.

The question may arise, What does wholeness mean? Wholeness, simply defined, is ultimate or total health of the three parts that make up an individual: the most important, the spirit; the soul, which includes the mind, will, and emotions; and the body. So to live in a state of wholeness is to be complete, not lacking anything in the spirit, which is the part of the individual which communes with God. To be complete in spirit is to have a personal relationship with the Living God who created us. This vital relationship with God will be addressed in detail in the chapter on spiritual health.

The next part is to be whole or complete in your mind, will, and emotions. This is really an extension of spiritual health, because one who has a personal relationship with the Living God will have the love, joy, and peace that God gives, and this will overflow from the spirit to the mind, will, emotions, and even the body. The love, joy, and peace that God brings is unlike any that the world could ever bring. God's love is one of self-sacrifice, as God gave His Son so that we may live abundantly and eternally with Him. The experience of God's love is wonderful because it is not dependent on us or what we do, but on Him and who He is. God is love. So when God lives in our hearts, we experience His love. God's joy is unchangeable. When we experience the joy of the Lord, it is not dependent upon our circumstances but on the God who lives inside us. His joy is there in the most unhappy and unlikely circumstances. His peace is the knowledge that He is with us and never leaves us nor forsakes us. He is our best our head. His peace goes beyond all human comprehension to guard our hearts and minds when we are in Him, that is, in a personal relationship with Him.

The last aspect is to be whole or complete in our physical bodies, and I will spend nine chapters addressing all aspects of physical health.

Dr. Keith J. Nemec

CHAPTER 1

HEALTH, WELLNESS, AND WHOLENESS

To begin any book entitled *Total Health = Wholeness*, we must begin with a definition of terms. First, let us define health. Dorland's Medical Dictionary defines it as "a state of optimal mental, physical, and social well being, not merely the absence of disease or infirmity." What we can conclude from this definition is that health is more than just feeling good — a lot more. I see this all the time at the Institute. A patient comes in with terrible lower back pain and can hardly move and after complete examination, is found to have a muscle strain. However, another patient comes in with minimal complaints of lower back stiffness and, after X-ray examination, is found to have severe degenerative arthritis and disc disease, on the verge of tremendous pain and disability. So what we see and feel is not always a true indicator of our health.

"I Feel Great"

This is a common expression of an average American who has no apparent health problems. When asked how do they feel, they respond "I feel great," or "good," or "OK," or something to the nature of being able to do what they want in life with enough energy and without pain. When looking deeper into the average person we start to see that "I feel great" type of people are not always what they appear to be and feel. Take for instance the person who has $^{200}/_{150}$ blood pressure. He outwardly might feel great, but inwardly, he is not. He is a time bomb ready to explode with a heart attack or stroke. Take the woman who says she feels great but has an undetected malignant tumor in her breast. Cancer doesn't hurt until it is in advanced stages. Or the man who says "I feel great" and has 90% occluded coronary arteries because of cholesterol buildup and is destined for a heart attack. How about children who are filled with energy, eating loads of refined sugar and progressively weakening their immunity and predisposing them to the number 1 disease that causes death in kids: cancer. Are you starting to get the picture? Health is far more than feeling great or good. All the time, people take caffeine, sugar, and nicotine, all stimulants, to keep them going with pseudo energy all day. They take pills for every symptom you can think of, and they feel okay. This is not health. This is chemistry. This is putting more and more Band-Aids over an ever-growing wound. This is running on empty and never knowing it until it's too late. There is a better way: to live in total health of body, mind, and spirit: to not only feel good, but to BE good. This only comes from energy and effort directed in the ways of producing total health. This is done by addressing the cause of heath problems instead of the effects. This is right now, today, starting to build a solid foundation of total health that will not topple like one built on sinking sand. How do you do this? By addressing every aspect of your health and working—yes, I said working—to optimize each area. This can be done by making changes in your life according to each chapter in this book. We address twelve areas of health:

Spiritual
Mental/Emotional
Nutritional
Digestive
Assimilative
Eliminative
Circulative
Immune
Oxidative
Nerve
Gland/Organ
Energy

This is the goal of this book: to lead you to higher levels of health, one step at a time, so you and your family will not only feel great, but you will actually BE great.

There are various aspects of our health picture. I will first divide them into physical (which can be further broken down into genetic, structural, eliminative, and cardiovascular), chemical, mental, and spiritual health. Our objective is that each one of these health components function optimally or to the best of their ability. Let us start with genetic health.

Genetic health

Genetic health is the inherent makeup that has been passed down to us by our parents, grandparents, etc. This is the only aspect of our health picture over which we have no control. If a man's father died of a heart attack when he was 50, and his grandfather died at the same age, chances are there is a genetic weakness of heart disease in his family which predisposes him to the same condition. This, though, should not depress us or give us a defeated attitude, because if we work on optimizing all the other aspects of our health picture, the chances of the genetic predisposition affecting our total health are decreased. Remember this: Our health is no one's responsibility but our own. We might not be able to change the genetic predisposition, but we sure can work to change our physical, mental, structural, chemical, eliminatory, and spiritual health. You might be asking, "How?" We will examine them one at a time.

Let us take the example of a man — let's call him George — who has heart disease running in his family. His genetic health factor is not very good. But let's move on to the next health factor: his structural health.

Structural health(Organ/Gland health)

Structural health involves our nerves and the organs and glands they supply, muscles, and bones.

The nervous system is the master control of all other bodily systems. If the nervous system malfunctions, it causes major imbalances in our health, much like the mass confusion that results when telephone lines go down, or the system malfunctions of a computer when the hard drive is faulty. So it is of utmost importance that we maintain a healthy nervous system, and to do that we must understand the No. 1 cause of nervous system imbalance and disorder: subluxation, or spinal bone misalignment pressing on the spinal nerve, causing anything from organ or gland dysfunction to pain, numbness, tingling, weakness, and/or burning.

If George had poor posture or at any time had structurally stressed his upper back (thoracic region), he could have misaligned or subluxated a spinal bone (vertebrae). This misalignment may press on the nerves in the spinal column that supply the heart and lungs. Misalignment can cause nerve irritation and impingement (pinching), which can cause decreased nerve energy going to the heart. This can cause George's heart to function much less than optimally, and possibly lead to problems which adversely affect his physical health picture. The effects of pressure on a nerve to an organ can be illustrated with the analogy of a dimmer switch: The more you turn the switch, the less electricity flows to the light bulb. Another analogy is that of a garden hose with the water turned on: If you step on the hose, less water will come out. Misaligned spinal bones similarly produce nerve pressure resulting in organ or gland dysfunction. So as you can see, structural health can be a positive or negative influence on George's *total health = wholeness.*

Circulative health

Circulative health, as defined in this book, is all that moves, primarily the circulatory system (blood flow) and the lymphatic system (lymph fluid flow.) The actual movement of our bodies with physical exercise is another component of circulative health.

The importance of this aspect of our health picture lies in the fact that it is through the blood and lymph flow that our body's immunity is maintained. White blood cells (WBCs) are carried through these systems to protect us from all foreign invaders (bacteria, viruses, fungi, and parasites) and invaders from within (mutant cancer cells). Every body produces cancer cells, but it is the job of the macrophage and the natural killer (NK) white blood cells to seek out, find, and destroy all cells that don't belong.

When I think of circulative health, I think of Dr. Joseph Janses' statement that "life is motion". To maintain optimum physical health, we must move or exercise. Movement not only strengthens our cardiovascular system but also affects every other system of our bodies. Physical movement or exercise causes our blood and lymph to circulate at a much faster rate, which brings more oxygen to all parts of the body and helps remove waste products and toxins at a greater rate. This faster rate of blood and lymph flow has an enormous health benefit with the immune system cells. For each 1-degree rise in body temperature, the speed and activity of the white blood cells doubles. In this way, fevers are one of God's mechanisms for destroying invaders to our bodies; therefore they should not be suppressed with medication. With a fever of 102.6 degrees, our WBCs are moving 16 times faster than normal, thus increasing our immune system response. Physical exercise also helps reduce the tension and stress that builds up in our muscles from our hectic lives. Needless to say, if George is on a three- to six-day-a-week aerobic exercise schedule (aerobic means elevated and sustained heart rate, not necessarily the exercise of aerobics) for 30 minutes per day, he is definitely going to get his heart muscle in better shape and will reduce his chances of his genetics catching up to him.

Chemical health

I have defined chemical health as simply "what goes in." Looked at from a systems perspective, this includes the digestive, assimilation, and respiratory systems. Digestion includes that which gets broken down to actually enter the body. Assimilation refers to what actually comes into the bloodstream as far as food and beverage is concerned. The last system included is the respiratory system, which brings life-giving oxygen and releases life-threatening carbon dioxide.

What I mean by chemical health is the effects of every chemical that enters our body, from the air we breathe to the water we drink to the food we eat. Once again, if George's job does not involve working amidst chemical fumes, he doesn't smoke, and he gets exercise in which he deeply breathes fresh air, this will be to his benefit. Also, if George drinks pure water (either reverse-osmosis or distilled water, rather than tap water), and if he eats a low-fat, low-sugar, low-salt diet which is high in fruits, vegetables, whole grains, seeds, nuts, and limited in red meats, chicken, fish, and dairy products, he is positively adding to his *total health = wholeness*.

Eliminatory health

Eliminatory health is defined as what comes out. This includes the five-organ system of liver/gall bladder, kidney/bladder, bowel, lungs, and skin. All these systems have an excretory element, ridding the body of unwanted waste products from cellular metabolism, internal toxic buildup, external toxic overload, and external chemical input. The reason this system plays such a vital role in our *total health = wholeness* picture is that no matter how much good you put in or how much of any of the other seven health categories you strengthen, if you are not eliminating waste products and toxins, you will become toxic and eventually ill. Imagine putting a small air filter in a room with a raging fire that is producing large amounts of smoke. The small air filter simply cannot keep up with the overload. Toxins and waste products must be removed, because any impairment in this area will lead to sickness.

Mental health

George's mental health can affect his *total health = wholeness* very adversely in that his mind does affect his body. The Bible says in Proverbs 23:7, "As a man thinks in his heart, so is he" (NKJV). This means that if George has become fearful that he will indeed suffer from the same fate that befell his grandfather and father, this fear can become deadly to him. The field of psychoneuroimmunology, or PNI has emerged on the clinical psychology scene powerfully, and research has proven that our thoughts and emotions do affect our physical body. Clinical psychologists in the field of psychoneuroimmunology are finding in cancer patients that they can sometimes pinpoint a traumatic or very stressful incident one to two years prior to the development of the cancer. So if George can know in his mind that he will not end up like his father and grandfather and has no fear of their fate, this again may have a positive impact on his overall *total health = wholeness* picture.

Spiritual health

The last aspect of our *total health = wholeness*, spiritual health, also comes into play in George's situation. If George knows that God loves him and that he has a personal relationship with his Creator, this will give him love, joy, and peace. Philippians 4:6-7 says, "Do not be anxious about anything, but in everything, by prayer and petition, with thanksgiving, present your requests to God and the peace of God, which transcends all understanding, will guard your hearts and your minds in Christ Jesus." God and His Word will give George peace and hope, which once again will add to his total health profile. As you can see from the example of George, the concept that a man reaps what he sows becomes evident when we know what we have to do to be in health.

Let's pause to define wellness. Much like our original definition of health — optimal physical, mental, and social well-being —wellness means to be well and not ill or compromised in any area of one's health profile. But whereas health is the individual parts, such as physical, mental, and spiritual health, wellness looks at all the parts and fits them together as a complete picture instead of individual components. In the wellness model, mental health and spiritual health are also included. Each part of the person's wellness counts equally, all adding up to his or her level of well-being, or wellness.

Again, our objective is to be in optimal *total health = wholeness* and to adopt a lifestyle that will keep us there — well and totally in health. Wellness can be described as a combination of hereditary, structural, physical, chemical, eliminatory, and mental health. Some wellness models include the spiritual aspect of health, but only on an equal level with all other aspects of health, where one adds to his or her level of peace by being in communion with his or her God. But I am proposing a new model which I will call the *total health = wholeness* model, which goes far beyond giving spiritual health an equal place in the total health picture, to giving spiritual health the place of utmost importance. The spiritual aspect far outweighs all the others. It acknowledges that God created man to commune with Him, to know and enjoy Him, and to glorify Him. In relationship with God, man draws strength for every second of every day. This was stated so clearly by Jesus: "I am the way and the truth and the life. No one comes to the Father except through me." (John 14:6) We will discuss this in greater detail in the chapter on spiritual health.

One final definition is of utmost importance in the understanding of health: that of the term wholeness. Wholeness is the state of being complete or one in body, soul, and spirit. The difference between health and wellness is that health refers to the individual parts and wellness to the sum of the parts — genetic, structural, circulatory, physical, chemical, eliminatory, mental, and spiritual. So to say I am healthy is to say my overall health (the positive and negative influences of these individual aspects of our health added together) is good.

Wholeness goes far beyond health and wellness; it goes into the realm that made health and life in the first place. The state of wholeness is achieved when a person's body, soul, and spirit are whole, or complete and lacking nothing. Wholeness is made possible by the Spirit of God, who dwells in our spirit, the two becoming one. In wholeness, life and strength and health flow from the Spirit of God into our spirit, then into our mind, will, and emotions and finally into our physical body.

How can we lack anything when we realize that the God who created the heavens and the earth is in us? God empowers us through His Spirit so that through the Spirit, life, health, and strength can flow to our minds, and can, in turn, flow to our bodies. To be whole is to be as God created us to be. The Bible says in John 6:63, "The Spirit gives life; the flesh counts for nothing. The words I have spoken to you are spirit and they are life." The God who created us also sustains us spiritually, mentally, and physically. We will cover more of this in the chapter on spiritual health.

health = each individual part

wellness = all parts taken as a whole, but all parts essentially equal in effect on health

wholeness = all parts taken together, but spiritual the greatest, strengthening mind and body

Let's look at how it all fits together:.

Vibrant Health	Apparent Health	Not well	Disease	Death
Total health = Wholeness	(no subclinical findings)	(subclinical findings)	(clinical findings)	

Health

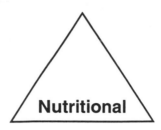

Wellness   # Wholeness

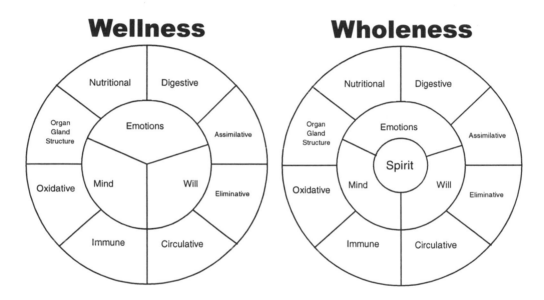

Most people address their health in a serious way only when disease has begun. Some seek diligently even when the first traces of not feeling well appear. How much more beneficial would it be if we were to begin *right now* to address our health from a wholeness point of view? The problem with some is they need "not feeling well" as a motivator, and most need disease to instill enough fear to motivate them to change their health. Why wait for sickness, disease, and fear to be the motivators? Rather let us listen to the Word of God which says, "Your body is the temple of the Holy Spirit." (1 Corinthians 6:19) Honor God with your body, and you will reap what you have sown — wholeness.

The wonderful thing in this health picture is that out of the seven categories, only one is unchangeable — genetic makeup, or inherited constitution. There is so much we can do for our health if we remember this fact: Nothing is impossible — nothing. I have seen healing miracles and do believe they are a part of God's plan for us today.

Let me just shed a few rays of hope on those of you who are sick. Did you know that your entire skeletal system is replaced in three months? Yes, I mean every cell is replaced in three months. Your DNA is replaced in two months — yes, all of it. Six weeks for your liver, one month for your skin, five days for your stomach. Your body is completely replaced in one year. Why is this significant? It means you can start making changes today that will benefit your body tomorrow. Remember you reap what you sow.

It is never too late to make a change. But there is one thing you will have to do, and this is intimidating to some people: *You will have to take responsibility for your own health*. There is nothing wrong with finding a doctor who is genuinely concerned about your health and who is willing to do alternative health care to coach you along back to health. In fact, I recommend the same doctor Thomas Edison recommended: "The doctor of

---

The Doctor of the Future

The doctor of the future will give no medicine but will interest his patients in the care of the human frame, in diet, and in the cause and prevention of disease....

— *Thomas Edison*

---

the future will give no medicine but will interest his patients in the care of the human frame in diet and in the cause and prevention of disease." But ultimately the responsibility is yours. Your body can heal itself every day if you give it a chance.

There are five areas that have to be addressed before one can truly walk in *total health = wholeness*:

1.) Fear vs. Faith
2.) Responsibility
3.) Change
4.) Knowledge vs. Ignorance
5.) All Things Are Possible For Him Who Believes

1. Fear vs. Faith

Probably the most devastating thing one can do to their total health=wholeness is to fear. Fear is an emotion that negatively stresses our body — especially our immune system. I believe when people are told they have cancer, the fear and emotion that rise up with the word CANCER do as much to shorten that person's life as the disease itself.

What is fear? It is a sense of total helplessness, knowing something is happening or about to happen that will have a potentially devastating effect on your life or the lives of your loved ones and you have no control over it. That is already occurring or about to occur. Fear is so devastating because on our Total Health=Wholeness Model it totally destroys our soul health (mind, will and emotion) as well as our physical health because the body is being driven on high speed with adrenaline production (due to the constant stress that fear is). This causing all systems of the body to eventually become exhausted and depleted. It's like running from a tiger who is trying to eat you 24 hours a day. Your body does not and cannot heal in this sympathetic nervous system stress. So under stress your body burns out, oxidizes and starts the progression of death, instead of entering the resting parasympathetic nervous system progression of healing and life.

This adrenaline production never stops because your mind never rests. Along with the complete fatigue of the system, especially the cancer fighting immune system (i.e., natural killer cells), you have the tremendous increased production of oxidant molecules. These molecules burn like a raging fire that's out of control and produce free radical molecules, which cause more cellular damage at other sites and starts new cellular fires throughout the body. This is very harmful because not only is the person who's living in a constant state of fear suppressing their immune system, they're losing their ability to fight the invaders. This constant adrenaline rush is so oxidative it depletes all one's natural antioxidant molecules. (see chapter 17)

This can be illustrated by people walking through a huge forest that has had no rain or moisture and is very dry, ready to go up in flames with the smallest spark. Now as these people are walking through the forest they are lighting matches and throwing them on the ground, which lights on fire immediately and starts to burn. Every time these fires start to burn, it rains just enough to put all these independent fires out. In this analogy the "people" starting the fires are the highly oxidative molecules that are being produced 24 hours a day in the person who is in fear and constantly secreting adrenaline because of this fear. The "fires" that are starting are sites of oxidative free radical damage starting to occur; being produced throughout the body. The "rain" that puts out the fire and stops them from raging are the body's natural antioxidants that are produced which in time eventually become depleted. Once this occurs these independent small fires start to rage uncontrollably and a cancer site begins to grow. So to sum this up when fear sets in not only does it stress and suppress your immune system and all other bodily systems (heart, GI tract, etc), but also gives rise to more cellular damage in these areas via oxidative free radical damage.

This means not only does fear cause a tremendous weakening of the body, but it also induces more damage while this weakening occurs. This is just on the physical or body side of health. The mind, the will and emotion side, is linked with this by the adrenaline response that occurs as previously mentioned. There are two ways the mind is affected by fear:

1. Emotions lead to constant adrenaline response ' oxidative molecules 'free radical formation ' cellular damage.

2. Will - when a person is confronted with a constant, great fear, it causes a loss of the will to live. This is seen by anyone who has the constant fear of living with cancer as well as the person who has the constant fear of living in poverty. The constant fear triggers a depression and a lack of desire to live. This can be devastating because in Proverbs 23: 7, "as a man think in his heart so is he." If we lose our desire to live we will die. "Hope deferred makes the heart sick." (Proverbs13:12)

Hope is tied to will because hope is knowing you will reach an expected end even though you are not there now. Hope says I know this is bad news, but Jesus died so that I may have an abundant full life. I know that "all things are possible for him who believes"(Mark 9:23.) So no matter how sick I am, how poor I am, or how lonely I am, I have health, riches and companionship that all come from the God who made me. And through His son, Jesus, His Holy Spirit dwells in me to give me the hope that "He will never leave me nor forsake me"(Hebrews 13:5). The hope that "when I am weak then I am strong"(2 Cor. 12:10). The hope that He will meet my every need according to His riches and glory. Hope is a sure thing, the only part of it that is unknown is the time period of waiting, trusting in Him. Hope is tied to the new covenant which says that all that is the Fathers is ours in Christ Jesus and also all that is ours is His. We are one — just like in a marriage where all resources collectively become each others.

Faith

Faith is a complete trust or reliance upon something or someone. In *Total Health= Wholeness*, our faith is in God and His word, His son and His Holy Spirit. As past evangelist Smith Wigglesworth said "God said it, I believe it, that settles it." Faith is to so completely trust or rely on something or someone that you can cease striving or rest in it.

Fear is simply a faith in the circumstances. When a doctor tells you that you have cancer and you have six months to live, your fear is really a faith in what he has said. You have trusted and relied on the doctor to know the truth and that this truth is unchangeable. Let me explain this with an analogy. If I were to tell you, "Get out of your house, a bomb is inside and it's going to go off in one minute," you have a choice. If you believe me, have faith in me, know my words be true, you will run out the door in panic. On the other hand, if you don't believe me, you will not run. You will not even move and your blood pressure and pulse rate won't go up one bit, because you know what I said to be untrue.

This is the same choice we have every single day of our lives, to live and walk in faith in a God who loves us, saved us from our sins, gave us eternal life, and rushes to meet our every need. Because He is love, and even placed His Spirit in our hearts so we could experience His love, His joy, and His peace every day, knowing that all things in this universe are upheld by Him, including ourselves.

Or do I walk in faith in imperfect man who only sees in part or knows in part, "Do I have faith in an imperfect world that is in a constant state of decline, physically, mentally and morally?" The answer is simple, who are you going to believe? God, who loves you and said he would never leave you or forsake you, or mankind and a dying world that will always leave you and forsake you, even try to destroy you? There is only one answer: I will trust in my God and His Word (Psalms 13:5, 25:2, 31:14,119:42) and

61

...ways be fixed on the author of life, the alpha and the omega,
...ng and the end, the first and the last, my eyes will be fixed on
...ng God. When my eyes are fixed on the God who created me, sus-
ta... ...ne, loves me and meets my every need — then my faith and hope will
rest in His love. Again faith is my response to what has been said, seen or
done. Hope takes that response and sustains it for what ever time period is
needed until the expected end is reached and His love binds it all together.

FAITH = My response to what has been said, seen or done
HOPE = Faith combined with an unknown time element (sustains for
however long because it is a sure thing)
LOVE = Binds Faith and Hope together

Now lets make this real with some real life situations. You find out you
have cancer and the doctor says you have six month to live.

1. *Faith* says "God made me, God sustains me, and even though I have
a terminal disease, God can and will sustain me as long as He wants me on
this planet. God can heal me, God can change all things." So I simply
choose to trust and rely on Him, not the disease or the words of the doctor.
I choose to believe, trust, and rely upon God and His words:

- I will never leave nor forsake you (Hebrews 13:5)
- I have come that you may have life and have it to the full, have it
  more abundantly (John 10:10)
- All things are possible for Him who believes (Mark 9:23)
- By His wounds I am healed (Isaiah 53:5)
- If He takes care of the animals and birds, surely He will take care of
  me (Matt. 6:26), the one who was made in His image (1Cor.11:7) and
  who His Spirit dwells in (1Cor. 3:16)

Rather this, than have fear which is to believe, trust and rely upon the
doctors words, this lump growing on my body and these pains I am having.

2. *Hope* says "I know God will make me whole, He will heal me, and
He will meet my needs. He will never leave me and He will give me a full
abundant life, but I don't know when." Remember, hope is a for-sure enti-
ty with an unsure time element attached to it. Hope is the fact that a mil-

lion dollar diamond is buried in your yard, but there is a time element before you find it.

This brings up questions that need to be addressed. The first is, if it is a given fact that a one million dollar diamond is buried in your yard, you will start to dig and dig and dig and dig. About six months later you will start to doubt if it really is there. If you still believe the truth, that there is a diamond there, you will not become discouraged that you will never find it.

This is when we realize that in all things God wants us to give Him the glory and wants us to grow or mature and become strong in Him. When we reach the end of our energy, strength, hope, and faith, that's when His strength, hope and faith are seen in us. "When we are weak, then we are strong" (2Cor.12:10.) When we reach the end of ourselves, that's when we are carried by Him.

I love the "Footprints in the Sand" poem that asks "Lord why are there times in my life when I only see one set of footprints?" His reply: "It is then that I carried you my child." You know it's hard to carry someone until they reach the end of their own strength and ability. So when our faith and hope are growing weak, this is when His faith and His hope that He placed in our hearts start to manifest and we can go on to receive all that He has promised.

There is another vital component to walking and living in His faith and His hope and being surrounded in His love. Not only has and does God speak to us through His word, the Bible, He also right here, right now, speaks to our hearts through His Holy Spirit. This same Spirit is with us every second of every day and has all the wisdom, knowledge and power that we would need in every situation.

Let me explain this with a story. A friend of mine and his wife had been out in the forest preserve on a picnic. After they had left, they realized that her wedding ring was missing. It had been on the blanket, and when the blankets were shaken to be put away her ring went flying somewhere into the grass. This is similar to the above illustration of knowing there's a diamond in your yard, but not knowing where. It was quite hopeless for this couple because they didn't have six months to a year or more to find her ring. So they prayed that God would reveal where the ring was. After talking to the woman's father, to whom the Holy Spirit had shown exactly where the ring was, they went to the spot and it was there, just as He said it was. It was a miracle, it was God's Holy Spirit speaking to His people. When they listen, miracles happen everyday.

So remember in this life we are called to have faith — total trust, and rely on one truth, that the Living God loves us. And in this love He meets all of our needs, hears all our prayers and speaks directly to us to lead us and guide us by His written word, the Bible, and His spoken word, the Holy Spirit speaking to our hearts right now — today. So let us live by "the faith" of the Son of God who loved us and gave His life for us (Gal. 2:20.) It's either that or live in fear everyday of our life of something or someone. The choice should be clear — choose life and to live in Him who created it.

2. Responsibility

The first step in regaining one's health is taking responsibility and to know that you have to take care of yourself because no one else will.

To take responsibility means to admit there are probably things you have done in your life and/or are still doing that are contributing to your present state of health. This is not in a negative sense to condemn you but more in a way to motivate you to change your mind set which will cause you to make lifestyle changes that can improve your *total health = wholeness*. Many patients are looking for a good doctor but how many of those patients know that the doctor is looking for a good patient, one who will follow his complete recommendations? It's not how strong we start a race that counts, but how strong we finish it. A question I ask my patients is "I know what I the doctor am doing to restore your health, but what are YOU doing to restore it"?

Responsibility not only says there are many things, habits and lifestyles that probably contributed to my present state of health, but responsibility also says that even if I've done everything right and still got sick — no one is going to take the responsibility to get me well except myself. Responsibility is a key in wholeness because without it we spend all of our time blaming someone or something for how we are. It started as early as the garden of Eden, when God called Adam to be responsible for his sin and he tried to pass the buck to Eve by saying "it was that women you gave me, she made me do it." It was not Eve's problem, it was Adam's. He directly heard the voice of God tell him not to eat of the tree of good and evil. Eve never heard God say that, she only heard it second hand from Adam.

It also was seen in David's life where after he sinned and the prophet Nathan confronted him with his own sin (although he didn't know it), when he said that that man will surely die — Nathan said to David "You are that man." (2 Samuel 12: 7-13.) David acknowledged, "I have sinned against the Lord." David took responsibility for his sin even though it cost him division in his family and the life of his first son. Psalm 51 shows David's confession of this sin — taking responsibility instead of trying to ignore it or pass it off on someone else. It is interesting to know that David was the central figure in the Old Testament that had a revelation of grace and mercy as opposed to law and justice. David did not receive what he deserved and neither do we who are in Christ. Responsibility says what ever has happened is already done and we can do nothing to change it, but we can do a lot to affect the present and future by taking responsibility for our health and our family's health. You are responsible for not only your heath but the health of your children until they become adults.

3. Change

Also closely linked with responsibility is the concept of change. By nature, we all like stability and knowing what today and tomorrow is going to bring into our lives. People do not like to change how they do things because sometimes that change entails more work in their lives. Change can also mean that perhaps the way we have always done something could have been wrong, and nobody likes to be wrong.

There's a story about a woman who was taught by her mother to always make meat loaf by chopping the ends off before cooking it. One day, the daughter asked her grandmother what significance there was to cutting the ends off the meatloaf. Her grandmother replied, "My pan was too short to handle the meatloaf, so I used to cut off the ends to make it fit."

It's easy to see how habits and ideas can be passed from generation to generation with no questions asked about whether or not we are doing something the best possible way. This is where I challenge you to be willing to change all your ideas and all the ways you presently live if in fact there is a way to do it better, or promote a healthier or more whole outcome. I call this having a mind of a child. Children are always open to learn, always open to change, and never set in their ways because they haven't yet learned that they are supposed to do things the way they have always been done, the stable, safe, predictable adult way. This is one of the reasons I think children can experience the Spirit of God so freely because they are so open to let Him do whatever He wants to do in their lives. They put no restrictions on God to move in their life. Once the mind becomes that of an adult we think we know the answers and become very closed to change. The adult mindset prefers the comfortable and predictable way.

They like to stay in their comfort zones and the thought of anything that brings them out of that zone makes them uneasy. We must always be open to change our ways of thinking and living in order to improve our quality and quantity of life no matter how strange or foreign it may seem at first. When I conduct food sensitivity testing at the Institute and consult with patients on removing items that are negatively affecting their health, this change doesn't always feel good in their mind or body right away, so resistance sometimes comes up. Many times the changes we have to make in our lives are uncomfortable, take more time or require more energy and effort. All this is necessary to achieve a higher quality of life. Again, many times change stretches our comfort zone so we must be committed to allow that stretching in order to achieve a greater level of *total health = wholeness*. Never be afraid to change, to have the mind of a child, it is a major ingredient in all success.

4. Knowledge vs Ignorance

Along with change is the concept or idea of knowledge vs ignorance. This can be seen in my life when I decided to change my diet to a totally animal free vegetarian diet, or vegan, as it is called. This choice was not made out of sickness or necessity, but out of a desire to increase my health and my families level of health. After researching all possible diets, there was no question that a diet void of all animal products was the most health promoting. During my research, I learned a lot more about how meat contains parasites, bacteria, hormones and toxins that are all cancer forming and health depleting. So, by free will, I chose to change my diet in order to achieve better health.

Many people today remain ignorant to this fact. Ignorance is defined as lack of knowledge. So people say, "I like meat," and "It doesn't matter what I eat, because when it's my time to die I will die." This is a person who is oblivious to the truth and chooses to live in ignorance rather than to acquire the knowledge that would help him, his family and friends. So choose to always keep an open mind, or the mind of a child to change and acquire knowledge on how to live to the best of your ability rather than living blindly in ignorance. As the scripture says "A fool in his heart says there is no God"(Psalm14:1), because anyone who has any reasoning can see by the creation of the world around us and by seeing the birth of a baby that there is an awesome creator behind creation. Let us not be fools in any areas of our lives, but be open to truth — all truth.

5. *All things are possible for him who believes.*

"All things are possible for him who believes" (Mark 9:23.) Remember, God is in control and nothing is finished until its finished. When we have a tumor and the doctor says we have six moths to live. When we struggle to make ends meet and see no possible solution in the future. When we sink into depression with no possible way of ever correcting it. When fear grips us so tight that we despair even to the point of life itself. We must always, always, always remember that the Lord said He would never leave us or forsake us. Remember that He promised to meet all our needs according to His riches and glory. That He said He came so that we could have life lived to the full and have it more abundantly. If He takes care of the animals and the birds then how much more does He love us who were created in His image, and even to the knowing every hair on our heads. He knows everything about us.

This is when we have to understand that all things are possible for him who believes. If we trust in our creator, He will never let us down. We might feel we are going through some hard times that don't seem fair, we might even shout, "Where are You, God!?" But this is when we will realize that we are walking through a wilderness on the way to the promised land. The wonderful thing about the wilderness is that we have to walk being empowered and strengthened by Him because we soon get to the end of our self and our ability. That is when His glory manifests and we mature in Him. That is "when I am weak then I am strong."

(2Cor. 12:10) starts to emerge. That is when I find out I am "more than a conqueror"(Rom.8:37.) Remember a conqueror has victory in his own strength or ability. A "more than a conqueror" has victory in God's strength because he came to the end of himself and called out to God, and that is where God met him. So when you feel like giving up, when the odds are too great, when you cannot go one step further, it's great, because that is when you are supernaturally lifted up by the hand of the Lord. That is when you find the new strength to go on that you never knew existed. That is when you receive the true revelation that He is with me, and He never will leave me or forsake me, "because He loves me"(Psalm 91:14.) So, for those of you who feel you've been stuck in something for such a long time, I suggest you compare yourself to yourself, and if you do you will find that you have indeed grown in Him and His strength.

You are not at your final destination yet, but at least you have left on the journey...and that is what our life is, a journey. A journey through the wilderness learning to trust Him everyday to supply our every need just as He supplied the Israelites with their daily food (manna). They could not store the manna, they had to have faith - trust and rely on God and the truth that He would meet their need every morning. And He did, He always does if we would just have faith in Him and turn our lives over to Him.

Remember, when you start this journey you will be walking 95 percent in your strength and five percent in His strength. Then, as you continue to walk in His strength through the wilderness of your life, you will slowly start to walk more and more in His strength and less and less in your own until one day you will arrive at the promised land, walking 100 percent in His strength, depending totally on Him and knowing it is only in Him that you live and move and have your being(Acts 17:28.) When you arrive at the promised land you will no longer walk in your own ability or desires (the flesh) but you will walk in His ability and His desire (the Spirit) and it will be wonderfully awesome, so get started today on your wilderness journey and know that "this is the day the Lord has made let us rejoice and be glad in it"(Psalm 118:24.) Never compare your journey to anyone else's, yours is the one God has you on which is very different from the journey of your friends, your family or others you know. So keep your eyes fixed on Jesus, the author, and perfector and finisher of your faith so you can cross the finish line in His strength, knowing you have fought the good fight, you have run the race, you have kept the faith (2 Tim. 4:7.)

I will close with a true story that opened my eyes to the reality that "all things are possible for him who believes." A certain man went to the doctor feeling very ill and upon examination it was found that he had a malignant tumor in his abdomen the size of a volleyball. Among the treatment alternatives discussed were surgery, radiation and chemotherapy, which all had a combined success rate with this particular type of cancer of little to practically none, but the man left the doctor's office knowing that "all things are possible for him who believes." He returned for examination three months later. Totally amazed, the doctor asked what the man had done because the tumor was gone and there was no sign of cancer in his body. The man replied, "I had everyone at my church praying for me, I changed my diet to a vegetarian one and I worked with alternative medicine doctor who put me on a detoxification program to get the chemicals and toxins out of my body while I worked on getting the proper nutrients for healing." As you can see, all things truly are possible for him who believes, for him who takes responsibility for his own health, for him who keeps an open mind to change, and for him who is led by faith and not by fear.

Chapter in review

Health is made of the following components:
genetic
structural, nervous system
physical
eliminatory
chemical
mental
spiritual

The five areas that need to be addressed to walk in *total health = wholeness*:

1. Fear vs. faith
2. Responsibility
3. Change
4. Knowledge vs. Ignorance
5. All Things Are Possible For Him Who Believes

Remember, all aspects of your health are changeable except one (genetic), and nearly every cell in your body is regenerated in one year. Therefore, there is great reason to hope that you will experience healing.

I appreciate the speech Winston Churchill gave to a graduating class. When the distinguished Churchill stood to give his words of wisdom to these young people going out to make a mark in the world, his speech was only seven words long: "Never give up; never give up; never!"

What powerful words if we could only incorporate them down deep inside of us. Instead of just retaining knowledge in the brain, we have to believe enough to make it part of us, so no person or thing can take it from us. We must own it. This is true revelation.

CHAPTER 2

DISEASE

What is disease?

Disease, simply put, is a departure from health. When your body is healthy, it functions just as God meant it to. This is truly amazing, because as we study the concepts of homeostasis, or balance, we see that our body is created to keep perfect balance. *Guyton's Medical Physiology* textbook defines *homeostasis* as "maintenance of static, or constant, conditions in the internal environment." Every second, countless chemical reactions are going on in your cells and are so orchestrated by God that they maintain perfect harmony and balance, each reaction affecting another. But if this homeostasis is broken, the body begins to go out of balance; breakdown, damage, and disease begin. If this normal balance is not regained, disease eventually leads to death, which is the cessation of all functions.

As we look further into what disease is, we can see that disease is the opposite of what God intended. In the garden of Eden, Adam and Eve were perfect. They walked and talked with God, and they were made in His image. God created them whole in body, soul, and spirit. They would have lived forever in this state, just as we will in heaven. Then came Satan, and along with the moral and spiritual fall of man came departure from the physical perfection and wholeness that God had intended. Once spiritually perfect, now spiritually dead; once a perfect mind, now corrupted with fear, self-awareness, and stress; once a perfect body, now imperfect and open to pain, sickness, disease, and death. So disease, in simple terms, is all that is opposed to God — as darkness is to light, so is disease to health.

In the same way that homeostasis is the perfect control mechanism that balances and checks all systems and functions of the body, disease is the breakdown of this perfection into the opposite — imbalance and imperfection.

A study of disease leads us to the modern germ theory, in which Louis Pasteur stated that specific diseases are caused by specific germs. This led to the consequent realization that specific drugs could destroy specific germs and eliminate the diseases they could cause. Additionally, it was discovered that simply washing hands between surgeries (which was never done before) drastically decreased the mortality rate.

We have lived the 20th Century with this theory, and the results of it have been tremendous, greatly reducing the number of deaths due to infectious diseases, especially bacterial. But now we have to rethink our theories of disease cause and correction, as the major causes of disease and death are now related to diet and lifestyle. The Number 1, 2 and 3 causes of death are heart disease, cancer, and stroke.[1] All of these can be affected greatly by diet and lifestyle changes, without drugs or surgery. In recent years, infections caused by new antibiotic-resistant bacteria have caused a surge in the number of people dying from infectious diseases that previously were under control. Why? Because we have overstayed the dominance of the germ theory and drug treatment for sickness and disease.

Pasteur's contemporary, Bernard, believed that it wasn't the germs that caused the diseases but rather the weakening of the tissues — i.e., the immune system. The two theories can be compared by a simple illustration: Let us call the garbage in a garbage dump the "weakened tissue" and the rats and flies the "germs." According to Pasteur, the rats and flies caused the garbage to appear; but according to Bernard, the garbage caused the rats and flies to appear. Bernard thought that it wasn't the seed (germs) but the soil (immune system) that caused the disease. This makes more sense as seen in all the successful alternative health-care treatments operating by this premise around the world. On the horizon is the dawn of a new form of health care that will focus its energy on the prevention of disease rather than its cure.

Doesn't it make more sense to teach people how to stay well or whole, as God meant them to be — rather than waiting for them to break down with disease, and then trying desperately to fix them with tremendous time, energy, effort, pain and suffering, anxiety, and fear? Doesn't it make more sense to teach our children not to touch the stove rather than being excited that we know a great plastic surgeon who can reduce the amount of scarring to the burned hand? It seems ridiculous, but this is what is happening in our country. People are doing whatever they want, eating whatever they like, and waiting until they break down; hoping it won't be them, or that their genetic constitution will be like the man who can smoke and drink and live to be 100.

Let us stop all this haphazard health-guessing and out-of-self-control foolishness, and start once again on our journey of health and wholeness. Not only will this add years to our lives, but it will also add life to our years. Also remember it is our responsibility to teach our children. "Train a child in the way he should go, and when he is old he will not turn from it" (Proverbs 22:6).

I believe the next twenty years will usher in the heyday of sickness and disease. AIDS is just the tip of the iceberg. Not only will viral diseases like AIDS and Ebola take a tremendous toll on life, but so will the already-mentioned increase in antibiotic-resistant bacterial infections. These will join heart disease, cancer, and stroke, already on the rise. There will come a day when doctors will have nothing to offer us, and we will be left with no alternative but to return to the plan God had for us, the plan of wholeness in body, soul, and spirit. This is when prayer, attitudes, decisions, commitment, lifestyle, and diet will all come together in achieving *total health = wholeness*. This will be discussed in more detail in subsequent chapters.

But let me just say that if our bodies are temples of the Holy Spirit, and we are called to take care of these temples, we can use God's wisdom in achieving the task. His wisdom started in Genesis, telling us how to eat; it progressed in Leviticus, teaching us how to prevent sickness and disease; in Psalms and Proverbs, it taught us that our minds, attitudes, and actions all play an important part in our total health. The new covenant erased the old in regard to our relationship with God — it was by grace and no longer by law — but it did not erase the wisdom in maintaining our health and wholeness. The spiritual plan was replaced in the new covenant; the natural plan was not. What was naturally good for Old Testament people, then, is also good for us today.

How sick are we?

We are not getting healthier, but sicker. Don't let that scare you, but educate you. My desire is that you would choose to improve your total health through an educated decision rather than through fear of either getting sick or, even worse, through actually being sick. In 1900 the United States of America was the healthiest nation in the world. By 1920 we dropped to No. 2, and by 1978 we had fallen to No. 79.[2] Why this decline?

Heart attack

Heart attack is the leading cause of death in the United States.[3] Over 1.5 million people have them[4], and over 700,000 people die from them each year.[5] If you are the average American, your chance of dying from a heart attack is about 50 percent.[6]

This drops to less than 4% if you switch to a vegan (no animal product) diet.[7] Much time and money has been spent to repair coronary artery blockage and damage caused by heart attacks through bypass surgery, but little has been done to address the cause of the problem in the first place. Treating the effects of heart disease with surgery instead of addressing the causes is like bandaging our fingers only to pick up the hammer and smash them again.

Dr. Dean Ornish has developed a program that prevents and reverses heart disease, which neither medication nor surgery can do. His program consists of a vegetarian diet, exercise, and relaxation and meditation techniques.[8]

Cancer

In 1900, three percent of all deaths in America were caused by cancer; by 1994, the percentage had risen to 22.[9] Today, cancer is the second-leading cause of death at 38% in the U.S. If deaths due to cancer continue to rise at their present rate, cancer will surpass heart disease as the No. 1 killer in America. In the U.S., more than one out of every three (38 percent) Americans presently die from cancer. In the next five years that percentage will probably rise to 50 percent.[10] Over one million people are diagnosed with cancer each year, and about 520,000 die from it.[11] An even more alarming fact is that cancer is now the leading cause of death in children ages 1-14 besides accidental injury.[12] How can this be? Why should this be? Children's bodies are so vital, so able to bounce back from sickness. Fifty years ago you rarely heard of children getting cancer. What is happening? Hopefully this book will not only answer that question but address what to do about it.

The parts of our bodies most commonly affected by cancer are the skin, lung, colon, rectum, and breast. In 1993, the top three types of cancer were lung, colorectal and breast.[13] These three forms of cancer combined to total almost 50 percent of all cancer.[14] Diet and lifestyle changes could reduce these three drastically.

The following factors can cause cancer, according to the National Cancer Institute:[15]

Diet — 35-60% (some sources say up to 90%)
Tobacco — 30%
Alcohol — 3%
Radiation — 3%
Medication — 2%
Air and water — 1-5%

Stroke

The third leading cause of death in the United States is stroke.[16] Strokes are caused by atherosclerotic plaquing and decreased blood flow to the brain, much like heart attacks. Every year, 550,000 Americans have strokes, or cerebral vascular accident (CVA). Of these, 162,000 die,[17] and many of the rest are left with significant disabilities.

The top three diseases — heart disease, cancer, and stroke — comprise about 88% of all deaths in this country. It is estimated that up to 90 percent of deaths attributed to these three factors could be eliminated through changes in diet, lifestyle, and attitudes. Remember, *total health = wholeness,* and when we improve the whole of our health, rather than just one or two aspects of it, we will be as God created us to be: WHOLE.

What causes disease?

Disease, or departure from health, begins when we no longer function as we were created in body, soul (mind, will, and emotion), and spirit. The seven general categories of total *health = wholeness* are:

1) Hereditary
2) Structural (organ /gland)
3) Physical -circulative
             -lymphatics
             -exercise
4) Chemical
5) Eliminatory
6) Mental
7) Spiritual

When any one of these parts is affected, the others are affected as well. As we weaken parts of our total health = wholeness, we become vulnerable to disease.

A brief introduction to each of the categories follows. In later chapters, they will be examined in more detail.

Hereditary

Some people are prone to heart disease because it is a genetically inherited weakness. The effects of heredity on total health cannot be denied; but since it is not a major cause of disease, and since we can do nothing about this part of our total health picture, we can only attempt to minimize any negative genetic influence on our health. If you are genetically predisposed to cancer, you are not without hope; there are many preventive measures you can implement. On the other hand, if your grandfather and father lived to be 100 while smoking, drinking, and eating meat and potatoes, you cannot assume that you will be exempt from disease and a shortened life span. Remember: you reap what you sow.

Structural (Organ/Gland)

Structural health refers to the neuromusculoskeletal system, or simply the function of the nerves, muscles and bones and how these control all

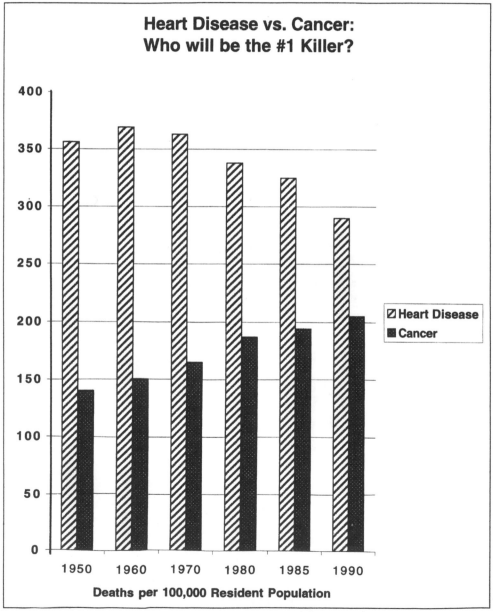

Heart Disease vs. Cancer:
Who will be the #1 Killer?

Deaths per 100,000 Resident Population

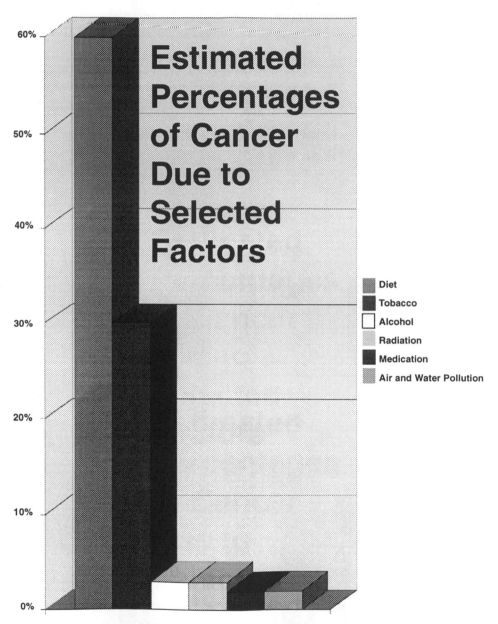

Estimated Percentages of Cancer Due to Selected Factors

Diet
Tobacco
Alcohol
Radiation
Medication
Air and Water Pollution

Source: National Cancer Institute, Cancer Rates and Risks (Washington, D.C.: 1985); also R. Doll and R. Peto, "The Causes of Cancer: Quantitative Estimates of Avoidable Risks of Cancer in the United States Today," J Natl. Cancer in 1981;66:1191-1308.

your organs and glands. You may wonder what these have to do with sickness and disease. The answer lies in the nervous system. God created us so perfectly that everything is in homeostasis, or balance. The role of the nervous system is to control all other glands, organs, and systems; it is a major concern when this master control malfunctions. A comparison can be drawn with a large business which relies heavily on computers; when the computers shut down, so does the business.

In my practice, I have seen many ailments of the stomach, heart, lungs, bronchi, kidneys, bladder, intestinal tract, reproductive systems, eyes, ears, nose, and throat respond very well once nerve pressure is relieved from the spine. The muscles and bones play a large part in this, as they support and protect the nervous system — i.e., the spinal cord and spinal nerves. The spinal nerves, which go to every tissue in your body, branch off the spinal cord and go through the hole in the spinal vertebrae joints called the intervertebral foramen (IVF). If the IVF is compromised or made small by spinal bones that have moved out of place, the resulting nerve pressure can lead to a host of other problems.

Physical

I classify physical health as movement, and I separate it into three areas: circulative, lymphatic, and exercise. The circulatory system deals with the movement of oxygen in from the the lungs and through bloodstream, along with all the nutrients to every cell in your body. The lymphatic system is the center of the body's immune system containing ⅔rds of the white blood cells or WBCs). It also includes exercise and the circulation of WBCs in the lymph flow as vital aspects of our *total health = wholeness*. Exercise is what moves the blood and lymph more effectively throughout the body.

The physical aspect of our total health is very important in the life of our cells, which need oxygen from respiration, and disease-fighting capabilities of the WBCs. Exercise also has many health benefits, but only if it is being done regularly and at the appropriate level. Inefficient oxygen flow not only leads to cell and tissue death, but also to anaerobic activity, which is a common environment for cancer cell growth. Lack of WBCs causes increased chances of everything from colds to cancer. All bacteria and viruses are consumed by our WBCs. We always have cancer cells in our body, but usually our immune system destroys them before they destroy us. Lack of exercise poses many possible health hazards, from a decrease in the number of circulated WBCs to fight off disease, to a decrease in the body's own detoxifying ability, to an increase in stress and tension.

Chemical

This category of health can be defined as what goes in — through air, water, food — and how we digest and assimilate it. The chemical area is a possible major source of sickness due to the high levels of poor, dead, cooked (not life-giving) foods, toxins, chemicals, polluted air, and water that goes in. Remember the computer axiom: Garbage in, garbage out. If we put chemical preservatives, pesticides, and artificial everything inside us, it is just a matter of time until our systems break down and disease sets in.

Eliminative

If the chemical aspect is defined as "what goes in," the eliminative aspect is defined as "what comes out." This is a key factor in health, because if our kidneys, liver, lungs, and bowel don't remove toxins, wastes, and poisons, then sickness will result. What happens when a person with kidney disease is taken off dialysis (machine filtration)? They die. Point made. The same is true with our liver, lungs, and bowel.

Mental

The mind is a key factor in health; if it is over-stressed or filled with fears and anxieties, all kinds of health problems can surface, because there is a direct link between the mind and immune system activations. This has led to the development of a whole new field of medicine called psychoneuroimmunology. If a survey were done across America to see what one ailment doctors would eliminate if they could, the unanimous answer would be stress, because it kills. Science is discovering what the Bible says in Proverbs 23:7, "As a man thinks in his heart, so he is" (NKJV.) We will explore in more detail later the ways in which the mind is very important to our *total health = wholeness*.

Spiritual

Some would ask, "What does your spiritual life have to do with your health?" A great deal, I would respond. God made us to be whole in spirit, soul, and body. The Word of God says that the "Spirit gives life." God breathed into Adam, and he became alive; the word for breath is *pneuma*, which means spirit.

How can the spiritual aspect negatively affect your health? If you do not have a clear and true revelation of the fact that God wants you whole in body, soul, and spirit — and if you do not recognize who you are in Christ, the love of God, and the new covenant — you will not know to reject illness because it opposes our salvation. The Greek word for salvation, sozo, means "saved and healed;" sickness opposes the wholeness that Jesus died for. Lack of understanding in this area can lead to debilitating, and even deadly, thoughts about illness: Maybe God is using this sickness to teach me something.

God does not teach through sickness but through His Word. I will tell my son, "Don't touch the fire; it is hot, and it will burn you." I don't have to stick his hand in the fire for him to learn. This would be an act of cruelty, not love. If we always remember that God is love, we will never question where problems come from. Although God never brings sickness, He can use anything and everything that happens in life to build us up and make us mature and complete, not lacking anything.

When my wife became ill, God did not dump it upon her. She, unknowingly, brought it upon herself with improper diet and high levels of stress until she broke down. But in it all God was glorified, because not only was my wife healed through prayer, but God opened our eyes to the importance of diet, detoxification, lifestyle, and wholeness so we could help others. My wife shares the perspective of Joseph found in the Book of Genesis: What man [and the devil] meant for evil, God meant for good.

Disease risk factors
Many factors affect the functioning of these systems and, therefore, the body:

Diet and nutritional risks
high animal fat and protein diets
pesticides
preservatives
drugs
hormones (estrogen)
caffeine
tobacco
alcohol
Chemical risks
toxic chemicals in food
toxic chemicals in water
toxic chemicals from smoke
toxic chemicals from fumes (i.e., exhaust, paint)
toxic chemicals from air pollution

Environmental risk
radiation from sunlight
radon gas from the ground
electromagnetic radiation from power lines and electrical devices
bacteria/viruses/parasites/fungi

Lifestyle risk
stress
fear

Diet and nutritional risk factors

The National Academy of Science estimates that nutritional factors account for up to 60 percent of the cases of cancer; some sources say as high as 80 percent.[18] Cancers of the colon, rectum, kidney, prostate, uterus, and breast are linked with the consumption of fat and protein, especially meat and animal fat.[19] In the book, Healing Nutrients, by Dr. Patrick Quillin, it is stated: "It has now been well accepted that proper nutrition could prevent 50-90% of all cancer."[20] Other sources say 90% of all cancer is environmentally caused and thus preventable. These environmental factors can be broken down into: 1) diet (35-60%); 2) tobacco (30%); 3) alcohol (3%); 4) radiation and sunlight exposure (3%); 5) pollution of air and water (1-5%); 6) medications (2%).[21] Of these, nutrition, or diet, is the most important cause.

It is amazingly good news that up to 90% of all cancer can be controlled by taking charge of our lives. It is our own responsibility to make choices in life that positively affect us. I am glad that my choices can prevent up to 90% of cancer that might otherwise destroy me.

Fat

Typical animal fat and even some vegetable fat are heavy stressors on health. Dr. John McDougall states in his book *The McDougall Plan*, "Of all the macronutrients in a rich diet, excess fat causes the greatest burden on the body. Eventually, the body fails to compensate from this burden, and disease results. After we eat a meal high in any type of fat, our blood cells actually stick together in clumps that plug the blood vessels."[22] This results in decreased circulation of oxygen (up to 25% for 4-6 hours), vital nutrients and disease-fighting white blood cells, along with increased blood pressure and chances of heart attack and stroke.

Countries with a higher intake of animal fat have a greater incidence of breast cancer.[23, 24] Japanese women who eat meat daily have a risk of breast cancer 85 times higher than those who rarely or never eat meat.[25] The Surgeon General's report on Nutrition and Health stated: "Indeed, a comparison of populations indicates that death rates for cancers of the breast, colon and prostate are directly proportionate to the estimated dietary fat intakes."[26]

How else does fat affect the body? Higher fat diets increase estrogen levels (female sex hormones) in the blood, which in turn increases the growth of breast tumors. Vegetarian women have much lower estrogen levels than non-vegetarians, which greatly reduces their cancer risk. Studies have shown, though, that when a strict vegetarian adds eggs and cheese to his/her diet, the cancer risk becomes almost the same as that of a meat eater.[27, 28]

How little fat should we have in order to avoid these risks? The National Cancer Institute has recommended no more than 30% of our total caloric intake be from fat. However, studies of the Japanese in the 1950s showed that cancer rates were very low when fat intake was limited to about seven percent of total calories.[29] Dr. McDougall recommends 10% calories from fat, all from vegetable sources.

It is important to remember that we need fat — the good fat which vegetable sources like flax seeds, olives, safflower, sunflower, and sesame seeds can provide. Without the essential fatty acids that these provide, many systems of the body no longer function properly, especially the nervous system which is coated with myelin sheaths, which need fatty acids. Diets too low in essential fatty acids have been linked to various diseases of the nervous system, especially multiple sclerosis. So remember, you need some of the right kind of fat every day.

Protein risk

Cells need protein to grow and maintain the body's health, but excessive protein has a reverse effect. When we eat too much protein, the excess has to be broken down by the liver and excreted through the kidneys as urea (This is very stressful to the kidneys potentially causing damage to the microtubules). Urea tends to pull more water out of your body acting as a diuretic, which causes the kidneys to excrete not only more water but more minerals, especially calcium. So not only does a higher intake of protein cause kidney disease but also osteoporosis. This calcium loss is also attributed to the calcium being pulled out of the bones to buffer (because of its alkalinity) the acid imbalance that the protein digestion leaves. A study of the African Bantus, who eat a low protein (47 grams/day) and low calcium (400 milligrams) diet, revealed that they are essentially free of osteoporosis.[30] Interestingly, the native Eskimos, who consume a fish-laden diet very high in protein (250-400 grams/day) and calcium (2,000 milligrams), have one of the highest rates of osteoporosis in the world.[31]

The high protein diets of most Americans, containing over 100 grams per day, causes calcium to be lost from the bone, and it ends up in the urinary tract as kidney stones. An interesting fact is that protein consumed in excess of our needs causes destruction of kidney tissue and progressive deterioration of kidney function. By the eighth decade of life, people of affluent societies commonly lose 75% of their kidney function.[32]

Pesticides

In the United States, farmers use 845 million pounds of the nearly 3 billion pounds of active pesticide ingredients every year, at a cost of about $5 billion.[33]

Pesticides pose a wide range of dangers, from cancer to birth defects, from damage to the nervous system to immune system deficiencies. In 1990, the World Health Organization estimated 3 million severe pesticide poisonings worldwide, 220,000 of which resulted in death. Some of the more recent studies estimate up to 25 million cases annually. These cases only include the ones that are obvious poisonings and does not consider all the symptoms that may not be thought to be related to pesticides, like general malaise (ill feeling), headaches, suppression of the immune system causing frequent illness, lack of energy, and other toxic-related symptoms.

In a study done by the United States Department of Agriculture in 1992, some unsettling news was discovered. In this study of pesticide residue in produce, the USDA revealed underlying potential health risks in the nation's produce supply. The reports findings were that even after washing and peeling fruits and vegetables collected in 1992, pesticide residue was found on about 60% of the 5,750 samples. Also stated in the report: Many samples contained multiple residues, with as many as eight found in one sample. Further facts revealed that 25 different pesticides were found in the apples sampled, 21 of which are either carcinogenic, neurotoxins (toxic to the nervous system) and/or toxic to the endocrine system. How can this be allowed? The answer was found when the food industry, which joined forces with the chemical industry on the pesticide issues, boasted that less than 2% of the washed, peeled, and cored samples violated current EPA standards. The problem is that the alleged "safety" provides a false security, because the standards themselves are not necessarily safe.[34] (See chart next page).

Preservatives/additives

Many chemicals are added to our foods to preserve the food and extend its shelf life, or to enhance flavor, thicken, emulsify (keep oil and water mixed together), pickle, or color. These are all chemicals that are not natural to the body. They have to be broken down by the liver and increase the toxic load and eventual buildup of toxins in the body. Your white blood cells have to remove them from your bloodstream by digesting them. This poses a major health threat, because if your white blood cells are wasting energy and effort eating your dinner or the preservatives and additives in your dinner, they cannot fight bacteria, viruses, fungi, parasites, and cancer. This opens your body up to all kinds of diseases, especially cancer formation. Here are a few to give you an idea of their effect on your health.

BHA

This additive is used to preserve food containing oil; it slows rancidity. In 1982 it was found to induce tumors in the stomach of rats. The International Agency for Research on Cancer, which is part of the World Health Organization, considers BHA to be possibly carcinogenic to humans, and the State of California has listed it as a carcinogen.[35]

BHT

This preservative is similar to BHA. Reports also show increased incidence of tumors with its use.

Artificial colorings

Synthetic food dyes have long been suspected of being a potential health hazard. Red Dye No. 3 has been banned for some purposes because it caused thyroid tumors in male rats. Yellow No. 5 is associated with allergic reactions in some people including hives, running or stuffy noses, and, occasionally, severe breathing difficulties. The Federal Drug Administration has estimated that between 47,000 and 94,000 Americans are sensitive to Yellow No. 5.[36]

Aspartame (Nutrasweet, Equal)

Aspartame is dangerous to phenylketonurics (PKU), or people who don't metabolize phenylalanine (which is in aspartame). High levels of this amino acid can lead to mental retardation.

Pesticide Rating Compared to Strawberries

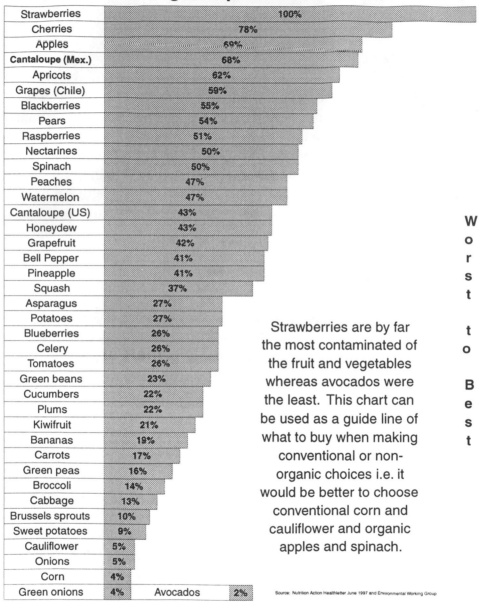

Strawberries	100%	
Cherries	78%	
Apples	69%	
Cantaloupe (Mex.)	68%	
Apricots	62%	
Grapes (Chile)	59%	
Blackberries	55%	
Pears	54%	
Raspberries	51%	
Nectarines	50%	
Spinach	50%	
Peaches	47%	
Watermelon	47%	
Cantaloupe (US)	43%	
Honeydew	43%	
Grapefruit	42%	
Bell Pepper	41%	
Pineapple	41%	
Squash	37%	
Asparagus	27%	
Potatoes	27%	
Blueberries	26%	
Celery	26%	
Tomatoes	26%	
Green beans	23%	
Cucumbers	22%	
Plums	22%	
Kiwifruit	21%	
Bananas	19%	
Carrots	17%	
Green peas	16%	
Broccoli	14%	
Cabbage	13%	
Brussels sprouts	10%	
Sweet potatoes	9%	
Cauliflower	5%	
Onions	5%	
Corn	4%	
Green onions	4%	Avocados 2%

W o r s t t o B e s t

Strawberries are by far the most contaminated of the fruit and vegetables whereas avocados were the least. This chart can be used as a guide line of what to buy when making conventional or non-organic choices i.e. it would be better to choose conventional corn and cauliflower and organic apples and spinach.

Source: Nutrition Action Healthletter June 1997 and Environmental Working Group

Other studies have shown other possible effects from aspartame use. They include altered brain function, behavior changes, dizziness, headaches, epileptic-like seizures, and menstrual problems. Even more alarming is the study that showed an increased risk of brain tumors.[37]

Nitrites and nitrates

Sodium nitrite and sodium nitrate are used to preserve meat and keep its red color. Nitrates are not harmful until they are converted into nitrites in the body; then the nitrites combine with another compound in the body called secondary amines to form nitrosamines, extremely potent cancer-causing chemicals. Philip Hartman, Ph.D., of Johns Hopkins University has stated that nitrites have long been a significant cause of stomach cancer.[38]

Additives and hyperactivity

In 1989, a study looked at children's behavior after making several dietary changes. The study involved 24 hyperactive boys between the ages of 3½ and six. All had sleep problems or physical symptoms such as stuffy noses or stomachaches. In the study, the children were fed a vitamin-rich diet including special food that was low in sugar, and food devoid of colorings, flavorings, MSG, caffeine, preservatives, chocolate, dairy products, and other substances that parents said might affect their child. After four weeks on the diet, 10 of the boys averaged a 45% improvement in behavior, and more than half showed some improvement.[39]

Hormones

Hormones are very definitely linked to an increase in cancer, especially of the breast.[40, 41, 42] As stated earlier, high fat-diets increase the amount of estrogen that the body secretes, which in turn promotes growth of tumor tissue especially in the breast. Hormones are entering our bodies at alarmingly high rates. Now beef and chicken and all dairy products contain BGH — or synthetic bovine growth hormone. This is given to increase the weight and milk production of these animals. But, once again, when we ingest these hormones through our food supply, our risk of getting cancer increases. Growth hormones make cells grow faster and this includes cancer cells which all people have in their bodies.

Have you ever noticed how the size of an average professional football player in the last 50 years has increased by at least 50 pounds? When we eat food containing growth hormones, we are going to grow, but this is endangering the normal hormonal balance of the body. If a man consistently takes testosterone to become more muscular or stronger, eventually his own body stops producing the hormone. The same is true with thyroid hormone and most others. God made our bodies to function perfectly in homeostasis, with nothing added. Why eat foods or consume drinks that increase your cancer risk and throw your body out of balance?

Caffeine

Caffeine is a stimulant drug and is found in tea, coffee, and cocoa. It increases stomach acid secretion and can raise blood pressure. It also can cause nervousness, sleep problems, nausea, and restlessness. Caffeine completely throws off the blood sugar balance and keeps the body from healing because it is kept in a constant state of stress and tension similarly to always running away from a lion. You cannot rest and heal if you are always running.

Caffeine can interfere with reproduction and cause birth defects. In animals, such defects as cleft palate, missing fingers and toes, skull malformation, and delayed bone growth increase when they consumed amounts of caffeine equaling that found in three cans of pop per day. Caffeine also can aggravate fibrocystic disease of the breast in women. There has been some correlation to the link between bladder cancer and caffeine intake.[43] Caffeine also acts as a diuretic, robbing the body of its needed water supply.

Alcohol

Alcohol has long been known for its damaging affects on the liver. All natural therapists agree that if the liver is not functioning properly, you will get very sick. Toxic load buildup is a great irritation on the system as a whole, as well as on the cellular level. Excessive alcohol consumption can lead to cirrhosis of the liver or actual death and scarring of the liver tissue. This irreversible damage leads to a premature death. It was the ninth leading cause of death in the United States in 1990.[44]

You will be surprised to know how much alcohol is too much. According to Nan Kathryn Fuchs, Ph.D., a healthy liver can handle only two to three teaspoons of alcohol per hour; it takes as long as 24 hours to eliminate the alcohol and the byproducts from just one drink.[45] One-third of all Americans drink, and 10 million are alcoholics.

Some of the effects of alcohol, besides liver problems, are as follows:

- Alcohol decreases the heart's work capacity. According to Nathan Pritikin, "Just two cocktails will cut it about 20% for about 24 hours. If you are a two-drink-a-day person, you have already deprived yourself of 1/5 of your heart."[46]

- Dr. Patrick Quillin reported in a study that the rate of strokes in drinkers is double that of non-drinkers. Heavy drinkers have more than five times the stroke risk of non-drinkers.[47]
- Excessive alcohol consumption raises blood pressure.[48]
- Excessive alcohol consumption has been shown to increase the likelihood of developing a variety of cancers, including cancers of the throat, mouth, larynx, esophagus, bladder, breast, lung, rectum, pancreas, head, neck, and liver.[49]
- Excessive alcohol consumption results in loss of white blood cells (which fight bacteria , viruses, fungi, and cancerous cells).[50]
- Excessive alcohol consumption depletes our bodies of Vitamins C and A, folic acid, B vitamins, potassium, magnesium, iron, and zinc.[51]
- Excessive alcohol consumption causes decreased absorption of calcium and causes calcium to be leached from our bones. Heavy drinkers are likely candidates to develop osteoporosis.[52]

Smoking

There are approximately 50 million smokers in the United States.[53] More than 85% of them want to quit this terrible addiction,[54] and 40 million Americans have already kicked the habit.[55]

Everyone knows smoking can be hazardous to health and can cause cancer, as the Surgeon General has stamped this statement on every packet of cigarettes. Let us look at the harm that smoking can really cause:

• **Cancer**. Tobacco smoke is made up of a wide array of harmful substances, many of which are carcinogenic. Some of them include benzopyrenes, formaldehyde, nitrosamines, hydrogen cyanide, aromatic hydrocarbons, phenols, and polonium 210 (a radioactive element).[56] Lung cancer is the No. 1 killing cancer today, and if you smoke two packs of cigarettes a day you increase your risk of contracting it by 15 to 25 times. Even one pack a day is likely to cut your life short by at least seven years.[57] The World Health Organization states that almost 400,000 Americans die each year because of smoking.[58]

• **Heart disease**. The nicotine in tobacco smoke stimulates the adrenal glands to secrete adrenaline, which is your fight, fright, or flight hormone. Adrenaline causes the heart to work harder and need more oxygen. Tobacco smoke contains carbon monoxide, which replaces the oxygen molecule in the red blood cell, causing oxygen deprivation.[59]

• **Chronic fatigue**. Because the heart is overworked and oxygen is replaced by carbon monoxide, it takes more and more energy for the body to do simple functions. This oxygen debt is extremely debilitating for people who have chronic fatigue, because in this disease the person already has a cellular metabolism which can produce only about 50% of the energy normally required for cellular function. These people get worse with exercise, because the body bounces back from the energy drain very slowly. An analogy is a very slow rechargeable battery. It takes a long time for the body to recharge, so it runs on low energy, resulting in significant problems. Smoking just destroys what little recharging ability their bodies have.

• **Chronic obstructive pulmonary disease.** This includes many lung problems like emphysema, asthma and bronchitis, most of which will eventually decrease life span and greatly decreases quality of life. If you have ever seen a friend or family member hooked up to an oxygen tank 24 hours a day, you know what I mean.

• **Secondhand or passive smoke**. In 1986, the eyes of the American people were opened to this health hazard when the U.S. Surgeon General, C. Everett Koop, wrote a report entitled *The Health Consequences of Involuntary Smoking.* In the report, secondhand or passive smoke was classified as even more harmful than primary smoke.[60] Passive smoke has been shown to contain twice the tar and nicotine and five times as much carbon monoxide as mainstream smoke. Also, nonsmokers sitting in a smoke-filled room inhale more than twice as long as those who are smoking.[61] In 1990, the Environmental Protection Agency stated that 53,000 non-smokers are killed every year due to the inhalation of passive smoke.[62] Children who live with smoking parents have a greater chance of developing respiratory diseases like asthma, pneumonia, and bronchitis.[63]

The devastating effects of smoking can be summed up by the following statements: "Cigarette smoking is the largest preventable public health problem currently existing in the United States" (Committee on Cigarette Smoking and Cardiovascular Disease.) "Smoking-related diseases are such important causes of disability and premature death in developed countries that the combat of cigarette smoking could do more to improve health and prolong life in these countries than any other single action in the whole field of preventative medicine" (World Health Organization.)[64]

Environmental factors

• **Sunlight**. Radiation from excessive sunlight exposure is becoming a growing cancer risk in America. Every year more than 600,000 people are diagnosed with skin cancer. Malignant melanoma is the fastest-growing and deadliest form of cancer.[65] Between 1973 and 1987, the rate of melanoma increased 83%.[66] Malignant melanoma is the leading cause of cancer in women ages 25 to 29, and is second only to breast cancer in women 30 to 34.[67] The National Cancer Institute predicts that one out of every six Americans will develop some form of skin cancer in his or her lifetime.[68] Here's a warning from Sydney Hurwitz, M.D., professor of dermatology and pediatrics at the Yale University School of Medicine: "Most skin cancers begin in childhood. The studies have shown that a history of sunburns during the first 20 years of life doubles the risk of skin cancer in later years."[69]

Diet is a key factor associated with sunlight. If you consume a diet low in hydrogenated oils and consume a lot of antioxidative foods containing natural beta carotene your chances of developing skin cancer greatly drop.

• **Radon**. Radon is a radioactive gas emitted from bedrock. It enters buildings through cracks in the foundation or holes in the basement floors and walls (drains, sump pits, etc.). Radon is an odorless, colorless gas that cannot be detected except by measuring devices. Radon is deadly and a very significant health hazard; it is the second most common cause of lung cancer. With lung cancer being the most common cancer of all and radon being the second highest cause of lung cancer,[70] you can see how very, very important this issue can be for your health. Fortunately radon can be easily and inexpensively detected with testing kits that can be purchased at your local hardware store. If the results are higher than the normal limits, you don't necessarily have to move or panic. There are companies that specialize in installing fans that aerate the gases under foundations, making these homes safe. Look under "Radon" in the Yellow Pages for listings. An easy safety precaution is to open all the windows in your house each day for half an hour to let the fresh air in and any potentially hazardous fumes and gases out. This includes basement windows or window wells. Also, seal any cracks in the foundation or walls.

• **Electromagnetic radiation**. Electromagnetic radiation is emitted by practically all electrical appliances and outside power lines. The longer you are exposed to low-level electromagnetic fields (EMFs), the greater the health risk, especially cancer in children. In a 1991 study done by the University of Southern California, 232 children in Los Angeles County who had leukemia by the age of 11 were compared to the same number of children who were healthy. The results showed that the children with leukemia were more likely to use 11 out of 15 electrical appliances (most significantly electric hair dryers and black and white television sets) as compared to the healthy children.[71] Dr. Robert Becker states that EMFs may be linked to chronic fatigue syndrome, AIDS, autism, fragile X syndrome, and sudden infant death syndrome. Also EMFs may worsen already existing conditions, especially those related to the nervous system, the brain, or mental illness — Alzheimer's, Parkinson's, depression, phobias, and addictive personality traits.[72] Doctors point to EMFs as a main reason for people having low energy, irritability, poor concentration, tension and stress. According to USA Today "EMFs are becoming the number one environmental concern in America." EMFs are also strongly emitted from power lines and may pose a health risk for people who live within 200 feet of the overhead lines.[73]

The best way to avoid EMFs is to avoid being close to any operating electrical appliance. The recommended distance is three to four feet. With large-screen TVs the distance should be increased to at least 10 feet. If you are really concerned, you can purchase a gaussmeter from an electronics store to measure the number of milligauss that are emitted from appliances. Most environmental experts suggest that your environment not exceed 1 milligauss, and 1.5 to 2 milligauss is significant enough to make changes in the household.[74] Recent results of a 25 year Swedish study involving 500,000 people exposed to sustained EMF levels revealed that the cancer risk for children continuously exposed to 2mG of EMF was 3 times higher than normal, while those exposed to 3mG showed risk for contracting leukemia 4 times higher than normal. Adults also ran increased risk of leukemia, lymphoma, and brain tumors.

Viral/bacterial/fungal/parasitic risk

A growing number of people are becoming toxic and developing weakened immune systems as a result of this group of health risks. AIDS is just the beginning of the infectious viral diseases that we will have to contend with. Bacterial infections are making a resurgence, and alarmingly, more strains are becoming resistant to antibiotics. Of the fungi group, candida has an overwhelming effect on the number of Americans it has affected. Parasitic infections can cause everything from poor digestion to bloating to headaches to a wide variety of health complaints. Intestinal parasites are particularly common, entering our bodies through our meat, chicken, and fish consumption. Learn more on these risks in the circulative and immune health chapters.

Lifestyle risk

Stress and fear are the two greatest lifestyle risks and probably negatively affect ones health more than any other group. We will address these issues in the mental and spiritual health chapters.

CHAPTER 3

MY HEALTH: WHERE DID I LOSE IT?

Let's look at the major components of health and alterations that can be made to improve our total health picture. Remember, nothing is impossible, or more exactly, everything is possible for him who believes. In this chapter, let's examine where and how we went wrong, as this is the first step toward correcting the problem.

STRUCTURAL /NERVOUS SYSTEM/ORGANS & GLANDS

Most people remain unaware of this category of health unless serious problems arise (i.e., paralysis after an accident due to a severing of the spinal cord). These extreme situations affect less than $\frac{1}{100}$ of 1% of the population. However, 90% of all Americans experience pressure on their nervous system causing one or more of the following symptoms: organ and gland dysfunction; pain, numbness, tingling, burning, or weakness of arms, legs, or any other part of the body. Does this high percentage surprise you? Perhaps it will help to consider the skeletal system and how it relates to the nervous system.

The spinal column is made up of 24 movable segments called vertebrae. Vertebrae are spinal bones that serve several purposes: They protect the spinal cord from injury and maintain a clear pathway for electrical impulses to flow from the brain through the spinal nerves to all areas of the body, so that your body can function as it was created to. If the foramina, or holes where the nerves exit the spine, do not remain open, nerve root irritation will eventually develop, leading to ill health of whatever organ, gland, or tissue that nerve goes to.

Think of the spinal nerve as a garden hose. If the water is flowing out of the hose and someone steps on the hose, the water ceases to come out. An outside pressure applied to the hose restricts the waters flow. In relation to the spinal nerve, this is called a subluxation. Another illustration of subluxation is a dimmer switch, which can either cause a light to work at 100 percent (fully lighted) or cause less light to be produced. In a similar way, nerve pressure due to subluxation can cause varying degrees of nerve pressure, resulting in impeded function.

The brain and spinal cord comprise the central nervous system. This system is the master computer that controls all other systems of the body. The cardiovascular, musculoskeletal and respiratory systems — all glands, organs, tissues, blood vessels — are supplied by nerves that come from the central nervous system. God had a tremendous plan when he designed our bodies, because the skeletal system not only gives us the ability to move, stand, walk, and run, but it also houses and protects the central nervous system, from the skull (protecting the brain) to the spinal column (protecting the spinal cord).

There is only one vulnerable spot in the spine, and that lies at the opening where the spinal nerve leaves the spinal cord and spinal column to branch to the arms, legs, back, neck, midback, and all internal organs, glands, and tissues. This is called intervertebral foramina (IVF), or the hole where the nerves exit the spinal canal. The vulnerability increases when the spinal bones are misaligned and are out of their normal position. This is called a spinal subluxation (similar to a dislocation, but to a lesser degree). It is subluxation that causes many of the problems associated with the nervous system or structural aspect of our health picture.

What causes these subluxations? The causes are many but can be grouped into four main categories: physical, mental, spiritual, and thermal stress. Let's look at each:

Physical stress is anything from an acute trauma like an auto accident to prolonged poor posture while sitting, standing, sleeping, or lifting. All of these will cause tension or strain in the muscles and stretching tension in the ligaments, causing laxity and eventual subluxation. The muscles and ligaments are the two supportive tissues that stabilize the joints and hold proper position in any point in the body. So if either of these has been irritated or injured due to a physical activity at one point in time or on a prolonged basis, subluxations will occur, eventually causing nervous system pressure.

Mental stress is very debilitating on the neuromusculoskeletal system because this stress does not go away if you rest or use proper posture. This stress comes from the pressures of life and lack of peace, joy and love. It can be caused by a high-pressure job with excessive demands, or a home life that is not peaceful. I have seen patients who in one day went from perfect spinal alignment with no subluxations to back spasms and numerous spinal subluxations due to one cause: Their spouse said, "I want a divorce."

Mental stress tends to be harder to remove in total health = wholeness than physical stress, because with physical stress all you have to do is teach a person what to do and what not to do. However, with mental stress and the mind, you are dealing with personalities and attitudes, which often are unchangeable or slow to change.

Spiritual health has the most negative or positive effect on our *total health = wholeness*. God created us and has a plan for our lives. He loves us unconditionally, will never leave us or forsake us, fills us with his joy, and gives us his peace. Without this knowledge, our mental health will decline, which will eventually have a negative impact on our physical health, causing disease. God created us and sustains us, and He alone gives us true purpose in life — to know Him and give Him glory. When we know Him and have a personal, living relationship with his Son, Jesus Christ, we will have in our hearts what He has: love, joy and peace. This is not dependent upon any circumstances, just Him. When one does not feel God's love, joy and peace in his life, it is the most stressful condition of all.

Thermal stress includes anything from cold (causing tightened muscles and misaligned spinal bones) to excessive heat (which does the same but for different reasons) to being affected by humidity and barometric pressure (both can cause swelling and fluid buildup around joints, causing pain, muscle tension, and spinal subluxation which can then lead to pinched nerves). Remember the pattern of stresses:

muscle tightening >subluxation > nerve root pressure> impingement > pain, numbness, tingling, burning, weakness, sickness or disease.

One's poor general state of physical health will also cause spinal subluxation.

How does subluxation lead to disease?

As far back as 1921, 138 out of 139 cases of cadaver dissection of people who had kidney disease showed atrophy of the spinal nerve leading to the kidney, due to spinal subluxation. This is not just stated by chiropractic profession, but even M.D.s are recognizing the correlations. R.F. Allendy, M.D., states, "It is possible that a slight irregularity in the disposition of the vertebrae by strangling certain spinal nerves at their exit from the spine can have considerable organic effects as the chiropractor school maintains."[1] Also stated by Ruben Herman, M.D., "It may never occur to them (his medical colleagues) that headaches, stomach trouble, neuritis, or nervous irritability they are attempting to cure may be due to nothing more serious than a displaced vertebrae."[2]

Brain Function and the Spine

Dr. Roger Sperry, a Nobel Prize winner for brain research found the more biomechanical faults (spinal misalignments or subluxations) that were present, the less energy that was available for thinking, healing and metabolizing. Dr. Sperry made another amazing discovery that 90 percent of the stimulation and nutrition to the brain is generated by the movement of the spine, similar to a windmill generating electricity. So anything that inhibits the movement of the spine would indeed decrease the power and energy to the brain to perform its complex function. So what inhibits movement of the spine and hence brain function?

1. Spinal subluxation, or misalignments of the spinal bones.
2. Lack of
   a. full body aerobic exercising (walking, swimming, etc.)
   b. rebounding (cellular exercise)

So, the best way to increase brain function is to:
1. Have your spine checked for subluxations and if present have them corrected. Chiropractic physicians are the experts in detecting subluxations and correcting them.
2. Start a regular full body aerobic and rebounding cellular exercise program consisting of a variety of full body movements to increases spinal mobility and flexibility. This should be done from three to seven days per week.

Dr. Ron Pero, Chief of Cancer Research at New York's Preventative Research Center and world renowned scientist in genotoxicology (study of environmental toxins) conducted a study of the immune systems ability to resist toxins and disease.

Three study groups were tested.

Group 1 Patients with good spinal movement that were checked regularly for detection and correction of spinal subluxations. These were chiropractic physicians' well patients who were on regular spinal maintaining care. Call this group chiropractic well patient.

Group 2 Non-chiropractic well-patients. This group had patients that felt good and had no health complaints who were not under chiropractic care.

Group 3 Non-chiropractic ill patients. These patients had some disease processes but were not under chiropractic care.

The results were as follows:

The chiropractic well-patients (Group 1) had a 200% stronger immune system than the non-chiropractic well patients (Group 2) and a 400% stronger immune system than the non-chiropractic ill patients (Group 3.)

Could there be a possible link between Dr. Pero's work and Dr. Sperry's work? Could spinal subluxation not only decrease brain function hence mind function, but also could this decreased brain function be contributing to the weakened immune systems of the non-chiropractic patient? Or is it that when we decrease brain power and energy (function) we actually cause the mind to negatively affect the body? And in this case the body is represented by the immune system.

For over 100 years chiropractic physicians have stated that the nervous system controls all other systems. When there is no pressure on the nervous system the body can heal itself maximally and when there is pressure on the system (subluxation) the body malfunctions and disease sets in. This is being substantiated by the work of Dr. Sperry, Dr. Pero and many others who have shown that spine affects the normal functioning of the brain and mind as well as the body.

Now, I am not saying that spinal subluxation and nervous system pressure and irritation is the cause of all sickness and disease, but I am saying that it is definitely a cause and should be evaluated if anyone is seeking optimal health. Who should be checked by a chiropractic physician? I think it would be safe to say, who should not? Who has not had falls and accidents, emotional stress and burdens, postural stresses, excessive weight, etc.? Even birth can be very traumatic to a baby's neck, as his or her head is being forcibly pushed into the pubic bone and pelvis with each contraction.

I am reminded of a true story told by one of my college professors about a chiropractic intern whose wife gave birth to their first child during his internship. The delivery was very hard, and upon delivery the baby's vital signs were irregular. Over the course of a few weeks more tests were done and treatments tried, but the child continued to get worse. Finally, out of desperation and stress, the intern went to his professor to tell him he was taking a leave from school because of the stress of seeing his son slowly perish. The professor's response was, "Did you adjust the baby (remove subluxation)?" The intern replied, "No," but he decided to see if it would help his dying son. So he went to the hospital and realigned the baby's very misaligned neck, and within ten minutes the baby's vital signs were normal, and he recovered totally.

ELIMINATIVE HEALTH

Simply defined, eliminative health is what goes out of the body, or the body purging itself of wastes, toxins, chemicals, and byproducts of metabolism. The avenues by which this most important task is accomplished are the bowel, liver,gall bladder, kidneys, bladder, lungs, and skin. If any one of these organs does not perform its function property, levels of toxins and waste products increase and start to circulate through the blood to all areas of the body. Left unchecked, these toxins and waste products start to deposit in tissues throughout the body, potentially causing a long list of health problems.

The first problem, a major key in health problems and toxicity, is impaired elimination. When asked what is the normal number of bowel movements per day, the usual response is one. But research among tribes who have almost no incidence of colon cancer and have great longevity and eat predominately fruit, vegetables, seeds, and nuts shows that they have a bowel movement after each meal. Why is it so important to our health to have this kind of regularity? Because in 1994 colorectal cancer was the No. 1 form of cancer in the United States among men and women as a combined group.

The major cause of colon cancer is constipation because of toxic buildup and inflammation of the intestinal lining. When we eat chicken, fish, or red meat, our intestinal tracts slow down greatly due to lack of fiber and the difficulty with which this heavy protein is digested. When comparing intestinal tracts of a meat-eating lion to man, we see the lion's is shorter and smoother for fast elimination time. On the other hand, man's digestive tract is longer and convoluted, showing it is designed to digest fruits and vegetables, whole grains, seeds, and nuts. But for meat, the transit time is too long, allowing greater chances of intestinal inflammation and toxic buildup.

Elimination is a key in the overall health picture, so I always ask people who consult with me about their ill health, "How often to you have a bowel movement?" The goal is three effortless and odorless bowel movements per day.

Again, consider our diets. White bread and pasta tend to constipate us. In fact, in the early part of this century, the prescribed treatment for diarrhea was to eat some white bread. Chicken, fish, and red meat are all hard to digest and hard to eliminate. Add some fat and you have a mess — sludge just sitting in you trying to squeeze its way through your intestine, moving very slowly. The standard diet of the average American consists of too much protein (90-120g opposed to the 30-50g necessary), too much fat, too much refined carbohydrates, and to little fruits, vegetables, complex carbohydrates, and fiber. So in working toward physical health, we have to look at elimination, primarily through the bowel.

The liver has a critical role in detoxing the body and is overburdened in today's society of high amounts of chemicals and toxins.

The lungs, the kidneys, and the skin also help eliminate waste products and toxins from the body and are all necessary to function optimally in good health. Dr. Alexis Castle at the Rockefeller Institute suggested the possibility that cells could live forever if kept free from their own waste and properly nourished. He set up an experiment in which the heart tissue of a chicken was immersed in a nutrient solution which was changed daily. He kept this tissue alive for 29 years. Shortly after the time of Castle's death, the attendant forgot to change the solution, and the tissue died. Who knows how long our bodies can live if cared for? I believe estimates of 120 years are not unreasonable.

The next elimination organ is our kidneys, which filter our blood to keep it pure. The kidneys have a tremendous role in elimination, because they excrete a number of toxic compound substances that increase the burden on the body and chances of tissue breakdown if not eliminated. As previously stated, the average American diet consists of 90-120 grams of protein per day, which is two to four times the daily requirement of protein. What happens to the excess? Protein is not stored in the body. If you cannot use it, it must be excreted, and the pathway of excretion is through the kidneys. This is very hard on the microtubules of the kidney and greatly increases the chance of kidney disease.

Our last elimination organ is skin, which releases up to 1.5 gallons of water each day.

The physical aspect of health correlated with circulation and elimination is breathing. So many people do not breathe deeply and properly. This is not only important in removal of CO_2 and other harmful waste byproducts, but it is also crucial in increasing the amount of oxygen we have in our bodies. (People who only chest-breathe never fill the lower part of their lungs, which supply up to 80 percent of the oxygen to our bodies). This is also seen in people who have asthma, emphysema, and other forms of chronic obstructive pulmonary disease. These people consistently cannot get enough oxygen into their bodies and have to take pure oxygen through respirators to make sure that the lesser amount they take in is enough to sustain the life of the body. Proper deep breathing also increases the normal lymph flow dramatically. In a research study conducted to analyze the flow of lymph (which is critical in the maintenance of a healthy immune system), the single most important factor in moving lymph was not massage, not exercise, but deep breathing. So deep breathing plays an important part in our health.

PHYSICAL EXERCISE

The other aspect of physical health that is often lacking is physical exercise to increase cardiovascular fitness, immune system response, elimination, energy, and mental clarity.

Exercise causes us to perspire and hence eliminate toxins and chemicals through our skin. It is also common for someone who is sick or toxic to have bad body odor, because he or she is eliminating toxins and chemicals through the skin. The average American gets little to no proper exercise outside of what they might do on their jobs. Many people are too tired before the day starts to get up and exercise before work, or they are too mentally and physically drained at the end of the day to go out and exercise. Our poor diets, chemical and toxic buildup, poor sleep (either quantity or quality), and stressful lives all lead to fatigue, which replaces our desire to exercise with a desire to just go to bed.

Exercise was much easier before everything became automatic. People used to walk more, ride bikes more, do more manual labor. Now we drive everywhere and do little physical work, but plenty of mentally-draining work.

Nearly four out of five adults get little or no exercise even though research has clearly demonstrated its positive effects on health. Also, studies have shown that if you do not get any exercise, your chances of having a heart attack more than triple.[3] In a study at the University of North Carolina, it was determined that an inactive person's risk of heart disease is the same as that of someone who smokes a pack of cigarettes a day.[4]

Another interesting study done among Harvard alumni tracked 16,936 graduates and found that those who burned 2,000 or more calories a week in exercise had a 28 percent lower death rate. Dr. Ralph Paffenberger stated in the study that for every hour you walk, you can add an hour to your life.[5]

Another exciting study, done on 4,500 people between the ages of 40 and 85 at Brown University by Vincent Mor, Ph.D., showed that those who remained moderately active by only walking regularly gained a 25-year advantage in performance over those who retired to a sedentary life.[6]

This and other research reports have shown that the greatest benefit from exercise was seen in the change from no exercise to moderate exercise — 30 minutes of walking daily, or three one-hour sessions per week. The health benefit from moderate to intense exercise was minimal. In fact it showed more chances of sudden cardiac disease — i.e., heart attacks — due to the level of exercise intensity combined with possible blockage of the coronary arteries. Remember, if we exercise very intensely but pay no attention to our diet, we are still at risk of cardiovascular disease. This was evidenced in runner Jim Fixx, who averaged ten miles of running per day but claimed that diet did not play as great a factor in health if one was exercising intensely. He died of a sudden heart attack in his 50s. So remember, a healthy diet combined with moderate exercise, such as walking daily or rebounding at a brisk pace progressively increasing to 30 minutes, will have great health benefits.

Another study by Dr. Steve Blair and his colleagues at the Institute for Aerobics Research, published in the *Journal of the American Medical Association,* showed how important moderate exercise really is. Dr. Blair tested 10,224 men and 3,120 women who appeared to be in good health. They participated in a treadmill test. Based on their levels of fitness, the participants were divided into five groups ranging from least fit (Group 1) to most fit (Group 5.) These people were tracked to determine the relationship between their level of physical fitness and their death rates. After eight years, the least fit group had a death rate more than three times greater than the most fit group. More important, though, was the finding that most of the benefits of physical fitness came between Group 1 and Group 2, especially in men. In other words, walking 30 minutes per day (the activity level of Group 2) reduced premature death almost as much as running 30 to 40 miles per week (the activity of Group 5.) Further, in Groups 2 through 5, deaths were lower from all causes, including heart disease and cancer, when compared with the sedentary people in Group 1.[7]

Similar results were found in 12,138 middle-aged men who participated in the Multiple Risk Factor Intervention Trial. The investigators, directed by Dr. Arthur Leon, divided these men into three groups based on level of exercise. During seven years of follow-up, those who exercised moderately had one-third fewer deaths from all causes (including heart disease), compared to those who were sedentary. Moderate exercise was defined as

at least 30 minutes a day of light or moderate intensity activi
walking, gardening, or home repairs. Mortality rates of those
levels of exercise were not significantly different from those w... moderate levels of exercise.[8]

Benefits of exercise
- Lowers death rate from all diseases, as demonstrated in the Harvard study previously mentioned
- Reduces risk of cancer
- Reduces risk of heart disease
- Lowers blood pressure
- Reduces stress
- Increases mental abilities
- Acts as an antidepressant
- Increases the immune systems response
- Reduces body fat. All sickness tends to thrive more in fatty tissue because it lacks a good blood supply, which carries the white blood cell defenders which rid your body of bacteria, viruses, and cancer.
- Reduces constipation. Colorectal cancer was the No. 1 form of cancer in 1994 among men and women as a combined group. Constipation is the major cause of colorectal cancer, and this can be greatly reduced through regular exercise.
- Increases blood flow, bringing more oxygen to the cells and ridding the body of more waste. Decreases the chances of toxic buildup in the cells, tissues, and organs because the amount of blood that is filtered by the liver and the kidneys increases.

Blood flow is sluggish through the tissues in people who perform no exercise. Exercise increases blood flow through all blood vessels, causing faster movement of oxygen and the essential nutrients into the tissues, along with waste products and toxins being moved out of the tissues. If you want an increase of white blood cells, which in turn increases your immune system's ability to fight off sickness and disease, then increase your blood flow with regular moderate to intense exercise for 30 minutes per day.

Exercise should be aerobic — sustained non-stop activity — to elevate the heart rate and maintain elevation throughout the workout. Lifting weights does not qualify as aerobic exercise; if we lift some weight, then rest a couple of minutes, then lift some more. What we are looking for is sustained elevated heart rate, as in walking, rebounding cellular exercise, swimming, bike-riding, jogging, or using a cross-country ski machine or step-climber machine.

From a structural point of view, the best exercises are the ones that are done in a non-bent position. Therefore, swimming and walking are better than bike-riding and other sitting exercises. The reason riding or positions in which the body is bent forward are avoided is because they increase the pressure on the lower back disks and, if continued over prolonged periods of time, tend to lead to back problems. Also, if you use a step-climber machine, do not lean forward when you begin to tire, but look up and stand upright. Some of my patients have even had some problems on cross-country ski machines because of the slight forward lean in the waist. The health-rider type exercise machines are good for the rowing or pulling-back motions, which are very good for posture and middle- and upper-back muscle toning, but the negative side is that the lower back is stressed by the sitting and leaning-forward position. The best exercise for the entire body is rebounding cellular exercise.

CELLULAR EXERCISE

Cellular exercise is one that utilizes the forces of acceleration, deceleration and gravity as it strengthens every single cell in the body at the same time. Cellular exercise, or rebounding, is the ultimate exercise for the immune system causing the circulating white blood cell count to triple. This threefold increase in WBC's literally means your immune system can consume cancer cells, bacteria, viruses, parasites and fungi three times as fast. I don't even have to tell you how important that is in preventing cancer from growing in your body or stopping it if it has already begun growing.

This form of exercise has many health benefits and virtually no risks if performed properly. It can be used by practically everyone no matter what age or health condition. It is very easy to start by just standing on a rebounder and gently health bouncing up and down to progressing to walking, jogging, running and even sprinting all to fit each individuals cardiovascular need. It produces little stress on the joints (up to 87% less than aerobics training),[9] so foot, ankle, hip, knee and back injuries do not occur. According to NASA report published in the *Journal of Applied Physiology* 49 (5); 881-887, 1980. The conclusion was that "The work output was greater while rebounding than running. The greatest difference was about 68 percent.[10] That sounds pretty impressive, an exercise that is 68 percent more efficient than running without any of the risks of injury of running and can be done in your own home 365 days a year. What are the benefits of rebounding?

1. Cellular exercise and strengthener of
    a. veins and arteries
    b. bones
    c. internal organs
    d. internal glands
    e. muscles, tendons and tissues
    f. eyes and ears
    g. skin
2. Increases lymphatic circulation
3. Increases strength
4. Increases endurance
5. Increases cardiovascular fitness
6. Increases weight loss
7. Increases balance, coordination, rhythm and timing

1. Exercises and strengthening all cells. According to Albert Carter, rebounding authority, "Your cells depend upon the diffusion of water through their semipermeable cell membranes to carry oxygen, nutrients, hormones and enzymes into the cell and flush out metabolic trash. The rate of diffusion of water into and out of the cells under normal conditions is 100 times the volume of fluid inside each cell each second. The oscillation of the cells between an increase G force and no G force 200 times a minute (with rebounding) increased the diffusion of water, into each cell at least three fold."[11] Also the strength of the cell is determined by the strength of its cell membrane. Sickly or weak cells rupture and die easily while healthy cells resist rupturing. Exercising at a higher G force causes the cells to naturally strengthen their membranes thus producing stronger and healthier cells.

2 Increased lymphatic circulation. This is probably one of the greatest benefits of all. Exercise can increase lymph flow by up to 30 times. The lymphatic channels are made up of one-way valves that open when the pressure below them is greater than above them and close when the reverse occurs. The up and down motion that occurs while

rebounding activates the one-way valves to their maximum and this happens one hundred times a minute according to rebounding authority Albert Carter.[12] The lymphatic system is the heart of the immune system and lymphatic circulation is vital to the movement of the white blood cells to destroy bacteria, viruses, parasites, fungi and cancer cells. If the lymph fluid moves slowly, the white blood cells cannot get to and fight the invaders or abnormal cancer cells quickly enough, so disease develops. It is also vitally important to know that the circulating white blood cell count triples after just one minute of rebounding. This means more white blood cells to eat cancer cells, bacteria, viruses, parasites and fungi.

3,4. Increase strength and endurance by exercising in a higher gravitational force atmosphere. Jumping on a rebounder can increase G forces up to 3.5, which means that your muscles adjust to an increased G force by becoming stronger.[13] This can be seen practically with Albert Carter, who's children had been rebounding before they could even walk. His son, Darren, was able to do 429 sit-ups in first grade and his daughter Wendie was able to beat all the sixth grade boys in arm wrestling although she had never arm wrestled before in her life. His three-and-a-half year old daughter could actually do one-arm push ups.[14]

5. As was stated above in a NASA report that rebounding is up to 68 percent more efficient than running. This rebounding developed more biomechanical work with less energy expended, thus less oxygen used and less demand placed on the heart. Also the ratio of oxygen consumption compared to biomechanical conditioning is sometimes more than twice as efficient as treadmill running.

6. Increase weight loss. Because of the NASA study that showed that rebounding was 68% more efficient than treadmill running it hits the 90% fat burning stage in less than half the time of regular aerobic type exercises.

With regular cardiovascular aerobic exercises like jogging, bike riding, aerobics, etc. the following time is allowed before we start burning fat:

First 10 minutes burns 90% glucose, 10% fat
20-30 minutes burns 70% glucose, 30% fat
After 30 minutes burns10% glucose, 90% fat

Because rebounding is 68% more efficient than the other cardiovascular aerobic exercises it hits the 90% fat burn stage in approximately 12 minutes instead of 30 minutes. This means it take less time to burn more fat.

Anyone who progresses to an intense rebounding exercise program will tell you that their increased heart and breathing shows them that one can become very fit on a rebounder. Silvia Ortiz took note that her cardiovascular and respiratory functions were even better than when she was running 50 miles every week and in just three months had lost 15 pounds.[15]

7. Increase balance, coordination, rhythm and timing. These are all naturally improved while one rebounds which is why it is ideal for athletes of all types, professional or novice.

To summarize rebounding, bouncing, walking, jogging or running on a rebounder is one of the best total health exercises available. Not only does it give a great cardiovascular workout even better that jogging with little risk of injury but it also exercises the lymphatic system which is the heart of the immune system. Rebounding cellular exercise also exercises and strengthens all the cells of your body by increasing the fluid exchange in and out of the cells three fold and strengthens the cells by strengthening the cell membrane thereby increasing the health of each and every cell.

Use these hints as a guide to customizing your own workout, whether you just like to walk 30 minutes per day, rebound or use exercise machines. Start slow — begin at five minutes per day — and add one minute each day until you reach 30 minutes. This should be done gradually over a four-week period. Remember, if you do have some blockages in your coronary arteries (it can happen in your 20s if your diet has been poor) the body makes alternative routes for the blood to flow. The small accessory arteries enlarge to take up the slack and become more major blood suppliers. This is why you need to ease into exercise if you haven't done it for a while. DO NOT go out and start walking briskly for 30 minutes the first day. Follow your doctor's recommendations only.

CHEMICAL HEALTH

I have defined chemical health as what goes into our bodies. I have broken this into three major groups — digestion, assimilation, and respiration — and will divide it further later in this book.

Digestion begins as the food enters the digestive tract and is broken down with digestive enzymes — in the mouth first, then in the stomach, where food is further broken down by hydrochloric acid. As the food enters the small intestine, further enzyme activity begins as the pancreas secretes amylase, protease, and lipase so that the starches, proteins, and fats can be fully digested and assimilated — or taken in — by the body. This process is helped by the excretion of bile from the liver and gall bladder. Bile helps emulsify or break down the fat that enters the intestinal tract. It also rids the body of toxic byproducts that were removed by the liver in the phases of liver detoxification. These harmful products leave the body as bile in the fecal matter.

Assimilation occurs next. Once food is digested, the small intestine must assimilate the nutrients from it. This is the key role of the small intestine, and if anything affects its ability to do this function, our level of health will suffer. The intestinal mucosal barrier has selective permeability, which means that it only lets through the substances that are good for the body and keeps out unwanted chemicals, toxins and larger food particles that have not been completely digested. I liken this to a mesh or screen with fine holes that only lets very small digested food components through, like the amino acids which are the building blocks of proteins. If the larger proteins themselves were allowed through this screen, they could potentially cause many allergic and autoimmune reactions, in which the body becomes highly sensitized to certain substances, or even to the body itself. This reaction is not possible when amino acids cross the mesh barrier, because basic nutrient components are not allergenic. Also larger food particles cause a weakening of your immune system because your white blood cells have to eat these non digested food particles entering your blood instead of eating bacteria, viruses, cancer cells, parasites and mold and fungi like candida. It may be helpful to imagine a piece of property on which no houses are permitted to be built; if they are, they will be demolished. However, it would be fine to put bricks, wood, nails, and other building materials on the property.

As I have stated before, we only want what is good for our health crossing this barrier (assimilating) after proper digestion. God made our bodies to deny the bad substances access into our bodies so they could not cross the barrier of selective permeability in the intestinal tract into the circulating blood which reaches every tissue, gland, organ, and cell. The first barrier of access is the intestinal mucosa, then the liver itself, which detoxifies the chemicals that passed through the intestinal barrier, or gut, or those that entered unchecked by our respiration.

Respiration often means the inhalation of chemicals and fumes that immediately enter our blood with no liver check first. Also, chemicals that come in contact with skin can have a similar effect. Anything that your skin touches enters your bloodstream in 20 to 30 seconds. This should make you think twice before touching chemical household products, even soaps and shampoos.

So in looking at the chemical side of our *total health = wholeness* model, we must remember to be cautious about what goes in our bodies.

MENTAL HEALTH

Our mind is a reflection of our spirit. If our spirit is alive because of our personal relationship with the Living God who created us, then it will overflow to our mind, and it will be filled with unchangeable love, joy and peace. So true mental health is inseparable from spiritual health.

SPIRITUAL HEALTH

This is by far the most important part of our *total health = wholeness*. God made us as a spirit with a soul that lives in a body. When Adam and Eve sinned, they became separated from God, and their spirits were no longer in communion with Him; in essence, their spirits had died, the direct communication line had been broken. Also as a result of their sin, the perfect world in which they had lived became an imperfect world. God, the Creator, gave His world to Adam, His creation. He told Adam to tend to the animals in the garden, to name them, and to rule over all of them. Adam and Eve were like owners of the world until the day they submitted to the lie of the Deceiver, Satan. On that day they broke their covenant with God and fell from perfection. On that day they gave the rulership of the world over to the devil, and he has had control ever since. Scripture calls Satan the prince of the world. But from the time man fell and turned the earth over to Satan and separated from God, God had a plan to regain the earth for His creation and, more importantly, regain the relationship, communion, and fellowship He had with His creation. This fellowship was to be even greater than that which He had with man before, because now He placed His own Holy Spirit within His creation so He could commune and walk and talk with man every second of every day.

Although Adam and Eve walked and talked with God, they did not have God living in them. Although Jesus walked and talked with his disciples, they did not have Jesus in them. That's why he told his disciples to wait for the Comforter, because when Jesus left, he would leave the Comforter, the Paraclete, with them. He told them God would be within them, and they would not worship at the temple, because the Spirit of Truth would be in them. Jesus made it clear there would be one provision: "I must go for Him to come."

When Jesus died on the cross, the disciples fell apart. Fear entered them because their strength and security, their Savior and Lord, their God had left them. Hence, Peter denied Christ, everyone scattered, and many considered returning to their former occupation as fishermen. Jesus appeared to them and reminded them to wait for the Comforter. What a change we see after the second chapter of the book of Acts in the Bible when the disciples received the Holy Spirit. No longer does Peter deny Christ, but he preaches boldly before the people and 3,000 receive salvation in one day. What was the difference? Before Pentecost, Peter operated in his own ability (in the flesh), filled with fear because his source of strength was gone. After Pentecost, he operated in God's ability, being filled and led by the Spirit. Peter no longer needed Jesus by his side; he had the Spirit of God dwelling within him.

What an awesome revelation this is to God's people. We are not just a people who know the risen Lord; we are not just a people who have received salvation and eternal life. We are a people who carry the Spirit of God around inside us wherever we go, whatever we do. He is with us, encouraging us, empowering us, giving us wisdom and knowledge. He cultivates His fruit in our lives: love, joy, peace, patience, kindness, goodness, faithfulness, gentleness and self-control. We do not practice these virtues to be like the Living God; these are the fruit that naturally comes when He dwells within us. A truth that has transformed my life is this: *We live from Him, not for Him.*

Our strength does not come in our trying our best to be better people or more like the Living God. This is in our ability or our strength, and no matter how noble the task, we will fail and come up short. Our strength comes from His Spirit living within us. The love we have for those who seem unlovable is not from us; we cannot produce it. It flows supernaturally from His Spirit within us. Our joy in the most trying times is not a product of our positive thinking; it is God within us pouring His joy into our hearts. So in our minds it seems almost incomprehensible that we could experience joy in the midst of painful or sorrowful times, but it is possible through God's Spirit.

When we are weak, He is strong; when we have nothing left to give, He lifts us up and carries us. When we feel inexplicable peace amidst the stresses and pressures of this world, it is His Holy Spirit touching our minds with a peace "which transcends all understanding, guarding our hearts and minds in Christ Jesus" (Philippians 4:7.)

So from the time Adam fell, God had a plan, a great plan, to restore and create a greater relationship with His creation. In order for this to occur, He had to send His Son to the world to regain what was lost and once again make our dead spirits alive. Jesus told the Pharisee Nicodemus that in order to enter the kingdom of God, one must be born again. What did he mean? He meant we had to be born of the Spirit and having our relationship and communication with God restored. Jesus came to restore the relationship between God and man and to place God's Holy Spirit within us.

What is the kingdom of God? According to Jesus, it is within you. If you have His Spirit within you, you have His kingdom within you. We don't have to live a life of misery waiting for heaven someday; heaven is within our hearts. The kingdom of God is within us. What could be better than living every day with the Living God inside you directing you, leading you, guiding you, empowering you, and giving you all His fruit, especially love, joy and peace?

How does all this fit into *total health = wholeness*? First of all, The Living God came to make us whole in body, soul and spirit. He came to heal the sick (make our bodies whole), to give us His mind (one filled with love, joy and peace), and to fill us with His Spirit (to make our spirits alive once again). He came to make the creation and Creator one, as husband and wife are one. To understand this, one must understand what covenant means. One also must have a revelation of the grace and love of God.

The following are basic to being in vital relationship with the Living God:

1. To know who you are in Christ and therefore to understand the new covenant;
2. To know the depth of the love God has for you;

3. To know the grace of God and understand what He did for the creation He loved;

4. To walk in His strength, not yours.

Receiving the revelation of these truths will transform your life. First of all, as we will see in the spiritual health chapter, the greatest part of your *total health* = *wholeness* is your spiritual health. Why? Because God said the Spirit gives life; health and wholeness flow from the spirit of a man to his mind (or soul), to his body. What is more healing to a person with cancer — to know that there is an 80%cure rate for this type of cancer with chemotherapy and radiation, or to know that the God who created him is inside him giving him strength, and to know that he will be with God forever?

We are here on earth for a split second of eternity. It is not whether we live to be 120 that matters the most, although God said we should in the sixth chapter of Genesis. But Paul said it best: "For to me, to live is Christ and to die is gain" (Philippians 1:21.) To Paul, living in communion with God by the Holy Spirit that dwelled in him, and doing what God called him to do with the power God gave him through the Spirit, was the only way he would live this life. But even better would be the day that he would be called home, finished with the race that the Living God called him to run.

What a comfort to know that the God who created you knows and loves you more than you love yourself. He who knows the number of hairs on your head has a plan and purpose for your life. As we sit at the feet of the Living God and come to know Him more and more, the world has less and less of a hold on us. Paul feared nothing because he walked empowered by the Spirit. If he was sick, he could be healed by the Spirit. If he was persecuted, he was strengthened, encouraged, and felt love, joy and peace supernaturally from the Spirit. Paul knew that no matter what trials or tests awaited him, it would just be another opportunity for God to be glorified by his triumphing in the strength of the Spirit. Paul said, "I will boast all the more gladly about my weaknesses, so that Christ's power may rest on me. ...For when I am weak, then I am strong" (2 Corinthians 12:9-10.)

So let's go back to our example of cancer. First we have to know that God wants us whole and healed. Jesus healed all the sick, all who came to Him in faith. The word for salvation is *sozo,* which means healed, delivered, saved. Some say that Jesus came only to give us salvation but not physical healing. In response to this, I quote Isaiah 53:5, "But he was pierced for our transgressions, he was crushed for our iniquities; the punishment that brought us peace was upon him, and by his wounds we are healed." Some say this means spiritual healing, not physical. This issue can be resolved by letting the Word of God be its own commentary. Matthew 8:16-17 reads, "When evening came, many who were demon-possessed were brought to Him, and He drove out the spirits with a word and healed all the sick. This was to fulfill what was spoken through the prophet Isaiah: "He took up our infirmities and carried our diseases." This is God's own commentary on His Word.

Second, God has given us natural medicine to heal our bodies: "Their fruit will serve for food and their leaves for healing" (Ezekiel 47:12.) These come in whole foods and herbs (leaves.)

Third, if all else fails and I die, I don't lose, I win: To die is gain. Can you imagine living in the overwhelming presence of God with all his glory? Imagine living in perfection with no sin, no hindrances, no pain, no suffering, no more trials, tests, or persecutions ... just enveloped in the glory of God and filled completely with love, joy and peace. I doubt very much if anyone who has ever tasted of this would want to come back and live a few more years on earth. Remember, earth is our playing field. All our victories and triumphs and overcomings in His strength will happen here, not in heaven. I think we will be watching rerun video's for eternity of how we stood in faith believing God for miracles that could only come when we were at the end of ourselves. Consider Paul, who received a stoning, but rose the next day and walked 30 miles to the next town. Or Stephen, who was filled with the Spirit of God as he spoke to the Sanhedrin (religious leaders of the day); as he was stoned to death, he saw heaven open and Jesus welcoming him home, and Stephen prayed for forgiveness for his killers. Or Peter saying to the cripple, "Silver and gold I do not have, but what I have I give you. In the name of Jesus Christ of Nazareth, walk" (Acts 3:6), and the man was healed.

We all have miracles of our own that have happened or are just waiting to happen, so let's enjoy the Living God, sit at His feet, run this race with joy, have fun while running, and when it's all over, receive the victor's crown from the Living God Himself in heaven, as Stephen did.

CHAPTER 4

THE INTERRELATION OF TOTAL HEALTH

All seven categories of our health interrelate. Each one touches all the rest. Let me give some examples.

Chemical to Structural

If we take in (consume or breathe) chemical substances that irritate our system, the body will, in response, go into a contractile, or tightened, state. It is the body's natural defense mechanism. If you burn your hand, you tighten up all your muscles in response to the thermal stress and withdraw your hand. This works with the sympathetic division of the autonomic nervous system. When stressed — whether thermally, chemically, structurally, physically, or mentally — your body goes into fight/flight response and secretes adrenaline, the hormone that prepares you for the encounter to either run or fight, in a sense.

When chemicals and toxins enter the body and adrenaline is secreted, your muscles are tensed. Sometimes they are so tense that they can pull spinal bones into misaligned positions, causing neuropathy or spinal nerve irritation. This causes a decrease in the functioning capabilities of whatever organ, gland, or tissue that nerve goes to, and results in pain, numbness, tingling, weakness, burning, or organ dysfunction (working at less than capacity).

I have patients who, when they eat foods they are sensitive or allergic to, like MSG, experience terrible back pain because of this cycle. So any offending chemical, toxin, or allergen can cause a contractile reaction due to the stress response and can lead to subluxation (misalignment of spinal bones which may cause pressure on nerves, which leads to pain or decreased organ function, and can eventually lead to disease).

Chemical to Eliminatory

As the toxic load on the liver increases, general toxicity throughout the body results and leads to many symptoms of illness, eventually culminating in disease. Chemicals, drugs, toxins and allergens enter the system through the digestive and respiratory tracts. If they enter via the digestive tract, they may lead to inflammation and the breakdown of the intestinal mucosal wall (our screen or selective mesh) which lets these toxins, chemicals, drugs, and allergens enter the hepatic portal blood supply to the liver. The liver cannot keep up with the additional work load (an analogy of a small air filter trying to filter the smoke pouring in from a fireplace with a closed flue, the air filter simply cannot keep up with the amount of smoke entering the room), and these substances enter the circulating blood and can affect all tissues and systems of the body, including the immune, neurologic (brain), and musculoskeletal systems. This can lead to a variety of toxin-related symptoms such as a suppressed immune system, poor memory, behavior changes, lack of concentration, joint aches and pains, and arthritis. As shown before, if the chemicals are inhaled, they enter these tissues much more quickly because the liver's primary detoxifying ability is bypassed (blood from lungs goes throughout the body before it gets to the liver to be cleaned).

The third possible point of entry for chemicals is the skin. The time it takes for chemicals to enter the body through the skin is 20 to 30 seconds.

Chemical to Physical (Circulation)

The chemicals, toxins, drugs, allergens and fats that enter the body can affect the physical health by decreasing blood and lymph flow and increasing cardiovascular risk. As will be seen later, dietary intake of the above slows blood flow greatly, and with decreased blood flow there is a greater chance of tissue and cellular damage due to lack of oxygen and inability of those tissues and cells to rid themselves of waste products. This also can cause an increased risk of thrombus or embolis formation (clots), which can lodge in the heart or brain causing heart attack or stroke. It is also known that decreased blood flow becomes a better medium for cancer growth. The slower the blood circulation, the less oxygen is distributed, and the more the cancer can spread unchecked by the white blood cells which are designed to devour these abnormal cells. Returning to our filter analogy, the higher the blood flow rate, the quicker the toxins and chemicals can be removed from the body. Many drugs and toxic chemicals cause the body to go into the stress response in which it secretes adrenaline and constricts blood vessels. This again might cause an increase in blood pressure and heart rate, and temporarily increase the normal flow of blood in the vessels only to try to filter these harmful substances into the liver. The reaction of this constant intake of chemicals causes stress that can lead to many other diseases, from gastrointestinal (ulcer, colitis) to cardiovascular (heart attack and stroke).

When the body goes into a flight/fight stress response, the blood flow is increased to the extremities (arms and legs) to prepare for action, but is decreased to the gastrointestinal tract. This regular decrease of blood supply for people who are under regular stress causes poor digestion, inflammation (colitis), and increased acid secretion (which leads to various ulcers). The increased adrenaline stress response on the cardiovascular system causes high blood pressure and overworking of the heart. This sustained high blood pressure leads to greater risk of heart attack and stroke.

The primary reason the cardiovascular system is at risk is cholesterol buildup and high fat diets. These narrow the coronary and cerebral arteries and can lead to insufficient oxygen supply to the brain or heart, thus causing strokes and heart attacks. It also leads to systemic hardening of the arteries and increased blood pressure.

The greater the resting pressure in the system, the greater the chance of many diseases developing, especially the blowout from aneurysms and loosened clots causing heart attacks and strokes, the No. 1 and No. 3 causes of death in the United States.

The relation between chemical and physical health can also be seen in lymphatic buildup or congestion. It is important to remember that whatever comes into our bodies via our lungs, skin, or digestive tracts that causes a slowing of circulation will also cause lymphatic congestion or buildup.

Let me explain what lymph fluid is, what it does, and how important it is in our total health = wholeness. (I will discuss the lymphatic system in greater detail in the Immune Health chapter.)

The lymphatic system is a system of channels like the blood vessels through which the white blood cells (WBCs) circulate. The body's immune cells congregate in the bone marrow, spleen, thymus, lymph nodes, and liver. Here the WBCs are made and stored. They circulate through the body from the blood vessels. When they get to the microvessels, the capillaries, they actually come out of the vessels and patrol the tissues looking for and being sent to areas of infection, or anything that does not have the right chemical code (antigen). Once these WBCs have eaten bacteria or viruses that have invaded the tissues, they re-enter circulation via the lymph channels, which have check points guarded by massive amounts of WBCs which kill the intruder, thus stopping the spread of infection. The stopping points are lymph nodes located in the abdomen, neck, armpits, elbows, groin, and knees. After going through the lymph nodes, some of the WBCs re-enter the circulating blood, while others remain in the particular lymphatic channel.

Lymphatic circulation is critical in maintaining a strong immune system because ⅔rds of your WBC's are located in your lymphatic system. This is why anything that causes lymphatic congestion is potentially devastating to the body. Imagine an army at war, with battles being fought at many locations. Now imagine that wherever the troops go to fight, their vehicles run out of gas and cannot return to fight new battles and cannot reload ammunition and supplies. This is analogous to what happens when our lymphatic channels clog or stagnate.

Cancer, soon to be the No. 1 cause of death in the United States, is a battle between the immune system and cancerous abnormal cells. The body can win this battle if the army works in perfect harmony, the troops are well-nourished, well-rested, and in excellent health, the ammunition is in great supply, and the vehicles are mobile and able to get anywhere they need to be in the least amount of time. Only in perfect harmony can your immune system fight cancer and win. A major part of this fight is efficient lymphatic flow.

So if lymph fluid is congested, the effectiveness of the immune system is reduced due to the decreased number of white blood cells circulating to destroy bacteria, viruses, foreign substances, and even cancerous cells. The fats we ingest will slow circulation and increase lymphatic congestion. This is especially true of animal fats. Therefore a diet high in animal fat will decrease circulation and increase cholesterol buildup in the blood vessels, causing:

- increased chance of heart attack
- increased chance of stroke
- increased blood pressure (which increases development of many diseases)
- increased chance of aneurysm
- decreased immune system response
- decreased lymphatic flow
- increased chance of cancer

Lymphocytes are a type of WBC that protect the body against anything that is foreign. All molecules in the body have a chemical code, or antigen, that the body recognizes as its own and does not attack. All other substances that don't have this code are treated as intruders and are attacked. This includes bacteria, viruses, parasites, fungi, pollen, and other allergens;

even foreign tissue from a transplant will be attacked if immunosuppressive drugs are not administered.

Chemical to Physical (exercise)

Some foods and chemicals we ingest even have a negative effect on our ability to exercise in order to remain healthy. The body treats white refined sugar as a stress, and our body responds to it with the stress adrenaline response previously described. Sustained ingestion of white refined sugar, then, can produce the symptoms of fatigue, sluggishness, and chronic tiredness. Needless to say, anyone feeling this way will not feel motivated to exercise much. So ingesting something that depletes your body of natural vitamins may cause a stress reaction, which results in altered blood flow to organs and can lead to chronic tiredness. It eventually stores in the body as fat, increasing blood pressure and the heart's workload. One can see that what we eat not only affects our ability to exercise, but can also affect our total health = wholeness.

This is also true with dietary animal fat which, when consumed, slows blood circulation, causes potential blockages of small blood vessels, and can reduce the amount of circulating oxygen in the blood. Again, with lack of circulation, sluggishness leads to tiredness, which leads to no desire to exercise.

Many other chemicals and additives have a similar effect on the body. Caffeine, also a stimulant drug, causes a temporary increase in the activity of bodily systems until the adrenaline cycle is depleted; sluggishness and fatigue follow this cycle, creating the need for more caffeine to jump start the systems again. Prolonged use of this drug in this way throws the body into great imbalance. Caffeine also is linked with certain cancers, like breast and bladder cancer.

There are many such examples to illustrate how chemical health correlates with physical health and exercise. Suffice it to say that we must do our best to monitor what we eat, drink and breathe.

Chemical to Chemical

What we eat, drink and breathe can affect our ability to digest, assimilate and eliminate properly.

As we have already discussed, the ingestion of certain substances causes inflammation of the intestinal mucosal barrier (the screen or mesh), leading to increased intestinal permeability (the screen gets too large, letting toxins and allergens into the blood stream), causing a condition called "leaky gut"(see chapter 13). Leaky gut is a major cause of overburdened liver function and toxicity, which affects the whole system.

As we have shown, toxicity can cause a whole gamut of diseases due to its ability to suppress the immune system, overburden the liver, settle in brain and nervous tissue, and so on.

The medical publication Lancet (341:49 1993), *American Journal of Physiology (258:603 1990) and the Annals Allergy (199)* mention the following agents which can damage the gastrointestinal mucosa and enter our body through the damaged screen:

- bacterial infection
- alcohol
- food allergy
- drugs
- toxic heavy metals (mercury, lead, etc.)
- stress
- poor diet
- parasites
- mycotoxins
- viral infections

Almost all of these are taken into our bodies through food, water, or air. Regular exposure to fumes and smoke, including tobacco smoke, leads in time to lung tissue damage, emphysema, chronic obstructive pulmonary disease and pneumonia. When lung tissue is diseased or damaged, it impairs the body's ability to take in the proper amount of oxygen and expel the built-up carbon dioxide byproduct. Again, this leads to a compromise of *total health = wholeness.*

Remember that anything that comes in contact with your skin — whether a hand lotion, shampoo, or oil and gas from working on a car — is absorbed through the skin and circulating through the blood in just 20 to 30 seconds. Be careful, therefore, about what you touch and what you let come in contact with your body. The general rule: If you can't eat it, don't put it on your hands or hair. This may cause you to consider using natural cosmetics and hair/skin care items.

Chemical to Mental

We can say that we are what we eat, drink and breathe. This can be taken a step further by saying that we act, behave and think as we eat, drink and breathe. There is a strong correlation between what goes into the body and our mental processes.

Dr. Ben Feingold postulates that additives, preservatives, and chemicals in food are the causes of many cases of hyperactivity. His clinic has had very good results putting hyperactive children on strict diets that limit artificial additives, preservatives, and chemicals.

A 1989 study on children's behavior and diet studied 24 hyperactive boys ages 3½ to 6. All of them had symptoms similar to food sensitivities, such as stuffy noses and stomachaches. Many also had sleep problems. In the study, the children were fed low-sugar, vitamin-rich diets that had no coloring, flavorings, MSG, caffeine, chocolate, preservatives, milk, or any other substance the parents thought might be contributing to the problem. After four weeks, almost half the boys showed almost 50 percent improvement.[1]

Dr. Alan Goldstein, director of the Temple University Medical School Agoraphobia and Anxiety Center in Philadelphia, states, "The typical diet of someone who comes to see us includes 8-10 cups of coffee a day, lots of sweets, and very few slow-release high-protein foods. Diet changes have shown benefit in some cases." One woman in Dr. Goldstein's clinic stopped drinking coffee and ate many small meals rather than three large ones, and her anxiety levels dropped in half.[2]

Studies have also linked hypoglycemia, or low blood sugar (common in people who consume a lot of refined sugar and carbohydrates), to phobias and alcoholism.

Dr. Jan Bancroft, associate at the University of Toronto, was one of the first people to conduct studies on music and learning. According to Dr. Bancoft "Right diet is one of the basics of good memory. If you don't eat properly, you don't nourish the brain".[3]

Structural to Eliminatory

As discussed, if a subluxation puts pressure on a nerve supplying the liver, gallbladder, kidney, bladder, intestinal tract, or lungs, the body will work at less than the 100 percent that God intended it to. This is analogous to stepping on a garden hose so the water doesn't flow or turning down the lights with a dimmer switch. Less electricity less light. This can lead to decreased elimination, greater toxic buildup, and eventual sickness and disease.

Structural to Structural

When one area of the spine subluxates, or misaligns, it becomes fixated, or does not move in its normal range of motion. The whole spine then compensates for this loss of motion. This leads to excessive motion (hyper-mobility) of other spinal bones and further subluxations. This process of one misaligned bone leading to others has a Leaning Tower of Pisa effect: If the foundation is off, the whole structure will be off. If a pelvic subluxation is left untreated and causes a low hip and functional short leg, many other subluxations will result. The misaligned spinal levels not only cause increased pressure on nerves and the possibility of pain, numbness, tingling, burning, and weakness, but can also cause organ dysfunction. We do not want any of our nerves pressed or pinched, as this can decrease the vital nerve energy that maintains the healthy functioning of organs, glands, and tissues in the body.

Structural to Physical and Chemical

Subluxation of the spine not only causes nerve irritation and organ dysfunction (which can result in major circulation, blood, lymphatic, digestion, assimilation problems), but it can also affect our *total health = wholeness*. For instance, subluxation of the thoracic spine and rib attachments (middle back) can decrease the ability of the lungs to expand fully. The ribs attach to the spine and move like a bucket handle. As the lungs expand with air, the ribs swing and allow further expansion. If the ribs are subluxated, they become fixated, or less mobile. When a breath is taken in and the expanding lung hits the non-moving ribs, it cannot expand further. Although the individual can still breathe, he is using much less of his lung capacity, which results in less oxygen entering the body and less CO_2 leaving the body. This buildup of acid in the system without adequate oxygen has far-ranging affects. Also, the lack of full lung expansion causes a decrease in lymph flow. Studies have shown the greatest benefits to lymph circulation are deep breathing with full lung expansion and increased circulation from cardiovascular exercise. Can you see how back and rib subluxation can affect the immune system due to a decreased lymph flow, thereby affecting *total health = wholeness?*

Structural to Mental

The two major arteries which supply the brain (which needs 30 times the amount of oxygen that the other organs need) are the carotid and vertebral arteries.

The vertebral artery goes though the spine in the neck and up into the skull, feeding the brain. A subluxation of any one of the upper cervical vertebrae can press on or kink the vertebral artery. This causes a decrease in blood supply to the brain and can lead to light-headedness, dizziness, mental confusion, memory loss, and headaches. Many of my patients have had dizziness and light-headedness alleviated through correction of their cervical or neck subluxations. Also, they often report feeling more clear-headed.

Eliminatory to Structural

Impaired elimination by liver, colon, gallbladder, kidney, bladder or lung dysfunction can set up a reflex arc that actually causes enough irritation to move back up the nerve root to cause a subluxation, as the muscles around that spinal segment tighten enough to pull the vertebrae or spinal bones into a misaligned position. This is nowhere near as common as the reverse, where pressure on a nerve from a spinal subluxation causes organ dysfunction due to the decreased nerve energy to maintain healthy organ function. So if one had a chronic subluxation in the lower lumbar spine affecting nerves sent into the intestinal tract or bowel, this could lead to impaired function> >dysfunction>disease. This could be the cause of many health problems. Remove the subluxations, and you remove the nerve pressure affecting the organ. The reverse occurs when an individual has, for example, an intestinal problem first (due to diet, stress, allergy, etc.) with no subluxation. He or she would eventually start to have back pain due to the irritation traveling backwards along the nerve from where it originated, causing spinal subluxation. People who have kidney problems tend to have increased lower back pain. People who have stomach problems tend to have pain between the shoulder blades.

As we close this chapter, I hope you are starting to understand that just as the proper functioning of all parts of your body is necessary for you to live and be as God created you to be, so it is with your *total health = wholeness*. All areas of your total health touch each other and are dependent upon each other — your liver is dependent upon your heart, and your stomach is dependent upon your lungs and your lungs are dependent on your ribs and your ribs dependent on your spine.

Your *total health = wholeness* interrelates, and that is how God meant it to be. So seek more than health, and more than wellness. Seek wholeness, and you will find it.

CHAPTER 5

WHOLENESS ASSESSMENT

The purpose of the Wholeness Assessment, or WA, is to be a measurement tool to chart your progress as you start your *total health = wholeness* journey. It is not designed to be an absolute or definitive measurement of one's health status, but merely a means of generally guiding you into greater and greater levels of *total health = wholeness*.

Also in everything remember we are comparing our self to our self, so do not compare any aspect of your health with anyone else. Just look to see if you have improved your *total health = wholeness* as compared to one year ago. In addition, do not live or walk in fear. If you scored in the "high priority" range it does not necessarily mean that sickness has occurred in your body (although it might have). Even so, you do not want to stay in this range for prolonged amounts of time because of the negative long term affects it can have on your *total health = wholeness*.

You should fill out the assessment once a month if you are presently ill in some way, or once every six months if you are just trying to improve your *total health = wholeness*. Remember, the man who thinks he can and the man who thinks he cannot are both correct. Also, success is measured by the journey itself, not just by the final outcome. Lastly, if we set a goal to shoot for the stars we might not make it, but we will achieve a lot more than the one who sets no goal at all. Set your goal on *total health = wholeness* and see just how much you can achieve.

WHOLENESS ASSESSMENT

The best total score for this assessment is 0, and best response to each question is 0.

Answer each question with a number from 0 to 3 depending on degree of response.

STRUCTURAL HEALTH

0=NO or not at all   1=mild   2=moderate   3=YES or very much

1. Joint, bone, muscle or nerve problems   ____
2. Back or neck pain   ____
3. Arm or hand numbness or tingling or weakness or burning   ____
4. Leg or foot numbness or tingling or weakness or burning   ____
5. Disc problems (past or present)   ____
6. History of auto or other traumatic accident   ____
7. Stiffness or limitation of normal movement   ____
8. Pain with movement   ____
9. Family history of back, neck or other joint problems   ____
10. Arthritis   ____
11. Pain or spasm in muscle   ____
12. Poor posture, i.e., sitting, standing, sleeping or lifting   ____
13. Do you daily perform spinal exercises: strengthening
    and stretching (0-yes.3-no)   ____
14. Are you regularly checked for spinal subluxations
    or misalignments? (0-yes, 3-no)   ____

                                                      Total   _____

NUTRITIONAL HEALTH

0=NO or not at all   1=mild   2=moderate   3=YES or very much

1. Do you eat refined sugar (i.e. cookies, cakes, candy,
    ice cream, soda, etc. more than once a week?   ___

2. Do you consume dairy products (i.e. milk, cheese, butter, yogurt)
    more than once a week?   ___

3. Do you drink coffee or tea (non-herbal) more than
    once a week?   ___

4. Do you drink alcohol more than once a week?   ___

5. Do you eat red meat more than once a week?   ___

6. Do you eat out at restaurants or have fast food
    more than once a week?   ___

7. Do you eat junk food (i.e., potato chips, cheese curls,
    corn chips, pretzels) more than 1 time/week?   ___

8. Do you eat less than 2 servings of fresh fruit per day?   ___

9. Do you eat less than 8 servings of fresh vegetables per day? ___

10. Do you drink less than 10 glasses of water per day?   ___

11. Do you drink tap water?   ___

12. Do you eat animal products (meat, chicken, fish, dairy)
    every day?   ___

13. Do you eat food with additives or preservatives more
    than once a week?   ___

14. Rate your diet from 0= (plenty of fresh fruits, vegetables,
    low fat, no sugar, whole grains, seeds, nuts, no meat, no eggs, no
    dairy, no animal products) to 3= (little to no fruits and vegetables,
    plenty of meat, fat, and sugar)   ___ x3 = ___

                                                   Total _____

DIGESTIVE HEALTH

0=NO or not at all   1=mild   2=moderate   3=YES or very much

1. Do you chew your food less than 25 times per bite?   ___

2. Do you burp?   ___

3. Does your stomach get upset often?   ___

4. Do you feel bloated after eating?   ___

5. Do you feel full for a long time after eating?   ___

6. Do you have indigestion after meals?   ___

7. Do you get tired after eating?   ___

8. Do you get intestinal gas?   ___

9. Do you get constipated?   ___

10. Do you get diarrhea?   ___

11. Do you get stomach pain right before or after meals?   ___

12. Do you have or have you ever had a stomach ulcer?   ___

13. Do you have black stools without taking iron supplements?   ___

14. Do you drink liquids with your meals?   ___

15. Do you eat too much, or mix to many foods with each meal?   ___

Total _____

ASSIMILATIVE HEALTH

0=NO or not at all   1=mild   2=moderate   3=YES or very much

1. Do you have known food allergies or sensitivities?   ____

2. Do you frequently feel fatigued?   ____

3. Do you frequently have headaches?   ____

4. Do you get neck, back, arm, or leg aches?   ____

5. Do you frequently have enlarged lymph glands in the neck?   ____

6. Do you feel tense, nervous or irritable after eating?   ____

7. Do you get eczema?   ____

8. Do you get hives?   ____

9. Do you get joint pain in multiple joints?   ____

10. Do you have to urinate frequently?   ____

11. Do you have any stomach or intestinal symptoms?   ____

12. Do you have any restriction in breathing (nasal passages,
    or throat is tight or mucous filled)?   ____

13. Rate your stress level from 0-none to 3-extreme   ____

14. Have you had more than one cold/flu in the last year?   ____

15. Do you drink alcohol?   ____

16. Do you regularly take medications, and/or drugs?   ____

17. Do you have any history of intestinal parasites?   ____

18. Have you taken antibiotics in the last 3 years?   ____

19. Have you ever taken antibiotics more than 10 days
    for any condition?   ____

20. Have you ever had a yeast infection?   ____

Total____

ELIMINATIVE HEALTH

0=NO or not at all   1=mild   2=moderate   3=YES or very much

1. Constipation ___
2. Less than two bowel movements/day ___
3. Bad stool odor ___
4. Light colored stool ___
5. Hard or pellet like stool ___
6. Greasy/oily food intolerance ___
7. White coated tongue ___
8. Green or black coated tongue ___ x2= ___
9. Sour taste in mouth ___
10. Bad breath ___
11. Body odor ___
12. Water retention ___
13. Skin problems ___
14. Pain on right side under rib cage ___
15. History of jaundice or hepatitis ___
16. Exposure to fumes/smoke/chemical ___

17. Cholesterol over 200 ___
18. Cholesterol over 300 ___
19. Infrequent urination ___
20. History of recurrent bladder/kidney infection ___
21. Painful or burning urination ___
22 Cloudy urine ___
23. Rose colored urine ___
24. Strong odor urine ___
25. Back pain in kidney area ___
26. Sensitive to exhaust fumes/smoke/chemicals ___
27. Dark circles under eyes ___
28. Regular headaches ___
29. Perspiration stains on clothing ___
30. Frequent fatigue or sluggishness ___
31. Feet or hands perspire excessively ___

Total ___

CIRCULATIVE HEALTH

0=NO or not at all   1=mild   2=moderate   3=YES or very much

1. Heart skips beats or has extra beats___

2. Heart pounds easily with little or no exercise ___

3. Rapid heart beat without exercise ___

4. Chest pain ___

5. Calf cramps when walking ___

6. Swelling of feet or ankles ___

7. Heaviness in legs ___

8. High blood pressure ___

9. Low blood pressure ___

10. History of heart trouble ___

11. History of artery or vein problems ___

12. Family history of heart, artery or vein problems ___

13. Fatigue with minor exertion ___

14. Do you exercise less than 30 minutes per day of continuos cardiovascular exercise like swimming walking, bike riding,etc.? ___

15. Do you eat red meat? ___

16. Do you eat dairy products? ___

17. Do you eat refined sugar? ___

18. You don't perform any deep breathing exercises daily? ___

19. Do you wear tight fitting under or over garments? ___

20. Do you sit at least 75% of your day? ___

Total ___

IMMUNE HEALTH

0=NO not at all   1=mild   2=moderate   3=YES very much

1   Do you eat refined sugar? ___

2. Do you eat white flour products? ___

3. Do you eat dairy products? ___

4. Do you eat red meat? ___

5. Do you take digestive enzymes? (0=yes   3=no) ___

6. Do you get more than one cold or flu per year? ___

7. Do you get more than one sore throat per year? ___

8. Do you get cold sores? ___

9. Do your gums bleed easily? ___

10. Have you been on antibiotics more than once
in the last two years?   ___

11. Do your wounds heal slowly?   ___

12. Do you have any enlarged lymph glands?   ___

13. Do you have allergies or sensitivities?   ___

14. Do you presently or have you ever had low thyroid function?   ___

15. Do you have any blood sugar problems?   ___

16. Do you feel nodules in your arm pit, on the inside of your elbow,
in your groin or behind your knees?   ___

17. Do you smoke?   ___

18. Do you drink coffee?   ___

19. Do you eat fried food?   ___

20. Do you eat food that has additives and/or preservatives?   ___

21. Do you feel fatigued regularly   ___

Total_____

OXIDATIVE HEALTH

0=NO or not at all   1=mild   2=moderate   3=YES or very much

1. Do you daily eat less than 5 servings of raw fruits and vegetables?   ___

2. Do you consume vitamins A,C, & E daily through your diet? (0=yes 3=no) ___

3. Do you eat hydrogenated fats and oils
(margarine, long shelf life food that contain)?   ___

4. Do you eat fried food?   ___

5. Do you eat foods with preservatives (longer shelf life)?   ___

6. Are you frequently fatigued?   ___

7. Do you feel your stress level is high?   ___

8. Do you take time to pray and meditate each day? (0=yes 6=no)   ___

Total   _____

ORGAN/GLAND HEALTH

0=NO or not at all   1=mild   2=moderate   3=YES or very much

1. Do you have a family history of disease (heart, lung, cancer, diabetes etc.)?   ___

2. Do you have any personal history of heart, lung, cancer, diabetes etc.?   ___

3. Do you have any weak or improperly functioning organs or glands?   ___

4. Is your thyroid function abnormal?   ___

5. Do you get cold easily?   ___

6. Do you have a resting temperature below 97.6 degrees F?   ___

7. Do you get hot easily?   ___

8. Do you get dizzy when standing up quickly?   ___

9. Do you feel weak, shaky or jittery when you miss a meal?   ___

10. Do you get headaches when you miss a meal?   ___

11. Do you have mood swings when you miss a meal?   ___

12. Do you become tired or sluggish 1-2 hours after a meal?   ___

13. Are you very thirsty throughout the day not associated with exercise or salt intake?   ___

14. Do your wounds heal slowly?   ___

15. Do you feel fatigued regularly?   ___

16. Are your eyes sensitive to bright light?   ___

17. Do you catch colds easily when the weather changes?   ___

18. Do you have problems sleeping?   ___

19. Do you have PMS?   ___

Total ___

MENTAL HEALTH

0=YES or very much 1=most of the time 2=at times 3=NO or not at all

1. How successful (not financial) do you see yourself? ____

2. How significant do you see yourself? ____

3. How fulfilled are you? ____

4. How satisfied are you? ____

5. How happy are you? ____

6. How much fun do you have? ____

7. How secure (not financial) are you? ____

8. How peaceful are you? ____

9. Do you see your life without stress? ____

10. Do you see your life without anxiety? ____

11. Do you see your life without depression? ____

12. Do you know your purpose in life? ____

13. Do you give affection regularly? ____

14. Do you receive affection regularly? ____

15. Do you have at least one relative you can rely on? ____

16. Do you have one or two close friends you can confide in? ____

17. Do you organize your time effectively? ____

18. Do you take quiet time for yourself each day? ____

19. Is your income sufficient to meet your needs, with extra to save and give? ____

20. Do you attend a fellowship or social activity regularly? ____

21. Can you speak openly when you are angry or hurt? ____

22. Are you a laid back person who if it doesn't get done today, tomorrow is another day? ____

Total _____

SPIRITUAL HEALTH

0=YES   1=SOMEWHAT   2=AT TIMES   3=NO

1. Do you have an intimate personal relationship
   with the Living God?   ___ x 7 = _____

2. Do you have NO fear of what lies beyond death?   _____

3. Does God regularly speak to you through his Spirit and through his Word?   _____

4. Do you talk to God daily?   _____

5. Do you listen to Him daily?   _____

6. Is God in love with you?   _____

7. Are you and God inseparable no matter what you do?   _____

8. Do you know God's plan for your life?   _____

9. Do you know your purpose in life?   _____

10. When you get to the end of your strength, do you feel
    God's strength carry you?   _____

11. Do you experience His strength in your weakness?   _____

12. Do you know deep in your heart that in your weakness,
    God's strength is unveiled?   _____

13. Do you know deep in your heart that everything God has
    He gives to you?   _____

14. Do you know deep in your heart that the Living God lives
    inside of you, walking with and talking to you everyday
    through His Spirit?   _____

15. Do you experience God's love daily?   _____

16. Do you experience God's joy daily?   _____

17. Do you experience God's peace daily?   _____

18. Do you love yourself?   _____

USE THIS SCALE FOR THE FOLLOWING   0=NO,NEVER   1=AT TIMES

   2=SOMEWHAT   3=YES

19. Do you feel your faith to believe God is lacking?   _____

20. Do you struggle with fear?   _____

21. Is your self worth based on what others think about you?   _____

22. Do you condemn yourself?   _____

23. Do you feel alone?   _____

24. Are you addicted or bound to anything?   _____

25. Do you feel like a failure?   _____

26. Do you feel you lack spiritually?   _____

27. Is it hard for you to forgive those who have hurt you?   _____

28. Do you feel fear regularly?   _____

29. Do you carry resentment towards anyone or anything?   _____

30. Do you criticize yourself?   _____

31. Do you carry guilt?   _____

                                                   Total _____

Wholeness Assessment Interpretation

Name _____   Date_____

Health	Whole	Priority	High Priority	Score
Structural	1 2 3 4 5	6 7 8 9	10 11 12+	
Nutritional	1 2 3 4 5 6 7 8 9	10 11 12 13 14 15 16 17 18	19 20 21 22 23 24+	
Digestive	1 2 3 4 5 6	7 8 9 10 11	12 13 14 15+	
Assimilative	1 2 3 4 5 6 7	8 9 10 11 12 13	14 15 16 17 18+	
Eliminative	1 2 3 4 5 6 7 8 9 10	11 12 13 14 15 16 17 18 19 20	21 22 23 24 25 26 27+	
Circulative	1 2 3 4 5 6 7	8 9 10 11 12 13	14 15 16 17 18+	
Immune	1 2 3 4 5 6 7	8 9 10 11 12 13	14 15 16 17 18+	
Oxidative	1 2 3	4 5 6 7	8 9+	
Organ Gland	1 2 3 4 5 6 7	8 9 10 11 12 13	14 15 16 17 18+	
Mental	1 2 3 4 5 6 7 8 9 10	11 12 13 14 15 16 17 18	19 20 21 22 23 24 25 26 27+	
Spiritual	5 10 15	20 25 30	35 40 45+	
TotalHealth Wholeness	10 20 30 40 50 60 70	80 90 100 110 120 130	140 150 160 170 180 190	Add up the 11 Scores and Place Here ⇩

Your goal is to be Whole. Priority Scores require action to be taken.
High Priority Scores require immediate action to prevent sickness or
disease from developing if they have not already begun.

Wholeness Assessment Score Record

Name_____   Case No._____

	Whole	Score #1	Score #2	Score #3
Date				
Structural	4			
Nutritional	8			
Digestive	5			
Assimilative	6			
Eliminative	9			
Circulative	6			
Immune	6			
Oxidative	3			
Organ/Gland	6			
Mental	9			
Spiritual	15			
Total Health= Wholeness	77			

CHAPTER 6

YOU ARE WHAT YOU EAT

The Standard American Diet — or SAD — is truly sad indeed. It consists of the meat group (2 or more servings per day), the milk group (3 or more servings), the vegetable and fruits group (4 or more servings), and the bread and cereal group (4 or more servings.)

Then there's the Revised American Diet, broken down into more categories and presented as a pyramid, with fats and sweets used sparingly. This diet includes the milk group (2-3 servings), the meat group (2-3 servings), the vegetable group (3-5 servings), the fruit group (2-4 servings), and the bread and cereal group (6-11 servings.)

The problem with both diets is the milk and meat. Let's take a closer look at the problems with both.

MILK

Dairy products form mucus, which coats the digestive and respiratory tracts. Milk is not easily digested, and it's also highly allergenic.

Here are some other facts about dairy products (milk, cheese, butter, ice cream, yogurt, etc.)

Most of the world is lactose intolerant. Most of us lose the ability to completely digest lactose by age four. As a result, many milk drinkers develop diarrhea, gas, stomach cramps, bowel inflammation and toxicity.

- Dairy sources are high on the food chain, which concentrates toxins, pesticides, and hormones.[1]
- More than 20 percent of dairy cows carry leukemia viruses. Sheep, goats and chimps that are fed cows' milk sometimes develop leukemia. There's a great possibility these viruses can be transmitted to humans too.[2,3]
- Casein — a milk protein — is a common cause of food allergies. Casein needs the enzyme rennin, to break down, but rennin isn't present in humans after the age of four.[4] Cows' milk contains 300 times more casein than mothers' milk.[5] Casein, which is very sticky, is a main component in popular nontoxic glue. Casein coats the digestive system, leading to leaky gut syndrome, malabsorption and/or constipation. These all lead to a weakened immune system

and toxic build up in the blood along with a host of other health problems that stem from the leaky gut syndrome (see the Assimilative Health chapter). Casein is extremely mucus-forming, due to its bacterial breakdown (putrefaction), our allergic response, and its glue-like nature.

- Pasteurization destroys all enzymes, including phosphatase, which is necessary to assimilate calcium, minerals and vitamins. During pasteurization, milk is heated to at least 115 degrees Celsius, causing organic calcium to become insoluble and therefore very hard to digest. Temperatures from 190 to 230 degrees Celsius are required to kill typhoid bacilli, coli, tuberculosis and undulant fever, but pasteurization temperatures only reach 145 to 170 degrees. Pasteurization kills some beneficial bacteria which normally keep the harmful bacteria in check. Within 24 to 48 hours after pasteurization, the amount of harmful bacteria doubles.[6]
- Cows' milk has twice as much protein as human milk, because a baby cow doubles its weight so quickly.
- Baby cows who drank pasteurized milk died in 30 days.[7]
- Homogenized cows' milk prevents cream from floating to the top. If raw milk is ingested, the enzyme xanthine oxidase is digested in the stomach. If the milk has been homogenized, fat globules from the cream encase the enzyme, which can pass undigested into the blood, attaching to artery walls and becoming abrasive. The body repairs these abrasions with cholesterol. The xanthine oxidase enzyme is a significant cause of heart disease in the United States.[8]
- Bovine growth hormone (BGH), also called *bovine somatotropin* (BST), stimulates milk production. Synthetic BGH/BST causes up to a 25 percent increase in milk production.[9]
- The reason you don't want to be consuming growth hormone which is in milk, chicken and all meat is because it does just that! It makes tissues grow, which includes cancer cells which are cells that have mutated and already started to grow at an accelerated rate. When growth hormone combines with cancer cells their already rapid growth rate increases. This causes a tragic scenario. The average American has a sluggish to very weakened immune system. The immune system (Natural Killer cells and macrophages) prevents the cancer cells which normally form in everyone from getting out of control. So if one has a weakened immune system the cancer cells

can multiply in greater amounts because the white blood cells aren't able to do their job of killing them as quickly. Now to this we add daily amounts of growth hormone from dairy products, meat and chicken, causing the cancer cells to form colonies faster. We call these *tumors* and once tumors have formed it is much more difficult for the white blood cells (Natural Killer cells and macrophages) to get at and destroy the cancer. Can you see how dairy products, meat and chicken can ultimately destroy your health?

- Dairy cows used to live 25 years. Now, few make it past four years because of the BGH they are injected with.[10]
- Even pasteurized milk can transmit papillomavirus, which may be involved in a number of human cancers.
- Milk may be related to the onset of childhood diabetes mellitus.[11]
- Antibiotics are common in milk, due to cows' udder infections. Those antibiotics are transmitted to humans, causing reactions in those sensitive or allergic to antibiotics, or causing the production of antibiotic-resistant bacteria in our bodies.[12] One of these is sulfamethazine, a suspected human carcinogen.
- Pesticide from cows' feed gets concentrated as it goes up the food chain to you and me.[13]
- Finland has one of the world's highest dairy intakes — and the world's highest death rate from heart disease. Finns consume 1½ times more dairy products than Americans; coincidentally, Finland's death rate from heart disease is 1½ times higher than that in the U.S. High fat, high cholesterol, and liquid meat (milk) diets are not conducive to *total health* and wholeness.

The fact that we need calcium is a poor reason to say we must drink milk because pasteurization or heat renders the calcium practically unassimilable and of very little use to the human body. The average American gets 807 mg of calcium a day from drinking milk. Compare that to daily averages in Spain (308 mg), Brazil (250 mg), Taiwan (13 mg) and Ghana (8 mg).[14] People in these countries get their calcium from other sources like broccoli, spinach, soybeans, kidney beans, almonds, rhubarb, collards, turnips, etc.

The amount of calcium we need is debatable. The Food and Nutrition Board of the Nation Academy of Science recommends 800 mg per day for adults, while the World Health Organization recommends 400 mg. But God made our bodies so amazing that we absorb more calcium when consumed in lesser quantities than when we consume larger quantities. In other words, our bodies know precisely what and how much they need.

The risk of osteoporosis (thin, frail bones) is nearly double in meat and dairy-eating people than in strict vegetarians. [15]

The African Bantu women consume a dairy-free diet, and they still get 250 to 400 mg of calcium daily — half that of Western women — from vegetable sources. Bantu women commonly have 10 children in their lifetime, and they typically breast-feed their children for about 10 months. Even with this tremendous calcium drain and relative low calcium intake, osteoporosis is essentially unknown among these women. [16]

If you still believe you must drink milk to make your bones strong, here's an interesting fact: The five highest dairy-consuming countries (Finland, Sweden, U.S., U.K. and Israel) also have the five highest rates of hip fracture — a sign of osteoporosis.

Here's another case point that shows how we assimilate more toxins as we move up the food chain, when we move from eating plants to eating meat:

The Environmental Defense Fund studied the breast milk of 1,400 women from 46 states. The study found widespread contamination of breast milk with pesticides. The levels of contamination were twice as high in meat and dairy consuming women as in vegetarians. Because pesticides are concentrated in animal foods, the study advises women who plan to breast-feed to avoid meat, some kinds of fish, and high-fat dairy products. [17]

Multiple sclerosis is more commonly found in areas of the world where infants and children are raised on dairy products rather than on breast milk and vegetable foods. [18]

To close on dairy products, I leave you parents with the following thoughts concerning your children.

- Dr. Dan Baggett, a pediatrician in Alabama, directly correlates cows' milk with the following conditions seen in his office: [19]

1) eczema
2) asthma
3) strep throat
4) rheumatoid arthritis
5) growing pains

All of these conditions began to improve when dairy products were eliminated from the diet.

MEAT

Animal fat should be avoided at all costs because of its concentration of pesticides and toxic chemicals, and because of its known contribution to our No. 1 killer, heart disease.

It is well-known that meat intake leads to increased cholesterol due to the high saturated fat content. This in turn leads to narrowing of the coronary and cerebral arteries, which can ultimately lead to heart attack or stroke.

Let me list the reasons you shouldn't eat meat, chicken or fish:

1) drugs/hormones
2) fat and cholesterol
3) pesticides/chemicals from fertilizers/PCBs
4) parasites
5) bacteria

1. Cows are injected with growth hormones like bovine growth hormone or BGH. BGH not only stimulates growth in these animals, but is also highly suspect in cancer production — especially breast and colon cancer — according to the International Journal of Health Services.[20] BGH is not only found in meat, but also in dairy products, because dairy cows are injected with BGH for greater milk production. This hormone enters into our milk, and then our bodies and our children's.

2. Fat and cholesterol buildup from meat consumption causes not only atherosclerosis and arteriosclerosis (hardening of the arteries), but also heart attacks and strokes — the No. 1 and No. 3 causes of death in the United States.

3. Additionally, cholesterol buildup results in a concentration of toxic chemicals, as we move up the food chain in our eating habits. This concentration of toxins reaches its highest level in man when we eat meat, chicken or fish. Dr. Joseph Weissman, M.D., writes in his book, *Choose to Live,* that "animal products are the single largest source of pesticides in the human diet. We obtain from meat 16 times the amount of pesticides we would from the equivalent plant food."[21] Chemicals and toxins are stored in animal fat. And all animals, including fish and chicken, have plenty of fat. So, the more meat you eat, the more toxic you become. Although fish do not have growth hormone injected into them, they make up for it by greatly concentrating in their tissues the toxic chemicals they live in. They have a great affinity for absorbing and storing these chemicals, also making them a poor food choice.

4. Parasites are also a major concern in our total health. In her book, *The Cure for all Cancers,* Dr. Clark says all cancers are caused by parasites, especially the human intestinal fluke. As Dr. Clark states, "You are always picking up parasites. You get them from other people. From your pets and undercooked meat. I believe the main source of the intestinal fluke is under-cooked meat." Once infected, this parasite can be spread through blood, saliva, breast milk and semen, and therefore transmitted by kissing, breast-feeding, and sex.[22]

This parasite causes cancer by entering the blood stream and establish-ing itself in the liver, our detoxifying organ. So, whether or not you agree with Dr. Clark's conclusion on the cause of cancer, at least use it as food for thought when making dietary selections, avoiding meat, chicken and fish. And if you do eat meat, make sure it is thoroughly cooked. However, this causes an increased cancer risk from the heat altering the protein and fat molecular structure. Overcooked meat can yield a potential cancer-causing product called arachidonic acid. So, beware when you eat meat.

5. Bacteria is a major problem in the meat industry today. More and more salmonella and E. coli outbreaks are causing severe sickness, and even death, due to ingestion of these pathogenic bacteria. Estimates of the num-ber of such cases range from 400,000 to 4 million annually, with up to 50 percent of the reported cases needing hospitalization, and 1-2 percent of reported cases fatal.[23] Strongly consider these statistics before you eat meat, chicken or fish.

Bacteria is not only a problem with our food, it's also a problem with the animals before they are slaughtered. There's a high rate of bacterial infec-tions among commercially-produced livestock. These animals are regularly fed antibiotic-laced feed, which accounts for more than half of the 31 mil-lion pounds of antibiotics produced in the United States.

Finally, there has been a concern about a connection between cows infected with bovine spongiform encephalopathy ("Mad Cow Disease") and Creutzfeldt-Jakob Disease, a 100 percent fatal human brain disease.[24]

SUGAR
Yet another problem with a typical American's diet is sugar. Sugar in all forms — except in its natural state in fruits and vegetables — should be avoided because:

1) It extremely weakens the immune system.
2) It depletes the body of valuable B vitamins.

3) It depletes the body of necessary minerals such as calcium, magnesium, etc.
4) Excesses lead to sugar diabetes, one of the top fatal diseases in the United States.
5) It causes weight gain and stress on the whole system, especially the heart.

Let's take a closer look at each of these points.

1) Sugar weakens the immune system.

Sugar puts stress on the immune system. Animal studies show that such stress results in a decrease in white blood cells (WBCs), which prevent bacterial, viral, parasitic and fungal infections, and cancer.

Our immune system's most important fighters are WBCs, which prevent us from getting cancer. We all have cancerous cells developing in our bodies, but a healthy immune system — with macrophages (Pac-Man WBCs) and natural killer cells — keeps cancer in check. But in today's toxic world, we are exposed to many cancer-producing agents from the outside, which weaken our white blood cells from the inside, a bad formula indeed.

In one study, three groups of mice were injected with an aggressive malignant mammary tumor. Prior to injection the dietary induced blood sugar was altered to three different levels; high blood sugar, normal blood sugar and lower blood sugar. After 70 days 66% of the high blood sugar group had died, 33% of the normal blood sugar had died and only 5% of the lowered blood sugar group had died.[25] This demonstrates that the less sugar in our system the more cancer and pathogen protective we become.

Remember this: Greater Toxic Load + Weakened Immune System (WBCs) = Disease (especially cancer)

Our motto in detoxifying is, "Get the bad (toxins/chemicals) out of the system and get the good in," such as nutrients, vitamins, minerals, enzymes, antioxidants and phytochemicals.

Look at the following chart:[26]

EFFECT OF SUGAR INTAKE ON ABILITY OF WHITE BLOOD CELLS TO DESTROY BACTERIA

Amount of sugar eaten at one time by average adult in teaspoons	Number of bacteria destroyed by each white blood cell	Percentage decrease in ability to destroy bacteria
0	14	0
6	10	25
12	5.5	60
18	2	85
24	1	92
Uncontrolled Diabetic	1	92

THE AMOUNT OF SUGAR IN A 12 OUNCE CAN OF SODA DECREASES THE ABILITY OF THE WHITE BLOOD CELLS TO EAT BACTERIA, VIRUSES, PARASITES AND CANCER CELLS BY 40% FOR UP TO 6 HOURS.

A 12-ounce can of regular pop can reduce the ability of WBCs to eat bacteria by 40 percent for up to six hours. That means that if you drink pop and eat other sugars, your body's defenses are down. If someone sneezes around you, or you rub your eyes or mouth with your hands, you're highly susceptible to contract the bacteria or virus. Similarly, cancer starts to grow when WBCs are being suppressed with sugar, other dietary factors, stress, etc.

2) Sugar depletes the body of valuable B vitamins.[27]

B vitamins are essential for many bodily functions, too many to list here. A vitamin B deficiency can cause many problems, including:

- neurological disease
- pernicious anemia (red blood cells affected)
- fatigue
- blood sugar problems

- congestive heart failure
- memory loss
- skin and tongue problems

- allergies
- depression

Whenever we strip our sugars and flours — the manufacturers call it "refining" — to make them white, we're taking away what God gave them to be a balanced food. Whole wheat, for instance, has B vitamins together with the starches that break down into sugar, so we do not become deficient eating it. On the other hand, white bread, like white sugar, has been stripped of essential B vitamins, so the body in turn draws them from other places — like nerves — to metabolize the refined sugars that have been eaten.

REFINING GRAINS

Grains are energy powerhouses and have an abundance of vitamins, minerals, fiber, phytochemicals, enzymes and bioelectricity. Grains should primarily be eaten sprouted and alive or by making sprouted grain uncooked bread that is dehydrated at a temperature under 110 degrees Fahrenheit. Grains can also be grown into greens like wheat grass and barley grass and then juiced for even higher contents of all of the above, along with a high concentration of oxygen that they bring to your body because of the live chlorophyll.

But how does the average American eat grains? They have been cooked, refined and processed to make refined breads and pasta. They have lost all their enzymes, bioelectricity, oxygen — the three most important elements in any food source, and nearly all their vitamin, mineral, phytochemical and fiber content. The manufacturers of these products then—to satisfy the consumer quest for trying to get enough vitamins and minerals— add back synthetic vitamins and inorganic minerals that at the very best are non-absorbable and at the very worst are toxic. You the unsuspecting consumer read the white or pseudo wheat bread package and it says "fortified" or "enriched" with 100 percent of the recommended daily allowance of all these vitamins and minerals and you think, "great, I am eating healthy bread." In fact you are eating a sticky gluey clogging anti-nutrient that will cause not only a slow decline of your general health, but that will cause very specific respiratory and digestive and absorptive problems due to the wheat gluten that remains after processing.

Here's what happens during the refining and processing of a grain:

> 90% of fiber is lost
> 75-88% of trace minerals are lost
> almost all vitamins are lost
> 100% of enzymes are lost
> 100% of bioelectrical charge is lost
> 100% oxygen content is lost

To make our bread and pasta look pretty, chlorine bleaches are added to make the flour nice and white — these toxic chemicals are carcinogenic. What you are left with is a potentially toxic anti-nutrient that gives you nothing but empty calories. What is an anti-nutrient? An anti-nutrient uses up your nutrients instead of giving you nutrients. An example is eating an English muffin versus eating a banana.

1. 200 calorie English muffin needs three micrograms of chromium to be assimilated into the body. It only has one microgram, so the total comes up to 1-3 micrograms chromium = -2 micrograms or it takes away 2 micrograms of chromium form the chromium store in your body.
2. 200 calorie banana has 150 micrograms of chromium. It needs 3 micrograms to be assimilated into the body so 150-3 micrograms chromium = 147 micrograms.

This means the banana actually adds 147 micrograms of chromium to the body instead of taking away as the muffin did.

All these reasons are why refined grains are not healthy, but actually slowly destroying our health. A general rule is the more food you eat in the way God created the food the better your health will be — uncooked and living is best. The best grains to eat are non-gluten, sprouted forms like quinoa, millet and amaranth. These grains rarely cause any allergy or sensitivity and were the staple diet of the Aztec and Inca empires. Quinoa has been called the "Supergrain" because of its being a complete protein having all the essential amino acids needed for human health.

3) Sugar depletes the body of necessary minerals.[28]

When sugar depletes our supply of valuable minerals like calcium and magnesium, this can result in osteoporosis, arthritis and a host of mineral-deficient symptoms like:

- leg cramps
- muscle tightness or spasms
- low blood sugar
- diabetes
- low blood pressure
- PMS
- low back pain
- learning disabilities
- ADD (Attention Deficit Disorder)
- depression
- asthma

In his book, *Rare Earth's Forbidden Cures*, Dr. Joel Wallach states that sugar loads increase the normal rates of mineral loss in sweat and urine by 300 percent for 12 hours.[29] So if you regularly eat sugar, no amount of supplementation or diet will allow you to keep up with your mineral losses.

4) Excess of sugar leads to sugar diabetes.

The average American consumes 100-150 pounds of sugar per year.[30] Consequently, diabetes is the No. 7 cause of death in America. Our sweet tooth has cost us dearly. Interestingly, studies of the world's people who live longest — such as Tibetans and Hunzas — indicate that degenerative diseases, including diabetes, are virtually unknown among these peoples. A probable cause of our high rate of diabetes is the high intake of refined sugar, in the form of white sugar (sucrose), corn syrup (fructose), and all others ending in "-ose." David Reuben, M.D., states that "there is no doubt that diabetes mellitus — otherwise known as sugar diabetes — is caused by excessive consumption of refined sugar."[31]

5) Sugar causes weight gain and stresses the whole system.

Sugar's empty calories quickly flood the bloodstream and are stored as fat, which can be a major contributor to the alarming number of obese adults and children in the United States today. This excess weight causes stress on the whole system, especially the heart, which has to pump harder to circulate the blood to all the "excess" tissue. The excessive weight also is a contributing factor in all major disease.

Bottom line: Cut down on the sweets and add some fruit to your diet. You should be aware that the fruit today is hybrid for sweetness, being 30 times as sweet as it was created to be, so do not over eat fruit or it could negatively impact your blood sugar and your immune system.

SALT

Salt is the common name for sodium chloride. Sodium is essential in the human diet to maintain osmotic balance in the blood, extracellular and intracellular fluids. The problem is what form the sodium comes in. All salt whether from the ground (rock salt) or from the sea (sea salt) is an inorganic form, meaning it is from the earth. Your body only properly utilizes organic sodium which comes from plant sources that have taken in the inorganic sodium from the earth up through it's root system and has made it alive in the cells of the plants as organic sodium. Potassium is another mineral essential in maintaining osmotic balance in the body. The ideal sodium to potassium ratio in the diet is 1:5, which occurs naturally in most fruits and vegetables. The average American's diet is reversed at a 5:1 ratio with almost all their sodium coming from inorganic non health promoting earth forms. As inorganic earth salt increases in one's diet and the osmotic balance is altered, a person starts to retain fluid to dilute the excessive earth salt. This causes major problems with the fluid balance inside and outside the cells of all glands, organs and tissues, leading to death of the cells. This retaining of water also causes an increased weight and blood pressure which greatly increases the chances of having a heart attack or stroke. These two combined kill 50 % of all Americans. A general rule of good health is try to never use table salt in your cooking and watch out for processed, canned and restaurant food. These all are loaded with inorganic earth salt. A general way to know if your meal has earth salt added to it is to see if you get thirsty after eating. Eating organic plant bound sodium in fruit and vegetable sources never makes you thirsty.

CHAPTER 7

WATER AND AIR

What are the two most important nutrients you can put in your body? The answer is oxygen and water. You can live 2 minutes without air, 5-6 days without water and 30 days without food. The oxygen we breath combines with the food we eat to form energy. This energy is called adenosine triphosphate, or ATP. Oxygen is the most essential nutrient to enter the body and when it is in low supply your internal system starts to become anaerobic which means low oxygen environment. Why is this a problem? Because most pathogens like many bacteria, viruses and cancer cells thrive in anaerobic conditions. Nobel prize winner, Dr. Otto Warburg demonstrated that the key ingredient for the formation of cancer is a decrease of oxygen on the cellular level. It is also important to know that when the sugar content goes up in the body, the oxygen content goes down. They are inversely proportionally. What kind of symptoms and problems develop with low oxygen content in the body? Dr. Sheldon Hendler, author of *The Oxygen Breakthrough,* says that "ATP is the basic currency of life. Without it, we are literally dead. Imbalance or interruption in the production and flow of this substance results in fatigue, disease and disorder, including immune imbalance, cancer, heart disease and all of the degenerative processes we associate with aging."

How do we become oxygen deficient?

1) Poor Quality Air
2) Poor Quality Food
3) Poor Breathing Technique

1) The air we breath has become so polluted and toxic from the chemicals in the environment that the oxygen content has become lower. This is caused by exhaust, emmisions and smoke along with all the other 70,000 toxic chemicals that have been released into the environment.

2) Most of the food eaten today is cooked and devoid of life giving enzymes, bioelectricity and oxygen. The highest content oxygen foods are living green plants like wheatgrass, sunflower sprouts and buckwheat sprouts, next come raw green vegetables like leafy greens; kale, collards,

dandelions, spinach and broccoli, the all raw vegetables, then raw fruits. Cooked animal products have the lowest oxygen of any food source.

3) Most people only use 15% of their lung capacity throughout the majority of their life. This leads to poorly oxygenated blood. When we chest breath we use only a small portion of our lung capacity. Stress induces us to automatically chest breathe and this causes lower oxygen levels in the blood which cause stress to the body which promotes further chest breathing--a vicious cycle. Deep breathing, or diaphragm breathing fully expands and contracts the lungs causing a huge increase in the amount of oxygen absorbed into the blood. We were born to diaphragm breathe as you can see every time you see a baby breathe their abdomen move up and down. The best breathing technique inhales maximally through the nose until the lungs are fully expanded then slowly exhales until the lungs are maximally contracted. Usually this is a slow count of ten in, a momentary pause, and then slow count of ten out.

There are three ways that vital nutrients and biochemicals enter our body: through water, air and food. We have already discussed possible problems with the food we eat, but what about water and air?

Every single cell in your body must receive oxygen and nutrients in which it metabolizes to maintain life. The waste products from this metabolism must be flushed from the cells. Only water can do this. If we do not keep up with our 1 quart of water per 50 pounds of body weight per day requirement then the cells start to die in their own waste products. The less water you consume the more toxic you become and the greater the chance of disease onset.

WATER

Our bodies are made up of almost 75 percent water, and to stay healthy, we must replenish the water lost from respiration, perspiration, and excretion of urine and feces.

In his book, *Your Body's Many Cries for Water,*[1] Dr. Batmanghelidj says most people are slightly dehydrated. He also says that for all the body's systems to work right, including the immune system, we need an ample supply of water — eight 16-ounce glasses per day or, more accurately, 1 quart per 50 pounds of body weight per day. When Dr. Batmanghelidj was in prison in Iran over an unjust political issue, a man was brought to him suffering from an acute asthma attack, which can be fatal. The doctor had no medicine, but told the man to drink as much water as possible. Upon doing this, the man's asthma attack subsided. Dr. Batmanghelidj was obviously on to something very important. As the body water content goes down the secretion of histamine (a bronchial contractor) goes up. This lower water intake predisposes one for possible bronchial contractions and asthma onset. Dr. Batmanghelidj also documented 3000 cases of patients who suffered from dypepsia (gastritis, duodenitis and heart burn) were all improved with nothing more than the very large amounts of water consumed. These findings were published in the journal of clinical gastroenterology.

Some of the other symptoms and conditions that can occur when the body becomes more subclinically dehydrated:
- pain of all types increases
- stress increases
- blood pressure increases
- body weight imbalances
- allergies increase
- more prone to tumor formation
- skin disorders
- immune dysfunction or weakness (more prone to bacteria, viruses, parasites, candida and cancer

Some other dehydrating agents include:
- salt
- caffeine
- sugar
- alcohol
- stress

Our bodies need a lot more water than we thought. Unfortunately, we're not getting enough of it. And what water we do get isn't necessarily the best.

Three categories of water drinkers:

1) Just do not drink much water

2) Drink water, maybe even a lot, but is not absorbed into the cells because all this water is going to dilute all the salt, sugar and chemicals in the diet. This group tends to retain water in the tissues just to dilute the excessive salt and chemicals. This water is non functional to the cells

3) Those that live in total health. They drink the allotted amount of water daily and are almost never thirsty because the foods they eat are high water content and do not contain salt, sugar or other chemicals that need to be diluted with water. These people drink water for the health of it and see

water as preventative medicine. They power drink their water drinking 32oz. at a time and drink no closer than 30 minutes prior to a meal and at least 1½ hours after a meal so not to interfere with digestion and assimilation.

The average American doesn't get even close to the recommended 1 quart per 50 pounds of body weight per day; I have many patients who don't drink water at all. Second, is the water that we're drinking safe? More than 700 contaminants have been found in public drinking water, including pesticides, solvents, metals, radon and harmful microbes. Unfortunately, the EPA has set legal limits on, or maximum contaminant levels (MCLs), for just 54 of the 700-plus contaminants. Still, these 54 include some particularly nasty chemicals like arsenic and benzene, both carcinogens.[2]

Here are some of the many chemicals polluting our water supply:

• Chlorine supposedly makes water safe because of its ability to kill bacteria, viruses, parasites, algae, yeast and mold. But when chlorine is combined with other compounds, it forms new ones called trihalomethanes (ThMs), such as chloroform, bromoform and carbon tetrachloride, all very hazardous to your health. Dr. Kurt Donsbach links a high incidence of kidney, bladder and urinary tract cancers in New Orleans with the fact that water there is chlorinated beyond government standards. The result: 66 new carcinogenic compounds. ThMs, along with cadmium and fluoride, are also known causes of atherosclerosis. Studies have also shown correlation between chlorination and colon and rectal cancer.[3]

• Fluoride has been added to our water since 1945 because dentists believed it helped prevent tooth decay. But those opposing routine fluoridation of water say it causes cancer and other diseases. Fluoride is probably a weak carcinogen; nonetheless, it shouldn't be added to our food or water.

In the book, Fluoride: *The Aging Factor,* Dr. John Yiamouyiannis describes a village in Turkey where residents age prematurely. Many villagers show signs of wrinkling skin and brittle bones, etc. in their 30s, and many don't live to the age of 50. The cause of this condition is a 5.4 ppm (parts per million) level of natural fluoride found in their drinking water.[4] Parts of India have this same fluoride level — with similar age accelerating effects.

It is also documented that bone cancer and bone tumors occur in laboratory animals that have been treated with fluoride. Another study, done in the 1970s, showed a higher rate of cancer in areas with fluorinated water than in unfluorinated areas.

In experiments with rats, Dr. Leo Pira found that fluoride interferes with the proper usage of B vitamins, damages the thyroid and kidney, and causes heart muscles to lose their tone and degenerate.[5]

Dr. Dean Burk, former chief biochemist at the National Cancer Institute, made the astonishing statement that more than 50,000 Americans a year die of cancer caused by fluoridated drinking water.

Dr. Yiamouyiannis says fluoride interferes with the body's use of oxygen and depresses the making of ATP, from which we receive all of our energy for body and mind functions.[6]

Meanwhile, it's interesting to note that Europe banned the use of fluoride more than 20 years ago.

How much fluoride is too much? The amount of fluoride in our drinking water is 1 ppm. And even at 1 ppm, the fluoride has been shown to cause such problems as birth defects, mental retardation, heart and kidney damage, allergies and cancer. Fluoride also decreases the migration rate of white blood cells, which leads to suppression of the immune system.[7]

One report (prepared by the Library of Congress Congressional Research Service for the United States House Subcommittee on the environment and the atmosphere) lists fluoride (along with chlorine, asbestos, nickel and mercury) as a pollutant, dangerous due to its adverse effects on the central nervous system and increased rates of cancer, heart disease, and genetic mutations. According to chemistry indexes, sodium fluoride is more toxic than lead, and only slightly less toxic than arsenic.[8]

• Lead is a major offender of the nervous system, causing impairment, especially in children. It is commonly found in very old houses in the plumbing.[9] Since lead can leach out quicker in water that it sits in, it's not a good idea to drink tap water. If you decide to drink from the tap or cook with the water, let the water run until it is very cold, which can take two minutes or more. Even very low levels of lead are very dangerous to children and unborn children.[10]

So, what's the best kind of water to drink? These kinds, in this order:
1) distilled
2) reverse osmosis
3) filtered water
4) spring water (filtered through carbon)
5) mineral water (filtered through carbon)

Distilled water is the best kind to drink. It has been boiled and the steam condensed down back into pure water with no contaminants (either inorganic or microbial) and no minerals.

The next best type of water is that treated with a reverse osmosis with carbon filtration system, which can be bought (they range from $500 to $800) and placed under your kitchen sink. A key advantage to this type of filtration is that it does get rid of some radioactivity, if any, while distillation does not. Reverse osmosis filters out most everything: inorganic contaminants, like the heavy metals mercury and lead; microbial contamination from bacteria, viruses, and parasites; and organic contaminants, like pesticides, solvents and other chemicals. But reverse osmosis also has its disadvantages. It uses a lot of water; it takes 10 gallons of regular water to make one gallon of reverse osmosis water. It's also a slow process, and for households that use a lot of filtered or bottled water, it will be difficult to keep up with the demand. Also the filters have to be changed on the set schedule or they can build up bacteria. This would cause the filter to not only fail to filter out toxins and chemicals but also put bacteria into the drinking water.

One controversy concerning distilled water is that mineral-less water is supposedly not good for you. But the answer to this lies in your pipes. Look at a cross-section of a pipe that's at least 10 years old. You'll see thick mineral deposits which narrow the pipe, causing the water pressure to drop and the flow of water to slow down — similar to the narrowing of an artery, causing blood flow to slow down. The same thing happens in our bodies with regular water. Not only do these minerals deposit in the body's tissues, but they're predominantly metallic minerals, which are absorbed in minimal amounts compared to the amount consumed. A 10 percent absorption rate would be considered high, which means that for every 500 milligrams of calcium taken in, maybe 50 milligrams actually is absorbed for use.

So where do we get the necessary minerals that distilled water lacks? Almost all our minerals should come from plants. These are called organic minerals (from live plants) rather than inorganic (from the earth.) In other words, inorganic is like getting it from dirt, while organic is like getting it from a vegetable. When a plant takes an inorganic mineral from the earth, it changes the mineral to a very small particle suspension (called a "colloid") that actually loses its conductivity in water — the sign of a true organic mineral. The nice thing about plant colloid minerals are that they are so small they can go everywhere in the body, and they don't deposit in tissues like metallic minerals do.

AIR

WHY DO WE NEED OXYGEN?

Oxygen is the single most important nutrient that enters our body. Up to 96% of our nutritional need comes from oxygen the other 4% comes from the food we eat. We can survive 30 days without food, 5-6 days without water, but only 2 minutes without oxygen. Oxygen is the spark that maintains the life of all the cells in your body. Oxygen causes a biochemical reaction in which adenosine diphosphate (ADP) is transformed into adenosine triphosphate (ATP). ATP is the energy that is required to run all the cellular functions of your entire body, and without it the cells will start to die, leading to organ malfunction, disease and eventual death. Symptoms of low oxygen content in the body include: low energy, fatigue, poor digestion and a lowered metabolism. A low oxygen environment in the body is ideal for producing cancer cells because cancer cells (unlike healthy cells) grow quite well without oxygen. *According to Dr. Otto Warburg, Nobel prize winner for physiology and medicine, oxygen deprivation is a major cause of cancer and with a steady supply of oxygen to all the cells, cancer could be prevented indefinitely. Dr. Warburg also showed that when oxygen supply is decreased as little as 30%, cells filled with excess protein (from our high protein diets) can become malignant cancer cells.*

If oxygen is this important how can we get the maximum amount into our bodies?

The most available sources are:

1.) Exercise with a rapid respiratory rate (deep breathing) especially rebounding, which is walking, running, and jumping on a rebounder. This increases cardiovascular fitness 68% more efficiently than running without the same risk of injury. Rebounding also increases the lymphatic flow (which circulates the most white blood cells to boost the immune system) more than any other exercise. All the cells of your body are kept healthy by the diffusion of water, oxygen and nutrients into the cells and the diffusion of waste products out of the cells. Rebounding, because of its ability to exercise the body in a higher gravitational force (G force), also causes the diffusion rate of getting the "good" nutrients and oxygen into the cell and getting the "bad" toxins and waste products out of the cell to increase 300%. This makes rebounding the best total body exercise because it is the only exercise that strengths and exercises every cell in every organ, gland and tissue in the entire body. Rebounding can be done at all ages, and will help with all health problems. It is minimal stress to the joints if done on the proper rebounder and can be done 365 days per year in a three foot square space in your house.

2.) Food- The richest source of oxygen in food is found in green plants that are alive and still growing. Wheat grass, barley grass, sunflower sprouts, and buckwheat sprouts all have between 55-70% crude chloro-phyll, which is the oxygen carrying molecule in plants. Chlorophyll is almost identical to the heme molecule in the red blood cell which carries oxygen to all the cells of man and the animals. The oxygen content starts to diminish after cutting, so it is best to eat and drink the juice of fresh live sprouts and grasses. The other advantages to eating and drinking live sprouts and their juices is that they contain the highest amounts of any food source of enzymes, bioelectricity, phytochemicals, vitamins and minerals. Next in oxygen content comes dark green vegetables like kale, collards, broccoli, dandelion, spinach, etc.

3.) Air- There are devices that increase the oxygen content of the air while simultaneously purifying the air. Along with these benefits, they also properly ionize the air for good health. These super oxygen generators work on the same principle that air is purified after a thunderstorm. Air smells cleaner and fresher after storms because lightning creates ozone (O_3) which is oxygen with an extra molecule. When the ozone (O_3) comes in contact with bacteria, viruses, mold, fungi or other odors or chemicals in the air, the extra oxygen atom breaks off and oxidizes the offender, caus-ing it to either be killed, if it is living, or neutralized, if it is a synthetic chemical, fume or odor. After this reaction has occurred the ozone (O_3) molecule is transformed to a pure oxygen (O_2) molecule which we can breathe. The air is sanitized so well it is what is used in hospitals where clean air is vitally important. The second important function of this air purifying system is ionization. The ionizer releases negatively charged ions into the air and attach themselves to dust, pollen, dander, molds, bacteria, viruses and odors transforming their negative charge to them. This allows either neutralization of the particles in the air as they are drawn back into

the unit or the negative charge causes them to fall to the floor
can easily be vacuumed away. It is important to know that n(
(which are put into the air with the air purifier) have the following beneficial effects:
- inhibit cancer growth rate
- inhibit respiratory tract infections
- increases ease of breathing for hayfever and asthmatic sufferers
- lowers blood pressure

4.) Oxygen Supplementation- Oxygenated essential fatty acids in liquid form can increase the oxygen content in the body and can be protective
against bacteria, viruses, fungi, parasites and cancer cells. This supplement
also strengthens the immune system by helping the white blood   cells
destroy the above pathogens. It is important to understand that although
oxygen sustains life, it also has the ability in the proper form to destroy life.
These supplements take advantage of the powerful oxidative effects of the
oxygen on bacteria, viruses, mold, parasites and cancer cells. This cellular
oxidative metabolic pathway provides billions of activated molecules to
attack and destroy all invaders for hours after ingestion, or absorption
through the skin.

Unfortunately, not much can be done about the outside air we breathe.
It is a tragedy to see how much garbage is pumped into our atmosphere. In
Southern California alone, the following was pumped into the air in 1982:[11]
1) arsenic — 60 tons
2) benzene and hexachlorabenzene — 20,000 tons
3) ethylene dibromide and methyl bromide - 3,770 tons
4) methyl chloroform — 17,700 tons
5) methylene chloride — 16,700 tons
6) perchloroethylene — 21,000 tons

If this wasn't bad enough, our inside air isn't much better. The closed
environments of our homes and offices expose us to many toxic chemicals,
including cleaning supply fumes, subtle carbon monoxide fumes from natural gas combustion, and one of the most serious threats of all — odorless,
colorless radon gas.
Radon is a naturally-occurring radioactive gas that can seep from the
ground into homes and offices. It enters through any opening in the ground,

ιke foundation cracks, drains, sump pits, etc. According to the EPA, eight to ten million American homes have unhealthy basement radon levels — greater than 4 pci/l (picocuries per liter of air). According to Richard Guimond, former director of the EPA Office of Radiation, "[Radon] is the second most prevalent cause of lung cancer."[12]

What can we do about the air we breathe?

1) Don't stay around fumes of any kind, whether exhaust or just funny odors.
2) Use proper ventilation to move any unwanted fumes out of the house or building.
3) Open all windows in your house at least ½ hour per day, year round, to let fresher air in and stale (and possibly toxic) air out.
4) Leave all bedroom windows cracked open at all times.
5) Invest in a home air purifier and move it from room to room.
6) Have your home tested by the gas company for odorless carbon monoxide.
7) Have your home tested for radon levels, especially in your basement.
8) If radon levels are above normal, have an environmental air specialist install a radon elimination system, along with sealing any cracks or openings through which radon can enter the basement.

CHAPTER 8

TOXICITY:
THE MODERN DAY CAUSE OF DISEASE

I believe toxicity is, and will continue to be for decades to come, one of the biggest causes of sickness and disease in our country. When a person is toxic, all systems of the body start to malfunction, leading to cell, tissue, gland and organ damage. Toxicity can ultimately lead to death if not addressed by regular "detoxing" of the body, and maintaining it in a cleansed state indefinitely.

What Is Toxicity?

What does it mean to be "toxic?" It's when chemicals have built up in the body to a point that the body can no longer metabolize them quickly, resulting in cellular damage and, eventually, damage and malfunction to tissues, glands and organs.

This damage comes primarily through oxidation, which causes cell membranes to become weak and porous. Cellular material then leaks out, and extra cellular fluid leaks in, causing the cells to rupture and die. Toxicity also damages cells by changing them into free radicals, which are very destructive cellular intermediates that can cause a chain reaction of oxidative damage — similar to the starting of a forest fire by the spark of one match.

A toxin is any chemical or substance that, once in the body, causes cellular dysfunction, damage and death. Toxins kill cells, tissues, glands, and organs — either quickly or slowly, depending on how strong the toxin is. Toxins include alcohol, chemicals, preservatives, food coloring, dyes, and hydrogenated fats and oils.

To help illustrate toxicity, look at the liver — the organ that detoxifies (or breaks down) harmful chemicals, turning them into harmless waste products for excretion. This is an amazing picture of the way God designed us. All chemicals and drugs we eat, breathe, or drink go to the detoxifying plant — the liver — where they are changed to harmless waste products and excreted.

Additionally, your body's metabolism regularly produces chemical byproducts. So your liver must handle not only the load that comes from outside your body, but also those chemical byproducts from inside your body.

Imagine that your liver is like a portable air filter placed in an enclosed room. Suppose there is a fireplace in this room, but the flue is closed, so that smoke cannot escape, entering the room instead. Under normal circumstances, the air filter can do its job, even filtering *some* smoke. But under these circumstances, the filter cannot possibly keep up with the demand, so the smoke fills the entire room.

This analogy applies to your liver. Like the overworked air filter, the liver cannot keep up once chemicals and toxins in the body reach a certain level. At certain levels, toxins start producing symptoms in many areas of the body, depending on where the toxins accumulate. Toxic buildup in one gland or organ can cause cellular damage, which can lead to tissue damage, which can lead to organ and gland and joint dysfunction — thus, ill health.

What Causes Toxicity?

The **primary** cause of toxicity is eating, drinking, and breathing toxins and chemicals on a regular basis — whether you know it or not. We live in a toxic world; chemicals and toxins are everywhere. Once they are in your system, you need a program for getting your body "detoxed" regularly so these chemicals and toxins never reach critical levels.

A condition called "leaky gut syndrome" is a prime example of how you can be toxic without knowing it. In this condition, which does not necessarily cause pain, the intestinal lining becomes inflamed from poor digestion and assimilation, parasites, pathogenic bacteria, virus, fungi-like candida, food allergies, sensitivities and drugs.

Normally, the intestinal lining is like a fine mesh, allowing only basic digested food particles (like amino acids and simple sugars) to pass through, ready to be assimilated into the bloodstream. At the same time, a normally functioning intestine "screens out" larger food particles and toxins, preventing them from entering the bloodstream.

But when "leaky gut" occurs, the bowel lining is like a large-holed screen. The "fine mesh" (selective permeability) breaks down, allowing the passage of larger food particles, which can produce allergy and inflammation throughout the body. Also, toxins and chemicals can now leak into the bloodstream and be deposited in any organ, gland, or tissue, causing damage and dysfunction.

The **second** cause of toxicity is not getting the bad out. Since chemicals are everywhere, we are always taking harmful toxins into our bodies. Since we cannot take these chemicals completely out of our air, water, and food, we must detoxify our bowels, livers, gall bladders, kidneys, bladders and blood. Remember the air filter analogy? We have got to clean our filters and put them on high speed to filter all the smoke from the room. But we have also got to open the flue so the smoke — toxic material — stops pouring in.

The **third** cause of toxic buildup is poor digestion (breaking down the food for assimilation into the cells). If we don't chew our food sufficiently (25 times minimum), if we don't secrete enough hydrochloric acid in our stomachs to break down the protein, if we don't secrete enough digestive enzymes in the small intestine to totally break down the food into all its component parts for assimilation, if we do not combine our foods properly (some foods digest better if eaten with other foods) — these all lead to maldigestion. Maldigestion causes low levels of inflammation of the bowel, which leads to an increase of intestinal lining permeability ("leaky gut"), which leaks large undigested food particles into the intestinal tract. This can trigger a host of autoimmune diseases — like rheumatoid arthritis and lupus — where the body attacks itself. Leaky gut also allows all the toxins to enter your bloodstream, which then can be deposited in any gland, organ, tissue, or joint.

The **fourth** cause of toxicity is poor assimilation (getting the nutrients into the cells), which has two major causes: "leaky gut" (increased intestinal permeability), and food sensitivity/allergy. With a food sensitivity/allergy, the intestinal lining is inflamed from the food eaten, causing a breakdown or "leaky gut." The most common offenders are dairy products, milk, cheese, cream and butter. As much as 60% of our diseases might be traced to food sensitivities/allergies.

The **fifth** cause of toxicity are pathogens in the body, causing waste byproducts to build up, eventually leading to cellular damage or even death. Pathogens excrete waste products, which must be filtered out to prevent further toxic buildup. Some pathogens include bacteria, viruses, parasites and candida (fungi), all of which can (and probably do) live inside you right now.

The **sixth** cause of toxicity is probably one of the greatest causes of ill health today: Mental stress and/or spiritual stress. This includes all types of mental stressors affecting your life, such as personality, problems with family, friends, job, health, finances, and memories. Spiritual stressors include fear, loneliness, feeling unloved, a lack of joy and peace, and a lack of a personal relationship with the Living God. All stressors cause excessive production of adrenaline, an extremely oxidative molecule which causes cell damage if secreted long-term, instead of the intended quick burst of energy in time of dire need. Adrenaline is the "fight-fright-flight" hormone that prepares our body to run or move quickly, as if a tiger were chasing us. The problem arises when we are stressed all the time, which causes adrenaline to fill the blood and start damaging cells, tissues, glands, and organs.

So the more we understand Jesus' exhortation to "cast all your cares upon me, because I care for you," the less stress we will have and the less adrenaline produced. Philippians 4:6-7 says, "Do not be anxious about anything, but in everything, by prayer and petition, with thanksgiving, present your requests to God. And the peace of God, which transcends all understanding, will guard your hearts and minds in Christ Jesus." The phrase "do not be anxious" also means "do not take thought" or "be careful for nothing." I like that: "Do not think about it and be carefree, because God is in control."

So toxins can be of two general groups: exogenous ("from outside the body") and endogenous ("from inside the body".) Exogenous toxins include air, water, food and most of what we described above. Endogenous toxins include regular byproducts from cellular metabolism: normal waste products from normal functioning cells, and waste products from pathogenic bacteria, viruses, parasites, and fungi.

All toxins, whether from inside or outside the body, must be detoxified in the liver, filtered through the kidneys and excreted through bile in the intestinal tract or through the urine. So our first goal is to get the good in, through vital nutrients from predominately uncooked raw, living foods, pure water. Our second goal is to get the bad out, through regularly detoxifying the colon, liver, gall bladder, kidney, bladder and blood. This is our key to vibrant physical health.

The big question is "What can I do about toxicity?" You will find the answer in the chapters to come. But here it is in a nutshell:

1) Get the good in, and get the bad out.

2) Drink and cook in purified water (distilled or reverse osmosis).

3) Avoid all fumes. Breathe the cleanest, purest air possible.

4) Eat whole foods with no additives, preservatives, or chemicals. Eat organic fruits, vegetables, grains, seeds, nuts, beans, and sprouts. Eat as much raw, living and uncooked food as possible. Read labels: If it's unpronounceable or looks like a chemistry set, do not eat it.

The reason I stress toxicity so heavily is because we live in a toxic world quite unlike we did 100 years ago:

- Cancer has risen over the last century from the No. 25 cause of death to soon to be the No. 1 cause of death.
- There has been a 46% rise in the cancer death rate since 1950.
- Cancer is the No. 2 cause of death in children, second only to accidental injury.
- The EPA has set standards on only about seven of the currently used 70,000 toxic chemicals
- Every year over 100 billion gallons of liquid wastes are absorbed into our ground water
- The average American eats their weight in food additives every year.

What is going on with all this? We are killing our environment with chemicals, so we are also killing ourselves. Toxicity is deadly because it attacks *all* systems of the body, making them all vulnerable to disease. Your immune system fights cancer with its natural killer cells, cells that seek and destroy cancer cells. Toxins suppress the immune system, giving cancer cells a foothold so they can multiply and form a tumor. Chemotherapy and radiation are not the answer; they treat the effect, not the cause. Prominent cancer nutritionist Dr. Patrick Quillen stated if you miss enough cancer cells (through chemotherapy and radiation) to fill a pin head, they can spread like seeds and start growths throughout the body.

The answer is to treat the cause of the cancer, which also is the cause of most diseases. Get the good in and get the bad out regularly, and then let your body — the temple of God's Spirit — heal itself. Getting the good in means not only the good vital nutrients from whole food but also the good thoughts through prayer, meditation and positive mental attitude. Getting the bad out means not only the physical toxins from one's body but also the mental and emotional toxins which include fear, stress, frustration, anxiety, resentment, guilt and low self esteem. The Living God said cast your cares upon Him. He desires to take them from you because they are too heavy for you to carry. Through prayer and meditation, living in faith and trusting in God, one can be released from these toxic emotions and thoughts. Detoxification must be as much mental/emotional as physical to achieve *total health=wholeness.*

CHAPTER 9

SPIRITUAL HEALTH

The most important part of total health is spiritual health, without a close communion with our Creator we have no true purpose in life, no true meaning, because He made us to know Him, to love Him and to be loved by Him. Without this union we will spend all are days searching for fulfillment and never find it. The most important first step in this journey is to learn to listen to His voice in stillness and quietness. The Living God will reveal Himself to you if you take the time to listen and wait upon Him.

Now that we've laid the foundation of why we are sick, from here on we will discuss how to get well — not just well, but how to be in *total health = wholeness*.

The next ten chapters deal with the ten most important aspects of your *total health = wholeness*. Remember, health and strength and life flow from God's Spirit into our human spirit then to our mind, will and emotions, and finally into our physical bodies. We cannot be in *total health = wholeness* unless our spirit, soul, and body are all in health.

God made us as a spirit that has a soul and lives in a body. The spirit is the part of us made in God's image. Genesis says God breathed the breath of life, or *pneuma*, into Adam. So without the spirit, we would just be dust of the earth. It is vital to understand the wholeness concept of body, soul (your mind, will, and emotions), and spirit.

Every man, woman and child has a spirit, which God placed inside of them. The spirit has four functions: a moral conscience, intuitive knowledge, maintaining wholeness, and communion with God. Let's take a closer look at each.

A Moral Conscience

The spirit gives us our moral conscience of right and wrong. We can deny it, we can deaden it, we can ignore it, but God gave us all a conscience of knowing right from wrong. This is why, deep inside, we all want to do the right thing. It feels good to do the right thing, because that is one reason God created us — to know and do what is right. In today's society, we often see little to no conscience in people. One may think there is no moral conscience inside of people, but that brings me back to God's Word, which says that in the last days, people will want to hear only what the itching ears want to hear, and their conscience will be seared by a hot iron (2 Timothy 4:3, 1 Timothy 4:2).

God made us to do what is right and good. Whenever we consistently step out of the will of God's purpose and plan, we won't be joyful, content or satisfied. We are God's perfect creation.

Just as a car comes with an owner's operating manual, so do we. It is the Bible — the holy, inerrant word of God. That awesome owner's manual shows us exactly why God created us and how we can live a life to the fullest, and more abundantly.

When you bought your first car, you probably read the manual. You wanted to take such good care of it, you changed the oil every 3,000 miles. You tuned it up according to the manufacturer's recommended schedule. Why? Because you knew if you followed the manual, that car would perform just as the manufacturer said it would, lasting many years. We are the same. We were designed by our Creator to know and glorify Him with our lives. When we fulfill these purposes, we will be filled with unspeakable joy — so much joy we won't even be able to express it. We'll also live an abundant life as stated in the manual, the Bible.

If you took that nice new car and started pouring kerosene in the tanks, you would soon find your car wouldn't run right, and would stop running altogether. We're no different. We were meant to have high-enzyme, high phytochemical, bioenergetic, vitamin-rich and mineral-rich food put into our bodies for fuel — as Adam and Eve did — to live the full life the manufacturer said we would live. Instead, we dump enzyme-depleted (by cooking), vitamin- and mineral-deficient dead food into our bodies and expect to live the full life God promised. I believe if we did what the manual said to do, we would not only live as long as the Bible says we should — 120 years, according to Genesis 6:3 — but that we would also have full, abundant lives, another scriptural promise (John 10:10). Why, then, is the average life expectancy 75? Because we aren't "maintaining our car" properly. We're not putting in the right fuel, and we're using our bodies for other than the intended purpose.

To live an abundant life is to know and love God. If we follow His plan, we experience love, joy and peace. But if we take that nice new car and not only put the wrong fuel in it, but also drive it in ways it's not meant to be driven, the car will eventually break down — and I mean *really* break down — and not last as long as it should. Cars aren't meant to be driven through deep water, or off of cliffs, or into tornadoes.

If we want to live up to the manufacturer's warranty, we need to: 1) use our vehicle for its designed purpose; (this is to know and love God); 2) use the right fuel so it can perform its designed purpose; (this is the genesis diet of living and raw foods for optimal health); and 3) have the scheduled maintenance checkup to keep it running as it was made to. This maintenance comes when we read the owner's manual (His Word), follow the directions, and talk to the manufacturer's representative (God's Spirit) about the car's maintenance and operation.

Every answer to every question in life can be found in two places — either in the written Word of God (the Bible), or in the living Word of God written in your heart by the Holy Spirit. When God saw that man had fallen and sinned (missed the mark), He designed a plan in which he would send His Son to save the world from its sin, and that through His Son, man would have eternal life and know Him (John 15). Jesus said, "I am the way, the truth and the life. No one comes to the Father except through me." (John 14:6).

Before Jesus died and rose again to sit at the right hand of the Father, He promised the Holy Spirit to those who believe. He said His Holy Spirit would be inside us, inside our spirit. So, instead of God walking *with* us, He would be *inside* us, in the Holy Spirit. And the Holy Spirit would guide us, teach us, help us, comfort us, reveal all things to us and empower us.

To seek the answers to the questions of the world look to either the written Word of God (the Bible) or the living Word of God in your heart (the Holy Spirit). If you can't find the answer in the manual, then go straight to the manufacturer — that is, the Holy Spirit inside of you.

Intuitive Knowledge

The second function of our human spirit is to give us intuitive knowledge. This is when we just *know* something, even if we can't explain it. Like a mother's intuition about her child; she just knows things that cannot be explained. When I was young, my mother went on a trip to Europe. While there, she woke up in the middle of the night with a fear that I was in danger. She actually saw me about to fall off of a rooftop. She immediately called home, where it was afternoon in Chicago. My grandmother answered the phone, and my mother said, "Mom, where is Keith?" Grandma said I was in the backyard by the neighbor's garage, but after calling me, she found out I was on the neighbor's garage roof. My mother then told Grandma to not alarm me, but to tell me to slowly come down. I did, and all was well. Thank God for the intuition He placed in our spirits.

Intuition can be seen in many ways, when we just know things we can't explain. We just have a strong feeling about someone or something, and it comes to pass just as we thought it would. This is intuitive knowledge.

Maintaining Wholeness

The third function of our spirit is to keep us whole — alive and well. Proverbs 18:14 says, "A man's spirit sustains him in sickness." The spirit of a man is designed to keep him as well as possible, with what he has to work with. Many people believe that "mind over body" is the way to health today; if we think we're healthy, if we have a positive attitude and always look at the good side of things, this will help keep us healthy. I agree — and I'll say more about this in Chapter 10 — but I think there's a greater influence on our health, and that's our spirit.

The path of wholeness and total health flows from spirit first, then to mind, then to body. Let me explain: When you cut your finger, do you have to think your self into healing for that finger to heal? Does a baby have to have a positive attitude to get healed from a cold? The answer to both questions is no.

We get well because the spirit inside us always works to keep us as well as possible — that is, with what we have to work with. But if we put junk food and dead food of little nutritive value into our bodies, our spirit cannot do miracles, not like God's Spirit can. So if the raw materials aren't there, our bodies will break down. Remember, the spirit sustains a man in sickness.

John 19:30 tells us that when Jesus died, he gave up his spirit (that which sustained His physical body.) According to Luke 23:46, Jesus' dying words are, "Father, into your hands I commit my spirit." James 2:26 tells us "the body without the spirit is dead."

Communion with God

The fourth and most important function of the spirit is to help us commune and communicate with God. In our spirit, true fellowship and communion with God occur.

Let me make the entire Bible and plan of God easy for you:

1) God made man to fellowship with, to walk and talk with. He made man to know God and glorify Him. God made man in His image, so He gave man a spirit, breathing the breath of life into the dust of the earth.

2) Originally, man did walk and talk and fellowship with God, communing with his Creator via his spirit.

3) Man disobeyed God and broke God's covenant (contract). The result of the broken covenant was that man would surely die (Genesis 2:17). At that point, man died spiritually; at least his ability to have communion with God in his spirit was broken. And though God didn't originally intend for man to experience physical and spiritual death, years later, man's physical body died. Man was created to live forever, communing with God forever.

4) God made a better way for man. He sent His Son to die for us, in our place and for our sins. So when we accept Him as Lord (Master, King) and Savior, we are saved from our sin and eternal separation from God. We become a new creation; the old is gone, and the new has come (2 Corinthians 5:17.) When Jesus Christ becomes our Lord and Savior, it means we have asked Him to come into our lives. It means we no longer serve ourselves, but Him. We don't only love ourselves; we love Him also. He is our King who has set us free from the bondage of sin and the law of sin and death (Romans 8:2). Also, since He is our King, our life is no longer ours but His, spent doing whatever He calls us to do. All we do is out of love for the Father, not out of a condemning conscience, thinking if we make a mistake, God will not bless us and might even curse us. The Bible says **God is love, and God is in love with you, His bride**.

5) When Jesus was resurrected, winning total victory over sin and the Devil, he ascended to sit at the right hand of the Father. He told his disciples that when he leaves, He will send us His Holy Spirit — the Spirit of wisdom and revelation, the Comforter, the Paraclete, the Helper, the Counselor, the Empowerer. When Jesus walked the earth — as great as that was — He could only be in one place at one time, so He could only minister to a certain number of people. But the Holy Spirit isn't bound by space or time. When we receive Jesus into our hearts as Lord and Savior, we receive the Holy Spirit, which is God living within us. Now we carry God with us wherever we go, no matter what questions or problems arise. The God who created the heavens and earth lives inside us, and will never leave us. How much better a promise is this than just being with Jesus? Now the Spirit of God lives in us, 24 hours a day, 7 days a week. Our spiritual life is getting to know the God who lives in us, learning to hear the voice of the Spirit. When we learn to spend quiet time alone with the Holy Spirit, He will speak to our hearts about anything we seek, if we just train our spiritual ears to listen.

So, to review the message of the Bible, God made man to fellowship with Him, to know Him and give Him glory. Man disobeyed God and broke the covenant. God made a new and better plan by sending His Son to pay for man's sin and the broken covenant. This was a better covenant with better promises. When one accepts Jesus Christ as Lord and Savior, he enters into this new covenant and God enters into him in the form of the Holy Spirit. So not only does the all-powerful, all-knowing and all-loving God live inside of man, He also has written His law on man's heart. So the old covenant was made obsolete, the new one replacing it.

The Bible is so simple. It is just God's love letter to us, and all it says is, "Come to me, all you who are weary and heavy laden, for I will give you rest" (Matthew 11:28). What more awesome a possession can you have than to know that the God who created the universe lives inside you, ready to solve all your problems and answer all your questions and take away all your fears as He wraps His loving arms around you, His precious, precious child. Remember, **God not only loves you, He is in love with you.** When you were first in love with your spouse, nothing mattered but your spouse. Time, the world, money — everything else was of no importance compared to your spouse. That is a tiny picture of how much God is in love with us.

The Bible says in 1 Corinthians 6:17 that the Holy Spirit and our spirit become one when we ask Jesus into our lives to become our Lord and Savior. When we have the Holy Spirit in us, all things are possible. We now have the answer to every question, the solution to every problem. Not only will the Holy Spirit speak to our hearts about these things, He will also empower us to do them. When the Holy Spirit enters us, God Himself enters us, and we have it better than any Old Testament saint — better than Moses, Abraham, Jacob, Joseph, Noah or Daniel. Better than any of them, because although they had the Spirit of God upon them, none of them had the Holy Spirit of God living in them. God spoke to all of these men, but none of them carried the awesome power, knowledge, love, joy and peace of God around with them 24 hours a day, as we now can.

This is why Jesus told his disciples it would be better if He left, because only then would the Holy Spirit of God come dwell in them. What an awesome — and I mean awesome — thing to know wherever you are, God is with you, ready to help you, ready to empower you, to teach you, to guide you.

The biggest part of living in communion with the God who created you, sustains you and loves you, is having a relationship with Him. This begins when we ask His Son, Jesus Christ, into our hearts to be our Lord (King) and Savior (setting us free from our sin.) Once we have asked Jesus into our heart and our life we receive His Holy Spirit to empower us, teach us, guide us, help us and love us. The Holy Spirit who then lives inside of us speaks to us as a part of that relationship.

What is a relationship? It is communication. It is when my wife and I became one and started a life-long relationship of growth by talking and listening to each other. My wife and I would not have much of a relationship if we only either talked or listened — we need to do both everyday to help our relationship grow. I need to tell my sweetheart my thoughts, feelings, purpose, dreams and goals. Then I need to listen to her wisdom and insight on them, and I also need to listen to hers and tell her what wisdom and insight the Lord has given me for her. This is how the two become one, always growing, always learning, always talking and most important always taking the time to listen.

One of the greatest weaknesses in a relationship is the inability to listen — and I mean true listening, not in one ear and out the other. This is the same weakness in our relationship with God. Most of us are pretty good talkers with God, we tell Him our list of all the things we need or want, and do this everyday, but how many of us take the time to be still before God in our busy lives and listen for His response to our requests? How many people have a revelation of "be still and know that I am God" (Psalms 46:10) and "you will seek me and find me when you seek me with all your heart (Jeremiah 29:13.)

Remember, God is a real person; His Holy Spirit is a real person who lives inside of you to give you wisdom and strength for every situation that comes up in your life. He does this by speaking to you through either:

1. His word, the Holy Bible (written word)

2. His voice spoken in your heart (spoken word)

The Holy Spirit speaks through His Word, the Holy Bible, by a revelation that hits you as you read his Word. This is seen when you open your Bible and start to read… when suddenly a verse or paragraph jumps off the page and causes a light to go on in your head. This is God speaking to you and he usually will confirm it with one or two other confirmations. Let me give you an example. One time while I was reading the word of God, the verse "when I am weak then I am strong" (2 Corinthians 12:10) seemed to jump out at me. I had read that verse many times before but it had never affected me like this before, so I started to pray and meditate about the verse. Later that day while in the car, I felt impressed to turn on the radio, which I usually do not do, and as soon as I did a man was reciting the exact verse "when I am weak then I am strong." This was the Holy Spirit confirming the word he spoke to me earlier. This is an example of how I heard God speak through his Word.

The second way God speaks is by His Holy Spirit into our hearts. This is when you are in prayer, talking to God and suddenly there are thoughts in your head that bring a sense of love, joy and peace. This is how you know it's from God: it will always bring love, joy and peace deep in your heart. Maybe you will not have peace in your head yet, but it will be in your heart.

Let me give you another example. My wife was driving along one day when the voice of the Holy Spirit spoke to her in her heart. He told her to ask Him for a particular piece of real estate. This was a total surprise because she never considered this or even wanted it but still she decided to seek God's further advice on the matter before presenting it to me. The very next week while I was talking and listening to God, the Holy Spirit spoke to me as a voice in my head saying that we should purchase a particular piece of real estate. I was also surprised and when presenting this to my wife she smiled and confirmed the message that the Holy Spirit told her a week ago.

This is how the Holy Spirit of God speaks to us. He speaks into our head in our own voice and confirms it with two or three confirmations just as my wife and I experienced. To add to this story, the Holy Spirit gave me an amount of a selling price for the property and when I called to see if it was for sale the owner replied it was and the selling price was the exact price the Holy Spirit had told me earlier. I do not believe in chance occurrences, but that God supernaturally confirms His words spoken to us.

Another point I would like to explain in listening to the voice of the Holy Spirit is that when the Spirit speaks He doesn't always make sense in our heads, but brings peace, joy and love in our hearts. This property that was mentioned made no sense at all in our heads because financially, we couldn't even afford it, but my wife and I had a supernatural peace in our hearts (both of our hearts) that was from God. When God gives a peace in your heart, He will make a way so that "all things are possible for him who believes."

So go before God and enjoy your growing relationship, remembering not only to talk to Him about everything in your day and life, but also taking the time to listen to Him for His response, His wisdom, His guidance. What would it be like if the only time I talked to my wife was to ask her for something and never listened to her responses or her needs? That relationship would soon die. Remember to talk and listen to God daily and watch your relationship with Him grow strong and mature.

EXPLANATION OF CHART (See Page 131)

The most powerful way to live and walk in the Spirit of God instead of the flesh of man is to take the time to meditate and listen to the Spirit of God, in quietness you will hear the Living Words of God spoken into your heart. They will bring love, joy and peace and will give you direction, new insights, revelations and answers to your questions. His voice is the quiet, still voice that speaks to your heart. Remember He said "if you seek me you will find me when you seek me with all your heart." So take quiet time to seek Him and have paper and pen on hand to write down any distractions (like things you have to get done that day) and also to write down your new ideas, insights, answers and so on. It is a wonderful thing to start growing in your communion and communication with the Living God, who speaks to us today, gives us insight and revelations today and empowers us today. This is why He is the *Living God.*

Our spirit is divided into four parts: conscience, communion, intuition and health sustaining. Our soul is divided into the mind, will and emotion. Our physical body is called our flesh. The choice we have in this life is to either live and walk in God's strength by His Spirit or to live and walk in our own strength or flesh.

The decision is the act of our will and it is our will that chooses which path we follow. Moses said, "Choose life," in Exodus and we also can choose life by living in the ever presence of God's Spirit, power, love, joy and peace.

We also can live in our own strength being led by the cravings of our mind (appearance, acceptance, acknowledgment and achievement) and craving of our body (food, drink, sex, drugs and entertainment). Also remember that any act done in your own ability whether good or bad is an act of the flesh. What dictates the decision of our will? It is influenced by our conscience which affects our mind, and intuition which affect our emotion and most directly the communion with God via his Holy Spirit living in our hearts will greatly influence our will. The opposing side affecting our will to walk either by the Spirit of God or by our own flesh is all the aspects of our flesh influencing our mind and emotions. No matter how weak we are His strength is there for us to choose life and live in the ever present Spirit of God. So remember no matter how great the temptation is, Jesus overcame all temptations so you could draw on His strength in time of need. When you reach the end of yourself, your strength, that is when you realize you have just begun to walk in Him and His strength.

HOW THE CHART IS USED

EXAMPLE: A man struggles with a weight problem he has had for years

The flesh (9) is a very strong factor in this problem. The flesh is the cravings of the body or mind. His mind (the mind of man) might say "I really want to lose this weight," but the flesh (9) overpowers most natural minds. So he struggles condemning himself and never solving his problem. His emotion (emotion of man) say "I am frustrated with myself, I have low self esteem because of this, I hate being like this, this is hopeless." The negative emotions are usually not strong enough to overpower the flesh. So this man is trapped in a cycle: Flesh (cravings of the body)(9) to the mind (6) to the will (7) and back to the flesh (9), 9>6>7>9. He also goes from the flesh (9) to the emotions (8) to the will (7) and back to the flesh (9), 9>8>7>9.

Now instead of addressing this problem from his own strength (which obviously has failed), he decides to address this problem spiritually. He will bring his problem before God each and every day in his quiet meditation time. He waits patiently for God to speak to his heart and give him new insight or revelation on how to solve his problem.

Now as he brings his problem before God daily he experiences the communion with God (2) which speaks the mind of God which says "I can do all things through Him who strengthens me." This is not him just memorizing a bible verse, but waiting for God to speak it into his heart so the words become alive, 9>7>2>1>2>6>7.

Next, the emotions of God fill his heart with such an overwhelming love, joy and peace that he takes his eyes off his weight and feels love and acceptance by his Creator, 9>7>2>1>2>8>7.

Then the Spirit of God starts to fill his spirit with new insights which then open his mind to possible diet modifications, exercise programs and stress reducing activities. But because these revelations came from God not from the man's own effort, they take on a whole new meaning and excitement. The man is changing his life in God's wisdom, strength and timing which makes it supernatural and the man feels God with him every step of the way. He is solving his problem with God by his side.

Lastly, God empowers this man through his own spirit to make the right decisions and choices through his will, 1>2>7. The end result is that he starts to live in the spirit, being led by God's voice and strength and begins the journey to overcome his problem. With God leading and guiding him he takes his eyes off of the desired end (ideal weight) and starts to enjoy the journey to get to the desired end because he feels he is not alone; God's presence is always with him filling him up supernaturally every step to the journey. He also gets the revelation that in overcoming this problem he will become so much more spiritually mature and his weakness will actually become his strength. He will then be able to give the gift away that he has received to another who struggles with problems in life, the gift of overcoming all things in God's strength: "for when I am weak it is then that I am strong." Also, once the man has learned to overcome any problem in life through God's strength, he can apply the same principles to all problems. The way to victory is the same no matter how the course has changed or how different obstacles appear, so once God shows us, and leads us to the victory or the promised land in one area of our life, we then apply it to all areas of our life and pass the wisdom and revelation on to others so they to can overcome all things in His strength. So the gift goes on and on and on multiplied throughout the world.

Our goal in life is to live and walk in the ever presence of God. In His love, in His joy, in His peace, in His strength, in His wisdom, in His Spirit and not in the flesh of the mind, emotions and body of natural man. Choose to live in the Spirit (7>2>1>2>7) and not in the flesh (7>9>7).

Spiritual Law vs. Natural Law

God created the heavens, the earth and everything in them. After doing so he instituted natural laws by which the universe and the earth are governed by. What type of laws? Here are but two:

1. Gravity
2. Second Law of Thermodynamics

Gravity

The law of gravity means that because you have weight or mass and the earth has a gravitational field, if you jump off a building, you will fall to

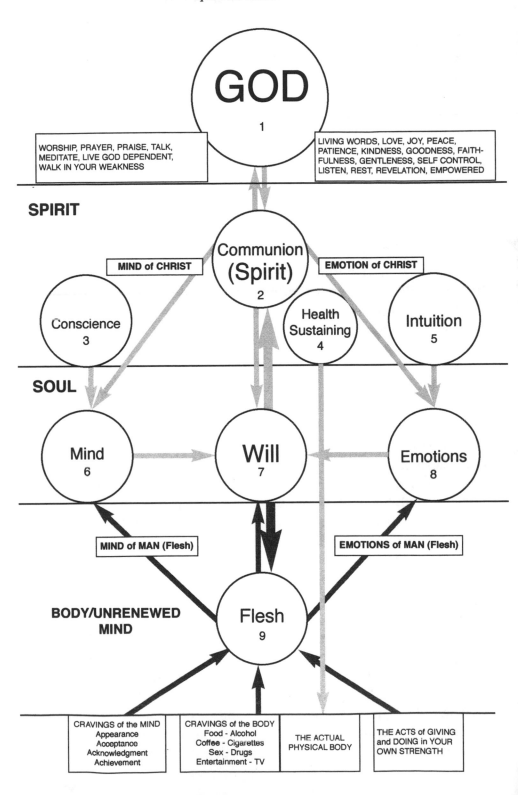

the ground every time at a precise set speed. Natural laws cannot be changed — they are as exact as the sun rising and setting everyday.

Second Law of Thermodynamics

This law states that everything (since the fall of man) is in a state of breaking down or getting more random. This means that everything is aging, not being renewed. For instance, when a child is born it grows, matures, ages and dies; not the reverse (old becomes young) and not a stand still (child never ages). This law totally excludes the possibility of evolution, a less-ordered creature evolving into the most-ordered, complex creation: MAN.

Spiritual Law

The Bible states in Romans 8:2: "the law of the Spirit of Life has set me free from the law of sin and death in Christ Jesus." This means that God created man perfect, holy and sinless and made a covenant with him. But man broke the covenant of life when he ate of the tree of the knowledge of good and evil. This set at least two new laws in effect, one spiritual and one natural.

The spiritual was the *law of sin and death*. The natural was the *second law of thermodynamics*. The spiritual law of sin and death began, meaning that the spiritual part of man that communed with God died. The mind, will and emotion of man in a sense died or became flesh (self-centered dependent instead of God-centered dependent) when man changed the meaning of life from God to himself. The first words out of Adam's mouth after disobeying God, breaking the covenant by sinning were, "I was afraid." So man's spirit died, his mind changed from one being filled with love, joy and peace to one filled with fear, anxiety and stress. The third result of the law of sin and death was that man's physical body would now age and die whereas before the fall, man was never meant to die. The only remedy for the new law of sin and death was that God made a way by sending His Son Jesus Christ into the world so all who would believe that He came to pay the price for their sins (all the way back to Adam) by dying for them and rising from the dead and being the lord over all. Then the "law of the spirit of life sets you free from the law of sin and death" (Romans 8:1.)

Once we ask Jesus Christ into our heart and our life, three things are regained. First, the spirit communication or communion is restored with God. Second, the mind, will and emotions starts the process of being transformed back to being God-centered and dependent instead of self-centered and dependent. As we start to grow in that relationship not only is the spiritual death lost in Adam renewed, thus the phrase in John 3: 3-5 Jesus said "You must be born again to see and enter the kingdom of heaven." Your spirit is made new or like being born again. This means you are restored into the family of God and no longer a lost sheep and you can talk and listen to your Father and His Son, Jesus, though the Holy Spirit, who now lives in you. This means because you personally know Jesus you will have eternal life (and be with Him in Heaven when you die.) Third is the progressive reprogramming of your mind to erase what the world, the flesh (mind without God, self-centered) and the devil has programmed into you. Roman 12:2 says, "Do not be conformed to this world but be transformed by the renewing of your minds." Once you enter a personal relationship with the Living God through His Son, Jesus Christ, and His Holy Spirit comes and lives in your heart. Then your spirit is one with His Holy Spirit and you must choose to believe what God says about you rather than what the world, your flesh and the devil say about you. Words like:

- you are a chosen child of God (Ephesians 1:5, John 1:12)
- you are a joint heir with Jesus Christ, sharing His inheritance with Him (Romans 8:17)
- you are righteous (2 Corinthians 5:21)
- you are holy and blameless before God (Ephesians 1:4)
- you are blessed with every spiritual blessing (Ephesians 1:3)

Once you truly start to believe what God says about you, then you will have victory in the soul (mind, will and emotions) and be set free living in the love, joy and peace God provides. That leaves the physical body, which is the temple of the Holy Spirit. We will receive a glorified body when we get to heaven. Perfect in every way and no longer susceptible to sickness or pain. But now presently our bodies fall under the natural laws which include sowing and reaping, and the wisdom and knowledge given in God's word (the Bible) that made the natural laws. Most importantly when it comes to our body these natural laws determine if we will live in total physical health or if we will slip into a progression of apparent health, subclinical symptoms, clinical symptoms and finally disease.

Sowing and reaping is a law whether we believe it or not. If we plant corn we will harvest corn every time. If I put live, raw, uncooked vitamin, mineral, enzymes, bioenergetic and phytochemically rich food in my body I will reap total physical health according to Genesis 1:29. If I sow dead, cooked, enzyme-absent, vitamin mineral deficient chemical and toxin-laden food I will eventually reap sickness, disease and early death. Many people think they can put whatever they want in their bodies and it will work fine. This is not so because it defies the natural law of sowing and reaping and also defies the word of God which says in 1 Corinthians 6:19, "Your body is the temple of the Holy Spirit - honor God with your body.

If you put regular gasoline in a high performance race car it would not run properly and neither will you with an average American diet. There are far too many people who spiritually are mature and who rest in God but who give no regard to what they eat or how much they exercise. They assume because they have such a wonderful relationship with the Lord that he will take care of the rest. I am not saying that at times he won't intervene and supernaturally override the natural laws because He will, but that is the exception rather than the rule. This is why I believe so many people die prematurely. To die in pain, suffering with cancer or to drop dead prematurely of a heart attack is not the way God intended us to depart this world and enter eternity with Him, but rather to live a full abundant life and the end of that life to fall asleep and enter his presence. This is how Moses died after 120 years, which should be our lifespan according to Genesis 6:3. Maybe not everyone will live to be 120 but I think we all should fulfill our purpose in life and know its time to go home because our work is done. This is how I believe every child of God should depart this world who walks in *total health=wholeness.*

I've talked about natural laws and the spiritual laws now I want to mention when one law supersedes another. A great example of this in the natural world is the law of aerodynamics. In this law, the law of gravity is superseded and a piece of steel weighing many tons called an airplane can fly: this is because one law overrides another for that point in time. As long as the engine is on and the plane is operating properly. The thrust and lift of the plane cause it to fly despite the constant gravity trying to pull it to the ground.

Another example of one law superseding another is when the spiritual law supersedes the natural law. This was seen when Joshua prayed that the sun would not go down before the battle was won and it stood still (Joshua 10:12-14). This can also be seen when the spiritual law supersedes the law of sowing and reaping. This can be seen when a person develops terminal cancer and by the power of prayer the natural law is reversed and the person is totally healed. This is a miracle and it comes from God. As wonderful as miracles are they are not predictable and it is better that we walk in the wisdom of God and take care of the temple of the Holy Spirit (our body) rather than waiting to become sick and then pray that God will heal us. It is far better to walk in the wisdom, knowledge and blessings of God than in the miracles of God when it comes to our physical health.

How should I apply the natural and spiritual laws to my life? First use the wisdom of the Bible to live by. Genesis 1:29 (a diet of raw fruits and vegetables, especially green foods) was the way mankind was meant to eat. The farther we deviate from this, the greater the likelihood of developing disease. This is the plain and simple truth. To this we add 30 minutes to one hour of vigorous exercise everyday. The reason exercise isn't mentioned much in the Bible is because it was assumed that when men worked the ground in farming and tending animals as most did before modern technology that they would get more that enough exercise. Today with all of our modern conveniences there are many who get absolutely no cardiovascular exercise at all in their lives. This has to be changed if we are to walk and live in *total health* = *wholeness*.

Second, after entering into a personal relationship with the Living God by asking Him into our heart, we can communicate daily with the Holy Spirit of God, who is the Spirit of all wisdom and revelation. No matter what challenge we face in our lives—whether it be a physical one of facing disease or a mental one of dealing with stress, fear, depression or despair or even a financial one trying to meet the needs of your family and keep a roof over your head and food or the table—the Holy Spirit has the answer. If we talk to Him and patiently take the time to listen and listen and keep on listening to Him, He will speak to our hearts and confirm His spoken word with either His written word (the Bible) or through others who have sought Him in prayer and confirm the words He has spoken to you. He may even confirm what He has spoken to you by placing it on the hearts of others to tell you something which just happens to be the same thing He has spoken to your heart, but neither one of you knew what the other was thinking or praying about. This is also a powerful and supernatural confirmation from God. When seeking the wisdom of the Holy Spirit on any issue in your life, some observations I have seen should be considered:

1. The Holy Spirit almost always speaks to your heart first about something you're praying about, then confirms it through others. Not the reverse.

2. Always have at least your husband or wife hearing the same word from the Holy Spirit and preferably have the whole family pray on all issues and make sure all are in agreement. The Holy Spirit will confirm the same word to all who seek Him. In our family when we bring up an issue or question we all ask the Holy Spirit to speak to us about the answer or action to be taken then we come together and ask each other "what did the Holy Spirit tell you?" If we are all in agreement then we do as He has instructed us. For those of you who are single you need to get together regularly with a small group of people (two or three) who have trained their spiritual ears to hear the voice of the Holy Spirit and try together to seek confirmation from the Spirit. If these are personal matters I suggest they be family or the closest friends that one feels comfortable in confiding in.

3. The Holy Spirit always brings peace in the heart when He speaks to your heart. This does not mean that it is always an easy decision or that it always makes total sense in your mind because it sometimes is not the case. Remember God's ways are not always your ways,His thoughts are not always your thoughts. Many times He has to stretch your mind by giving you peace in your heart first, then as you step out in faith trusting Him and His word, you start to see Him move supernaturally in your life. You will begin to live and walk more and more in the Spirit (speaking to your heart) than the flesh (trusting in your own self and own mind). When God told Abraham to sacrifice Isaac, his son who all the blessing and promises would flow through, it made absolutely no sense in his mind, but in his heart he knew that what God had spoken about his descendants would be fulfilled so he had peace in his heart as he faithfully obeyed the Lord, even though his mind was in turmoil. So remember: the Holy Spirit brings love, joy and peace in your heart. This is how you will know it is him who is talking to you.

4. Keep in constant communion/communication with Him, always talking to Him and taking the time to listen to His response. Allow for course corrections. Don't just hear His voice one time on an issue and take action. Regularly seek Him up to the time a decision has to be made to make sure the path you are choosing is really where He

wants you to be. God's ways are not our ways so sometimes He might have you choose a very unlikely course which makes no sense in your mind but there are things He wants to show and teach you as you mature spiritually in Him, always giving Him the glory, honor and praise for His strength to see the course to the end.

Let us use this decision making process of seeking the wisdom of the Holy Spirit, and the knowledge of the spiritual and natural laws in a real life situation like terminal cancer. *(See chart on page 139)*

Condition: Terminal Cancer

SL- Law of the spirit of life SD- Law of sin and death SR- Law of sowing and reaping.

SR - Ate average American diet along with getting little exercise which led to declining health, eventual sickness.

SD-1. Spirit
Separate from God because of Adam's original sin and have never accepted God's one and only provision, His son Jesus "I am the way the truth and the life, no one comes to the Father accept through me." (John 14:6)

2. Mind, Will, Emotion and Soul
Without the Spirit of God living in him to renew and reprogram his mind and fill his heart with the emotions of love, joy, and peace, he is very stressed which all contributes to a weakened immune system and the onset of cancer.

3. Body
His body, like everyone else's, is in a process of aging or decline. This cannot be stopped but can be slowed if the SR is properly applied in accordance with Genesis 1:29 along with daily exercise.

SL-Can supersede both the physical part of SD and SR.
This comes not from anything you do but rather from Him who created you. So if sickness knocks at the door, use the following checklist:

1. Is Jesus my Lord and Savior? If not, ask Him into your life not only will you experience His love, joy and peace here but you will for eternity.
2. Seek the Holy Spirit of God who lives inside you to see what is course of action you should take to rid yourself of this sickness:
   a) Undergo standard medical treatment
   b) Make major diet and lifestyle change along with other natural healing methods and natural detoxification programs
   c) The need to address issues of forgiveness, fear, guilt, self-criticism, resentment
   d) Know your purpose in life—your mission statement
   e) The need for demonic deliverance (rare but can cause disease)
   f) Trust in God for a divine miracle of healing
3. Continue to seek Him daily to see if there is any change of plan

He will speak to you with one or a combination of these and will rid you of your disease. But remember, don't make your decisions just in the mind, but let the Holy Spirit speak to your heart, which will bring peace with the decision. Also get confirmation from your spouse and other loved ones or close friend who hears the voice of the Holy Spirit.

To live and walk in wholeness of spirit as Jesus wants us to, ten revelations are needed:

1. Repent
2. Be baptized
3. Be led by the Holy Spirit
4. Live by faith not by fear
5. Live in hope not hopelessness
6. Live by grace not by law
7. Live in freedom not bondage
8. Live and walk in the Spirit and not in the flesh
9. Live in love, being God-centered not self-centered
10. Give what you have received

1. Repent

This word simply means to change one's mind or to change how you see or view life or its many facets. The church equates *repent* with confession of sin; that is not a complete definition. God repented in the Bible, which is to say He changed His mind (Gen 6:6-7) most commonly because of His

God's Way versus Our Way

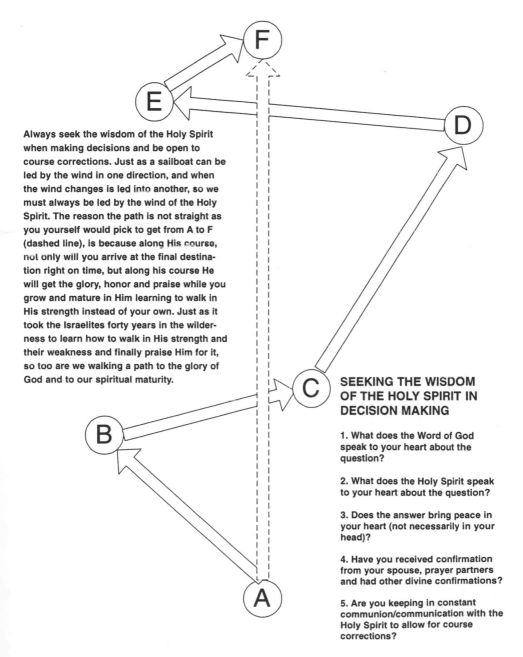

Always seek the wisdom of the Holy Spirit when making decisions and be open to course corrections. Just as a sailboat can be led by the wind in one direction, and when the wind changes is led into another, so we must always be led by the wind of the Holy Spirit. The reason the path is not straight as you yourself would pick to get from A to F (dashed line), is because along His course, not only will you arrive at the final destination right on time, but along his course He will get the glory, honor and praise while you grow and mature in Him learning to walk in His strength instead of your own. Just as it took the Israelites forty years in the wilderness to learn how to walk in His strength and their weakness and finally praise Him for it, so too are we walking a path to the glory of God and to our spiritual maturity.

SEEKING THE WISDOM OF THE HOLY SPIRIT IN DECISION MAKING

1. What does the Word of God speak to your heart about the question?

2. What does the Holy Spirit speak to your heart about the question?

3. Does the answer bring peace in your heart (not necessarily in your head)?

4. Have you received confirmation from your spouse, prayer partners and had other divine confirmations?

5. Are you keeping in constant communion/communication with the Holy Spirit to allow for course corrections?

peoples' prayers to Him (Gen 18:24-33.) To repent in today's world is just to have a mind open enough to be able to change a fixed or stagnant way you have always seen something. This applies to all areas of our lives. In healing sickness, I try to open peoples' minds up to change their views on diet, nutrition and the cause and prevention of disease. If we are open minded or if we have the mind of a child (which is not fixed or stagnant), we will always be growing, learning, maturing. The same holds true in the spiritual realm. God sent His Son, Jesus, to this world not to condemn it, but to save it. In the most awesome display of grace, God made the way so that all could come to Him and live in oneness with Him on this earth, and then live for eternity with Him in Heaven. How is this achieved? For it is by grace you have been saved through faith, this not of yourselves; it is a gift of God not by works so that no one can boast. (Ephesians 2:8-9.) Grace means a gift. How do we receive eternal life and all the blessings of being called one of His children? Simply by faith receiving the free gift given to you. To come to know Jesus as your Lord and Savior is to simply receive the free gift God has given you in His Son. Like all gifts, they cannot be earned; they are a gift. At your birthday party you receive gifts not because you earned or deserved them, but simply because those who love you want to show you by giving you gifts. Religion calls for work to make oneself worthy of God or to come into a right standing. Relationship says, "Come as you are. God's love accepts you just the way you are, no matter how broken, messed up or bad you have been or presently are." The only prerequisite to entering into His family for all eternity is that you change your mind on how you see life. Know that you cannot live this life apart from Him and that without Him you can never be free. We were all sinners who couldn't help or save ourselves until Jesus came and died for all of us and wrote on your account, "paid in full." He wrote a check to clear your account and signed it in His blood. The wonderful thing about this is that no sins past, present or future would be held to your account because "as far as the east is from the west, is as far as He has separated sin from you." Also "God made Him who had no sin to be sin for you so that you might become the righteousness of God." (2 Corinthians 5:21.) So open your mind and heart to Jesus, the one who saved you from your sin and gives to all who come to Him by professing with their mouth and heart, "Jesus is my Lord and my Savior" the gift of eternal life. This means not only to be with Him for eternity and live in heaven, but also to walk empowered by Him and His Holy Spirit on this earth.

2. Be baptized.

The physical act of baptism truly means that when you are submerged, the old nature—the part of you that lived independently of God— died and the new you that comes out of the water is the you that is Christ-centered with His Spirit placed in your heart. Baptism is a public profession of your faith in Jesus Christ as your Lord (King) and Savior (saved you from you sins). It is a public burial of the old you, the you who lived in your own strength and ability, and a public announcement of your new birth as a new person, now living and walking in God's strength, ability and wisdom. The meaning of baptism is that God's Spirit now lives in you to lead you, guide you, empower you, teach you and comfort you. No longer will you ever be alone, for the God who created you has now come to live in your heart. And where He is, there is love, joy and peace to fill every part of you.

3. Be led by the Holy Spirit.

After you have asked Jesus into your life and your heart, His Holy Spirit comes and takes up residence inside you. There is no greater or more awesome event than knowing the God who created the heavens and the earth, who creates all and sustains all, who created and sustains you, lives inside you. He comes as one to guide you, teach you, to empower you, to strengthen you, to comfort you, to help you in every circumstance of life, and to love you. This is the mark of a believer. God said that He would place His seal of ownership upon us by putting His Spirit in our hearts. To be led by the Spirit means in all circumstances of life you have God Almighty with you to help you through it, and not some far-off distant God, but one who lives inside of you who loves you so much that He meets your every need. Sometimes these needs are not met when you think they should be, but in His wisdom as He sees the whole picture of your life, rather than just seeing an immediate need as you perceive it. He said He would never leave or forsake us (Hebrews 13:5), and that we should cast our cares upon Him because He cares for us (1 Peter 5:7). Remember no matter how bad things appear, He is with you giving you the strength to go on and in it all you will give Him glory for the victories of life as you grow and mature in Him.

4. Live by faith not by fear.

Always remember it's God who made you and it's God who sustains you. Living by faith is simply living by the truth God has revealed in His written word, and the truth He reveals as He speaks by His Spirit into our hearts. Life is filled with decisions, and the greatest decision to make after one has decided to ask Jesus into their heart is to live trusting Him by faith rather to live trusting the world by fear. When you lose your job or you find out you have cancer or your spouse leaves you, your foundation is rocked, but if that foundation is set on the rock of the Living God and faith in Him and His Word, His Spirit who lives inside of you will truly be unshaken. The best way I can describe this is if in all these despairing situations of life Jesus were to physically appear to you and say, "Don't worry, I am with you and will lead you through all of this," you would totally relax because the Lord of Lords told you so and you physically saw and heard Him. Jesus did physically appear 2,000 years ago and did say He would never leave or forsake His brothers and sisters. Even to the ends of the world He would always be with us and so that we would always know, He said He would place His Spirit in us so that the peace He brings would always be there for us. Faith is simply taking God at His Word, where fear is believing the world or what men say above what God says. The choice is yours, but remember He lives in you and the faith you have is His faith (Galatians 2:20 KJV). So when you feel you're jumping off a mountain, you are really just jumping into His arms of love.

5. Live in hope not hopelessness.

God's hope is not like the world's hope which says, "Maybe it will happen or there is the possibility it could happen." God's hope is linked to God's faith. Hope is a sure thing. The only difference is the time period before the sure thing manifests. Faith is now — right now I trust God for my finances, my health, my family's well being. Hope is tied to the new covenant which says it is yours, all the promises are yes and amen in Christ Jesus. Hope takes now faith and adds a time period before it is fulfilled. Hope is a sure thing. Abraham trusted in God and became a father at an age of 100. "Against all hope, Abraham in hope believed and so became the father of many nations" (Romans 4:18).

Hope says, "God said it, I believe it and I will wait on His timing for it to be fulfilled." Hope is ultimately linked to the Holy Spirit who speaks to our hearts today, right now. If it is a fact that you have one million dollars buried in your back yard, hope is the patience and endurance linked with faith to see the promise to fulfillment. The Holy Spirit will guide you so you can stay on course to the final destination, the fulfilled promise. Not only does hope allow you to keep digging for the treasure, the Holy Spirit speaks to your heart, and guides you so you don't have to dig for your entire lifetime. The world's idea of hope is very much an uncertainty, whereas God's hope is an absolute truth that you can live by and He will never let you down. He loves you more than anyone ever could because He made you His very precious child.

6. Live by grace not law.

As previously stated, grace is God's gift to you; never earned or deserved, just received by faith. It is by grace that we enter into a personal, intimate relationship with our Heavenly Father, through His Son, Jesus Christ. It is also by grace that we continue to live in that relationship. Grace means God loves you no matter what you do because you're His child. In an earthly way you who are parents love your children not because they are perfect or because they always do or say the right things, but because they are your children. Nothing can ever separate us from the love of God. Grace simply means YOU ARE FREE TO FAIL AND GOD WILL LOVE YOU ANYWAY. You don't have to keep a list of rules for Him to love you. It does not matter what you do, because His love is not dependent upon you, but upon Him. When I was married I didn't receive the 500 commandments of marriage because if I would have I would have tried to keep them in my own strength and eventually would have failed. But instead, I loved my wife. So out of my love, I naturally keep any commandments because I want to, not because I have to. Jesus came with two new commands which entail the hundreds of old testament commands by simply saying first, "Love the Lord your God with all your heart, and with all your soul, and with all your mind, and with all your strength." And secondly, "Love your neighbor as yourself" (Mark 12:30-31). Remember, grace gives you the freedom to fail, but also gives you the freedom to succeed.

7. Live in freedom not bondage.

This is intimately linked to the grace of God. When Jesus set you free from your sins you have the free will to continue in it or turn from it. If you continue in it, God loves you no less; it just grieves Him to see his precious child living a life so much less than he or she is capable of. When you turn from it in His strength you experience true freedom and prosperity in everything you do. Prosperity means living in the ever presence of God and being blessed in all you do. An example of this is Joseph in the Bible. His life wasn't always perfect but he prospered in whatever he did. When he was a slave in Potiphar's house he became the head slave; when he was imprisoned he became the head of the prison and then eventually the second most powerful man in the world. This was about 17 years after he had the dreams of his brothers and father bowing down before him. It didn't happen over night, but God's promises are always fulfilled. To live in freedom is to know deep in your heart that you are accepted and approved by God because of Him and you always will be whether you stumble through life or run a victorious race to the finish line. He always loves and accepts you.

8. *Live and walk in the Spirit and not in the flesh.*

This means we are in the process (after receiving Jesus into our hearts, which is the salvation of our spirit, knowing we have a personal relationship with Him and will be with Him for eternity), of getting our minds renewed for the salvation of our soul (mind, will and emotions). When we ask Jesus into our lives to take over, we receive a new born-again alive spirit that communes with God, but we do not instantly receive a new perfect born-again mind or body. This is why we can say we are saved, we are being saved, and we will be saved; pertaining to spirit, then soul, then body. So in this life we renew our minds to Him and how He sees us, as we believe what He says about us instead of what the world or other people say about us. We start to live more in the Spirit's wisdom being led, guided and empowered more and more by the Holy Spirit who lives inside us and less and less in our own abilities and strengths, and knowledge. As we live more in the ever-presence and light of God, the flesh (which is the cravings of our body, and mind, and the self-centered ability) has less and less a place in our life. To walk in the Spirit is to walk, more and more, by His faith, His hope, and His love and less and less in our fears, our uncertainties and our self centeredness. As we walk more and more in the Spirit and less and less in the flesh, the faith of the Spirit becomes more evident in one's life. Love, joy and peace prevail more and more in every part of this person because he rests in the God who created and sustains him, as a baby rests in the loving arms of his mother. To walk in the Spirit is a lifetime of spiritual growth and learning to give more and more control of your life over to God. As you do this you will rest more and more in His love and peace, experiencing joy in all that you do because you will know you have or will have the victory over everything in His strength. Remember, you are *more than a conqueror* when you walk in His strength.

9. Live in love being God-centered not self-centered.

What is love? Is it a feeling or emotion? No, love is what Jesus did at the cross. He loved us and His father so much that He laid down His life for us. Love is defined as self-sacrifice. Love is the opposite of selfishness or self-centeredness. Love thinks of others before thinking of one's self. Love gives out of joy, not out of commitment. Love is the supreme act of this life because God is love and anyone who lives in love, lives in God. It is very important not to love in the flesh but in the Spirit. What this means is that if I love you in my own ability or strength, no matter how noble a task it might be, it will fail because God is love; I am not. True love flows from the Spirit that lives inside of us. True God's kind of love loves the unlovable, or enables one to love when it is hard to love because God's love in God's Spirit flows from you to touch another human being. I believe the reason there is over a 60 percent divorce rate in America is because so many are living a life in the flesh, being self-centered and experiencing only emotional love, instead of living in the Spirit, in the ever presence of God and letting that Spirit of love flow and touch whoever He has called us to love — in His strength, not ours. This God kind of love never fails. Our human, emotional love will always fail, but when husband and wife live in this love the two truly become one being bound by the Spirit of love.

10. Give what you have received.

Once you walk in the ever presence of God and in His love, your needs will all be met. You will cease your striving to get what He has already given you — His love, His joy, His peace, His rest. Once your needs are met in Him, you can freely give what you have freely received. It is the Dead Sea Principle. The Dead Sea died because water flowed in but none flowed out. We are to be a constant flow of His love and His light to a dead and dying world. Jesus said inside of His believers there would flow streams of living water. This was the constant flow of love that would fill every part of our being and flow out into the lives of those around us. As this love and life flows out of us, His Spirit fills us constantly so His Spirit can always be poured out to touch everyone He has brought into our path. There is no greater joy in life than to experience an intimate daily personal relationship with the God who created us, and also to live and walk in the strength of His Spirit and change the lives of those who surround us. As Jesus said, the greatest two commandments are:

1. To love the Lord, your God with all your heart, soul, mind and strength.
2. To love your neighbor as yourself.

If you experience these in the strength of His Spirit and not in your own ability, you truly will rest in him.

I will finish this chapter by saying this: Every man, woman and child has a spirit created in God's image — a spirit that has moral conscience, intuitive knowledge, and tries to keep you whole in body, soul and spirit. But the communion-with-God part of your human spirit is dead, separated from God by your sin. Once Jesus comes into your life and you turn everything over to Him, that part of your spirit becomes alive and in communion and communication with God. And if that wasn't enough, God actually comes to live inside you in the Holy Spirit.

The possibilities in your life are unlimited with God living in you. The ability to know the will of God for your life comes as easily as asking and listening to His voice inside you for the answer — the answer to every question, problem, or concern you will ever have.

Thank you, Father, for sending your Son. Thank you, Jesus, for sending your Spirit. Thank you, Holy Spirit, for living in us.

CHAPTER 10

MENTAL HEALTH

The mental health part of our wholeness involves the soul, which is a combination of our mind, emotions and will. This is the pivotal point of our entire wholeness because our will chooses if we live and walk empowered by the Spirit, (which is the key to total health of spirit, mind and body) or if we live in the flesh of the natural man, living in the cravings of the mind and body, never being fulfilled, never being touched by God's love, never experiencing God's joy or God's peace. The choice is ours and the choice comes from our will.

The Mind

The mind consists of thoughts, reasoning, and intelligence. It is where all information is processed before decisions are made. Some say the mind is divided into two parts — our conscious mind and our subconscious mind. Our conscious mind is what we are aware of — information coming in from our eyes, ears, nose, taste, and touch. The subconscious mind, meanwhile, continually processes information we are not aware of.

Another view, supported by Pastor Paul Yongi Cho, says the subconscious mind is actually the spirit of the person. With this view, the subconscious mind flows with our observations in the previous chapter on the spirit's functions of 1) moral conscience, 2) intuitive knowledge, 3) maintaining wholeness, and 4) communion with God.

In this discussion, we will concentrate on the "knowing" conscious mind, where we process information in making decisions, thinking, and remembering. Most of our life is spent in the "mind realm" of the soul. Unfortunately, since the fall of Adam, man has made himself his own god, and in doing this, his mind has become an avenue to get what he wants out of life.

Usually, the ones who were smarter in school went on to be doctors, lawyers, and businessmen, while those with less intelligence often ended up with more labor-intensive blue-collar jobs. Our soul equates intelligence with success. Therefore, people try to achieve all they can with their minds. The thinking goes, *I can have all I want, or be all I want to be, if I only put my mind to it.* This thinking isn't entirely wrong, for the Bible says in Proverbs 23:7, "As a man thinks in his heart, so is he." But this is much more than just positive thinking. This is taking what is in the spirit and bringing it into the soul or mind realm. (I will discuss this more later.)

The problem with man's dependence on his mind is that he thinks he can do anything in his own strength. This is quite the opposite of Scripture, which says, "I can do all things *through Christ* who strengthens me" (Philippians 4:13.) The difference between the power of positive thinking and the power of the Holy Spirit in us is unfathomable. One can lead to an atheistic or no-need-for-God mindset, whereas the other means total dependence on the God who created us. Paul said, "I know nothing... except Christ crucified" (1 Corinthians 2:2.) Paul said he didn't come "with eloquent words or persuasive speech, but with a demonstration of the Spirit's power" (1 Corinthians 2:4.)

The creative mind is really not the mind at all, but the spirit of man made in God's image. As we have seen, one component of the spirit is intuitive knowledge, and creativity is born out of intuitive knowledge. This is true not only of a man who is saved (by asking Jesus into his heart and professing Christ as Lord and Savior), but also of the unsaved man who has never trusted in Jesus as Lord and Savior. Why? Because all men — even unregenerate men — are created in God's image in His Spirit. Just as God is a creative God, man is a creative spirit.

Another problem with our mind is when we relive the past, playing reruns of how we were abused, hurt, rejected and alone. Scripture addresses this too: "Therefore, if anyone is in Christ, he is a new creation; the old is gone, the new has come!"

(1 Corinthians 5:17) Paul said "the old is gone" — all the negative, painful hurt of the past is gone when the Living God comes into your life and His Spirit dwells in your heart.

Many people have told me that after they accepted Jesus Christ as their Lord and Savior, they still struggled with old bad habits, thoughts and feelings. They condemned themselves after reading this verse, thinking, *What kind of Christian am I if I continue to think these thoughts and have these feelings?* Romans 12:2 gives the answer: "Do not be conformed to the pattern of this world, but be transformed by the renewing of your minds." How do you renew your mind? Simple. You start reprogramming your memory banks to the facts: You are a loved, blessed, chosen child of God, because He is inside you. You need to erase those recordings that said you were a failure, a nothing. All the old hurt and pain must be erased and

reprogrammed with what is now in your spirit — which is the
of perfect knowledge and wisdom.

We are how we see ourselves. If we see ourselves as a failure, surely we
will fail. If we see ourselves as a success, chances are good we will succeed. But if we know Jesus personally and his Holy Spirit dwells in our
hearts, then we will see ourselves as we truly are. We will see ourselves as
God sees us — "unblameable, unreproveable" (Colossians 1:22), perfect
sons and daughters of God. If our Father in Heaven sees us this way, what
difference does it make what anyone else thinks or says about us? A gold-
en nugget to live by is, ***Don't live in the "if only" past or the "what if"
future, but live in the "what is" present.*** "What is" is what God our Father
says about us in His word. Remember when God spoke to Moses? God
didn't say His name was "I was" or "I will be," but the ever present "I AM"
(Exodus 3:14). He was saying, "I AM the answer to all your problems and
questions in life."

How can one break free from a past that binds them? The Word says,
"He who the Son sets free is free indeed" (John 8:36). You see this in an
animal that have been caged up its whole life. When you open the door, the
animal acts as if it's not even open. It has been programmed to become
used to confinement. Even when the door is opened, it doesn't realize it has
been set free. Thanks to Jesus, we never have to live in the bondage of the
past again.

Turning your life over to the Living God gives you the power to forgive
those who hurt you in some way — and really mean it. Forgiveness heals
the pain of the past so it cannot have a hold on us. God chose to forget our
sins; He also commands us to forgive: "If you do not forgive, then neither
will my Father forgive you" (Matthew 6:15.)

God loves us, and our sins were forgiven the second we asked Jesus into
our lives. But if we don't forgive those who have wronged us, we will
become bitter, hard-hearted, angry people who cannot feel God's love and
forgiveness. This anger and bitterness can actually cause all kinds of diseases, including cancer, and can also make our quality of life very poor.
Jesus said, "Freely you have received, now freely give" (Matthew 10:8.)
We are forgiven and blessed children of God. We need to also freely forgive to continue to operate in wholeness.

We also need to be led by and listen to the Holy Spirit. If there is any
reason to go into the past — and I think it would be rare — let the Holy
Spirit bring it to your attention at His timing, not yours or a counselor's.

The God who made you knows how to sustain you. He knows what you need before you need it. And He loves you more than you could imagine, because He is love. If God loves you that completely, then He will lead you down a path of wholeness if you will just listen to His infinite wisdom. This is the key to success in all great men and women of God. They hear His voice and do what He tells them to do. Remember, God is always on time, never early and never late. His timing is perfect. So ask the Holy Spirit if there is something in your past that needs to be addressed; most of the time it will be nothing but forgiving those that hurt you. He will tell you if you listen. He will also confirm it through the Word, through other people or events.

One last note on hearing the voice of the Holy Spirit: He is a Spirit of love and not condemnation. "Therefore, there is now NO condemnation for those who are in Christ Jesus" (Romans 8:1.) One thing the Spirit does is speak to our hearts about righteousness, which we always are when we are in Christ. The Spirit does not speak to our hearts about unrighteousness. So if you hear a voice that is condemning you or pointing out your unrighteousness, it is from the Evil One. Rebuke it.

One last comment on the past: Since we are new creations and the old is gone, the "old you" died when you gave your life to Jesus. You are now a new creation. And being new, the only reason to look to the past is to recount past victories in Christ. I like to keep a prayer journal, and when the prayer is answered, I highlight it and date it. That way, whenever I think God doesn't hear me or isn't helping me, or if I get a little down, I just flip through my prayer journal to see "what a faithful God have I, faithful in every way." I won't stay down for long. As Paul said, "Forgetting what is past ... I press on to the mark for which I was called — the prize" (Philippians 3:13.)

Another problem with the mind is living in the future. As I've stated, this is living in the "what if" instead of the "what is." Now, it's not wrong to dream and have goals and desires for your future. This is fine, but we don't live there. If you ask anyone who has attained a very high goal, they will say the journey was as important as reaching the goal itself. Look at the Israelites, when Moses led them out of Egypt. Because of their unbelief, God made them wander in the wilderness for 40 years until two things happened: 1) the unbelieving generation died, and 2) the present generation knew nothing but to depend on God for their every need.

Once they knew deep in their hearts that God was their source and their shining light, there was nothing to fear. And 40 years later — after the report filled with fear of giants in the Promised Land — there was a different attitude, the same attitude that would be in David, the boy who killed a giant, Goliath. The Israelites learned in their journey that God was sovereign and their protector, and always will be. No matter what the odds were, it was OK, because God was on their side.

So, if they had wandered in the wilderness just thinking about the Promised Land, they would not have learned the lessons of depending on God for everything. And they would have died in the wilderness, just as the previous generation did. We cannot live in the future. We can dream of the future, but "this is the day that the Lord has made; let us rejoice and be glad in it" (Psalm 118:24). Let's rejoice in *today*, not the future. Also, remember that we know what our future holds if we love Jesus. Paul said it best: "For me to live is Christ and to die is gain" (Philippians 1:21.)

Our future is glorious — being filled with the light and glory of God where there is no darkness and His love consumes us in a way we cannot even imagine. Heaven is our future, and a wonderful one at that. But until it's our time to go home to be with God, we have a purpose, and we are to fulfill it right now in this place: To know God and give Him glory. What else could we do but give Him glory, when we know He got what He didn't deserve, and so did we. God got the sin of the world and didn't deserve it, and we got eternal life and didn't deserve it. **That is love. That is grace.** So dream dreams, but enjoy the journey, because your best friend is with you every step of the way.

Mind/Body

Medical science has physically proven the existence of your brain, but cannot prove you have a mind. Your brain automatically regulates your body without you even thinking about it. For example, breathing – you don't think about it but your brain and nervous system automatically control it. Another example is putting you hand on a hot coal, you automatically pull it away without thinking about it.

After spiritual health the next most important component of your total health = wholeness is your mental/emotional health or soul health. Your mind, although it cannot be proven, makes the difference in regaining health or succumbing to disease.

This mind aspect of curing disease can be seen when patients with illness are prescribed placebos, which are nothing, more than sugar pills and 30 percent of these patients report a cure or substantial improvement. The mind so powerfully affects the body that attitude might have more importance in healing than any medicine, chemical therapy or radiation therapy.

The example of how the mind affects the body can be seen analogous to the operating of a large company. Your brain will be called the General Manager (GM) who basically operates the company day in and day out and keeps everything running smoothly. Your mind can be called the Chief Executive Officer (CEO). Now although the GM operates the company very capably, the CEO can at anytime step in and intervene and change the operation to however he sees fit. He needs no approval from the GM. Can you see how an extremely talented CEO can add to the company whereas a poor CEO could financially ruin the company? This is true in life and in health. Your brain runs the show, but your mind can be a great asset or be a great detriment to your total health = wholeness. Remember, the brain automatically caused you to pull your hand off the hot coal, but there are people who can control their mind to hold the hot coal and not feel the pain. This is mind over brain and mind over body, and our minds might be a major factor in who gets sick and who gets well. So to combat disease, you need a healthy brain and a right attitude mind.

Where does the brain get its energy from? According to Dr. Roger Sperry, Nobel Prize recipient for brain research, "90 percent of the stimulation and nutrition to the brain is generated by the movement of the spine". This is similar to a windmill generating electricity. Dr. Sperry also found the more biomechanical faults (spinal misalignments) the less energy was available for thinking, healing and metabolizing. For this reason and also that 9 out of 10 people have these spinal misalignments and aren't even aware of it, everyone should have their spine examined and if necessary corrected by the spinal structural specialist – the chiropractic physician.

This will ensure maximum energy made available to the brain so it can perform its proper functions. This same energy also helps operate the mind and its many functions.

Chiropractic physicians have helped many people with symptoms of brain fog, depression, anxiety, attention deficit disorder and in improving these various mind related symptoms. Attitudes also improve as well as general health because spirit directly affects the mind and the mind directly affects the body and the total health of the body. How important is attitude to general health? It may be the single most important factor after spiritual health in making us live in, walk in and enjoy total health = wholeness. Charles Swindoll said it best, " the longer I live, the more I realize the impact of attitude on life. Attitude, to me, is more important than facts. It is more important than the past, than education, than money, than circumstances, than failures, than successes, than what other people think or say or do. It is more important than appearance, than giftedness or skill. It will make or break a company, a church, a home. The remarkable thing is we have a choice every day regarding the attitude we will embrace for that day. We cannot change the inevitable. The only thing we can do is play on the one string we have, and that is our attitude. I am convinced that life is 10 percent what happens to me and 90 percent how I react to it, and so it is with you....we are in charge of our attitudes."

Emotions

Emotions are our feelings, how we react to situations in life. Emotions can be broken down into two categories — beneficial and detrimental.

Beneficial emotions are those that our Lord Jesus had. Like sorrow and compassion, as He wept with Mary and Martha over Lazarus' death (before He raised Lazarus from the dead.) Like anger, as He turned over the moneychangers' tables for making God's house a marketplace. Like joy, as the little children came to Him. And like love, evidenced by everything He did.

Emotions are good when they are rooted in who we are in Christ, and in God's Word. Let me explain: Fear of the Lord is good, because what it means is a holy reverence for His awesomeness. But fear of anything else is spoken against: "The Lord did not give us a spirit of fear, but of love and of power and of a sound mind" (2 Timothy 1:7.) Instead of fear, God gave us LOVE, which is Himself. He gave us power, which is His Holy Spirit within us. And He gave us a sound mind — a mind that knows God is always with us, because we are His blessed children, and all that He has is ours.

So if an emotion flows from the love of God or the love of your neighbor, if an emotion flows from the Holy Spirit inside of you, or if an emotion flows from the sound mind that Jesus gives you, those are wonderful. But if emotions flow from anything but the truth, they are major stresses to our *total health = wholeness*. For example, if I told you that you just won the lottery, your reaction would be one of extreme happiness. But when you found out it wasn't true, you would again feel down, depressed, or angry. If I told a parent their child was just hit by a car and killed, immediately their heart would pound, tears would pour, and deep sorrow would overwhelm them — even if it wasn't true, just because they believed it.

The point I am trying to make is that emotions should only be a reflection of the truth, not of lies. So if people tell you you're no good, you shouldn't react with negative emotions, because you know you are perfect — unblameable and unreproveable — in God's eyes. Who are you going to believe, God or man? If someone says, "You'll never be able to do it," you don't have to feel inadequate or sad, because you know you can do "all things through Christ who gives you strength" (Philippians 4:13.) If you feel down because you lost your job, the higher truth is that according to His riches and glory, He will meet your needs (Philippians 4:19.) God said he would never leave you or forsake you (Deuteronomy 31:6). He knows what you need before you know, and how much more precious are you to Him than the lilies of the field and the birds of the air (Matthew 6:25-33.)

To summarize, if your emotions are based on the highest truth — God's Word — then they are beneficial to your *total health = wholeness*. But if they are based on situations, people, places, and things, they can be detrimental to your *total health = wholeness*.

The Will

The last part of the soul, and the most important, is the will. Your will is your choice. When God made you, He did not make you a robot, but a living spirit in a body with a free will to choose — right from wrong, to obey or disobey, to choose whatever direction you want your life to go in.

The will is like a switch, deciding whether we walk in the strength of the Spirit or in the strength of the flesh. Living in the flesh means you depend upon *your* ability, *your* strength, *your* discipline, *your* self — without God. Living in the Spirit is to live totally dependent on God — depending on *His* Word, *His* Holy Spirit, *His* power, *His* self control. These are fruits of the Spirit (Galatians 5:22-23.)

Picture the will as a fork in the road. One path — dependence on God — leads to abundant life, love, joy and peace. The other path — dependence on self — leads to a stressful roller-coaster life of ups and downs. Someone asked me, "How could a loving God send people to hell?" I responded by saying that people send themselves to hell. God made a way so that all could come to Him through His Son, Jesus Christ. Jesus said, "I am the way and the truth and the life. No one comes to the Father except by me" (John 14:6.)

Scripture says, "My people shall perish from lack of knowledge" (Hosea 4:6.) Scripture also says, "There is a way that seems right to a man, but in the end leads to death" (Proverbs 16:25.) God sent His only Son to die a terrible death, so you could go to heaven with the account stamped, "Paid in full, by the blood of Jesus." If you were offered the key to the door of life and you choose — by using your will — not to take it, don't blame God for your eternal separation from Him. You were given the choice, so choose wisely, because that choice is for eternity.

God gave us His Holy Spirit to guide us. He gave us His Word to instruct us. With these two, we have all we need to choose — via our will — the right path that God has laid out for us. But God is love, and He leaves the choice up to us. I say *CHOOSE LIFE*. Choose to walk according to the Spirit and not the flesh. Once you make that decision, God will back you 100 percent.

Your Mission In Life

Everyone of us has a reason, a mission, a purpose for which God created them. This is God's will for our life. When and if we come to that place in life when we discover God's will for us, we will soar higher than anyone else, because whatever specific task He has created us for no one else can do this quite like us. When we do it, we actually do it effortlessly, and with timelessness. Effortlessly because it is natural to us; it is what we were created for and when we are operating in the purpose we were designed for there is no effort, it just flows. Timelessness because when we are performing the call for which we were made, it is pure joy, not work. When you are having fun time flies as if there was no time. When we are doing the exact thing God created us for, we also live and walk supernaturally in each moment. God releases supernatural gifts that enable you to perform your call like no one else in the world can. Things become naturally right when you are living your purpose, events just happen to move you forward in your purpose: doors open, contacts are made, timing is right; these are not coincidences they are divine appointments.

Unfortunately, many never find what their true purpose is, they never align their will with God's will for them. They do not seek Him and wait to be directed by Him. Instead they get a job or enter into a lifestyle that seems right to their mind. They settle because of what the world or their natural (without God) mind says when God has so much more for them. They end up living an ordinary life, missing out on the blessing of living a supernaturally extraordinary life. How do you find out what God's will is? Take time in meditation and prayer to listen every day. He speaks if you are listening, but He speaks to the heart and not to the head. Sometimes what is in your heart seems crazy to your mind. Continue to seek Him; if it is from Him the love, joy and peace will grow in your heart. This then will give you strength to overcome your mind and step out of your comfort zone to God's greater blessings, living your purpose in life. Most all the great people in life that accomplished something to change the world, to further humanity in some way are those who DID discover their mission statement, their call, their purpose. It is then that the spirit, soul (mind, will and emotion) and body connect together in perfect balance and supernaturally the world is and can be changed like never before. God has placed this inside everyone of us, but so few of us take the quiet time in prayer and meditation to discover this gift God has given each one of us. Take the time and then begin to live the life you were created for.

Now, let's put them all together.

The flow of life is always from the spirit of man (filled with the Holy Spirit) to the soul (mind, will, and emotions) to the body. "The spirit gives life, the flesh counts for nothing. The words I have spoken to you are spirit and they are life." (John 6:63)

The two avenues affecting the will are:

1) SPIRIT renews the MIND and the MIND influences the WILL

From the Spirit, Soul and Body diagram from the Spiritual Health chapter (Page 131) the path is (1>2>6>7).

2) SPIRIT empowers the EMOTIONS and the EMOTIONS influence the WILL

From the Spirit, Soul and Body diagram from the Spiritual Health chapter the path is (1>2>8>7).

1) Our renewed mind is reprogrammed with what God says about us, instead of what people and the world say about us. This renewed mind is totally fixed on Jesus, the Author and Finisher of our faith, and His words. This renewed mind doesn't go into the past to see what we used to be or used to think, because that person is gone, dead, no longer existing. A new creation has taken his place with a live spirit that can commune with God. This renewed mind knows that God can never lie, and if God makes a promise to His children, He will deliver it. If He says you are perfect, holy, unblameable and unreproveable, then no matter how you see yourself, or how other people see you, you truly are as God says you are. All you have

to do is understand that it really is true. This comes by faith — not your faith, but the faith of the Son of God who lives in you in the Holy Spirit.

What is faith, anyway? It can be defined as our response to what God has done. If I tell you there's a million dollars buried in your backyard, you can respond to what I said, or you can reject it. If you really believe it, you'll start digging and won't stop, no matter how long it takes. This is where patience comes in, a gift of the Spirit. Abraham, through faith and patience, received God's promise. Patience says it's there because God said it's there, and I won't give up or stop until I get what God promised me.

So the renewed mind sees things the same way God sees them, not the way a man sees them. Once our mind is renewed to what God says about us, and about all things, then our will aligns with that new mind. Just as the man who believes a million dollars is buried in his backyard, if he really believes and knows it's true, then his will takes over and says, "I will never stop digging until I find it, no matter how long it takes." When this will is empowered by God's words about you, your will becomes supernatural, and even when you get weak — "I cannot dig anymore" — then God becomes your strength to go on. This gives God glory when you know "I can't do it in my ability or strength, but I did it with the Holy Spirit's power."

2) Our other situation is our emotions affecting our will. This is usually the wrong avenue to affect the will, because many emotions of the world and of man, without the Spirit, are based on how we perceive situations instead of on the truth. Our example of someone accidentally telling the wrong mother that her child was hit by a car. This evokes all kinds of strong emotions, but all based on untruth. So we have to be very careful to not be led by feelings, but by the truth.

There are instances, though, that emotion can positively impact the will — if the emotion is brought on by God and truth. An example is when Jesus returned to Martha and Mary's house to find Lazarus dead. Scripture says Jesus was moved with compassion and raised Lazarus from the dead. Many other times, the Bible states that compassion moved Jesus to heal the sick and feed the hungry.

Can you see the difference between having our will moved by God and having our will moved by our own emotions?

Let me leave it by saying this: Smith Wigglesworth, a famous evangelist, once said, "GOD SAID IT, I BELIEVE IT, AND THAT SETTLES IT." Remember, all that we are in Christ Jesus is only ours if we believe it our-serves. If God says you are holy and perfect in His eyes, and you still see yourself as an imperfect person who still sins, then you will not live in the promise, "As a man thinks in his heart so is he."

Your heart is a combination of your spirit and soul. So it's not so much what you know or believe, as it is what truly is in your spirit — what God says about you. How can we know what God says? We can find it either in His written Word or through His spoken Word — the voice of the Holy Spirit inside us, who guides us into all truth.

The Apostle Paul says that we have the mind of Christ. We are to be made new, to put on the new self, to understand that we are created to be like God — righteous and holy. Mental/Emotional health is an outpouring of spiritual health. If Jesus is our Lord and Savior, then we have His Holy Spirit living inside us. And the fruit of the Spirit is love, joy, peace, patience, kindness, goodness, faithful, gentleness and self control (Galatians 5:22-23.)

So, to experience true mental health, we must let the Spirit of God fill us with His love, joy and peace. True health of the soul (mind, will and emotions) can never be attained outside of a personal relationship and communion will the Living God. That's the way He made us — to know God and give Him glory. Anything outside of that leads to emptiness and false love, false joy, false peace.

Many people believe that if they work hard enough and make enough money, they'll be happy. But it doesn't work. Some of the richest people in the world would say they're also the unhappiest, because they've found that true joy does not come from material riches. A bigger house, nicer car, better toys — none of it brings God's love and joy and peace.

Happiness comes and goes, depending on what's going on around you. If you get a promotion, you're happy. If you get fired, you're unhappy. If you get a good report from the doctor, you're happy. If you find out you're sick, you're unhappy, even fearful. When you marry the man or woman of your dreams, you're happy. When you find out they want a divorce, you're unhappy, maybe even suicidal; your life is broken. The point? You were never meant to look for happiness in a person, a place, or a thing.

Joy comes from the Spirit of God, and it never changes, no matter what happens. This kind of joy is empowered by the Spirit of God, who lives inside you when you know Jesus Christ as Lord and Savior. The Spirit is there through thick and thin, because God said, "I will never leave you nor forsake you" (Deuteronomy 31:6.) The Holy Spirit promises to comfort, guide, teach, help and empower you.

The Apostle Paul knew that his peace wasn't dependent on his circumstances. That's why he was filled with joy, singing songs of praise, while spending the night in a Philippian jail after being beaten nearly to the point of death. Despite his suffering, Paul sang and praised God. Why? Because joy is a fruit of the Spirit, which never leaves us. Paul knew the Spirit's joy.

Paul also knew the Spirit's power. Right after midnight, a supernatural earthquake shook the jail. All the cells opened. Paul then led the jailer to a personal relationship with Jesus Christ, and that very night, the jailer and his household all became believers.

How do you walk in the Spirit? By listening to and asking your Guide, the Holy Spirit, about everything you do. Walk in His strength, not your own; remember, when you are weak, He will be strong. This is glorifying to God. People notice things like this. It's not normal to sing praises to God when you're almost dead. This is supernatural. People will be curious. Tell them, "It's all the Living God, not me." And whether or not they believe in Jesus, they can't deny what has happened in your life.

I'd like to say one more thing about God living in us via the Holy Spirit. Some New Age religions say we are gods. But Christianity says God lives inside of us; we are not God, but He's always with us. New Age philosophy also says we can do anything we put our minds to. But Christianity says, "I can do all things through Christ who strengthens me" (Philippians 4:13.) It is not us, but Jesus that empowers us through His Spirit.

New Age thought says man is his own god and needs no other. Its teachings are all about self-improvement, that with your mind, all things are possible. But in Christianity one walks in weakness, depending on God's strength, wisdom and guidance.

On the surface, New Age religions and Christianity may seem to have some similarities, but really they are directly opposed to each other.

Remember: True mental/emotional health can only be attained when we *know* the Living God. The word "know" is used in the Bible for the most intimate of relationships. Adam "knew" his wife Eve, and she conceived a child. The Bible speaks of their relationship as "two becoming one" (Genesis 2:24.) God wants us to have the same kind of relationship with Him. To know Jesus is to have the most intimate relationship with God, and to give Him all the glory, honor, praise and recognition He deserves.

Then — and only then — will our mental/emotional health be whole.

Mind /Body medicine and therapy is on the rise as an important avenue to improve one's health. Many ask how can I help my mind to heal my body? The two most important things one can do in this regard are:

1) To have a personal relationship with the Living God and spend time each day in meditation and prayer, seeking His wisdom and revelation so you can live empowered by Him and His Spirit, which lives inside of you. This will impact your physical health more powerfully than any thing else you can do.

2) Next, take quiet time in prayer and meditation to discover your mission statement, your call, your purpose for which God created you because in that purpose you will find fulfillment.

Other steps that will help you decrease your mental/emotional stress thus help you more positively improve your total health = wholeness are:

1. TIME MANAGEMENT
2. ORGANIZATION
3. PERSONAL TIME EACH DAY
4. DON'T OVERCOMMIT
5. HAVE FUN
6. LAUGH
7. VISUAL IMAGERY/DREAM
8. JUST LET GO
9. PROPER DIET, EXERCISE AND DETOXIFICATION

1. TIME MANAGEMENT

Time is a precious commodity and it has wings to fly. We all have 24 hours in a day, so how we effectively use that time can either give us more time to spend with God, our spouse and family, or take away time so as to stress us and steal from all of these.

Two techniques that can be very helpful in managing or controlling time are:

1. A Schedule

Make one and stick to it. Do all similar activities at the same time. Let me give you and example. If a businessman is in his office starting to read through a contract and the phone rings, this interrupts him and takes his focus off his work. If his employees come in to ask him questions, again he is distracted, if he starts thinking of other things he has to get done once again another distraction. Now lets say this same person schedules a certain time for taking and making phone calls, a certain time for staff meetings and has a paper at his side at all times to jot down other things to get done, so he can keep his mind on his work. He will accomplish twice as much in his day.

2. Make A List Of The 7 Most Important Things To Get Done For The Day

Make a list of only seven things for that day and start with the most difficult or time intensive one first. When it is done your feeling of accomplishment will help you to breeze through the next six. Remember, no one remembers everything. If you don't write it down, don't expect it to get done!

2. ORGANIZATION

This goes along with time management. When everything is in the proper place, work becomes highly more time efficient. When time is both managed and organized, it frees up more time to be used wisely. An example of the importance of organization is if we had one million files in file cabinets that were just randomly put into the cabinets how long would it take to find the file we are looking for? Hours and hours of time would be wasted. Now if the files were filed alphabetically how long would it take to find a particular file? Maybe a couple of minutes. To be organized is to be time wise.

3. PERSONAL TIME EACH DAY

Besides having prayer/meditation quiet time each day which is vital to *total health = wholeness*, personal time is also important. Take at least 30 minutes each day for yourself. This can be used to listen to music, to knit, to exercise or just to taking a relaxing bath sipping some herbal tea. This time is best when it is uninterrupted and has no pressing time commitment following it. People who take time for themselves each day enjoy their days more because they always have something to look forward to.

4. DON'T OVERCOMMIT

Remember how precious time is. Keep your priorities in the proper order: Spiritual communication/communion (talking and listening to God) and family are always first. Then comes your personal quiet time, then your occupation, then extras. If you over commit things in your schedule, you invariably end up taking time away from the top priority commitments – Your relationship with God and your family. So before you commit to anything, pray on it and have your family pray on it with you. Make sure everyone is in agreement with the decisions. Do not major on the minors in life. Major on the majors, God and family.

5. HAVE FUN

Life is a journey, so enjoy it! If you're not, do something to change it so you are. I have told many people to quit their jobs because the stress would eventually cause them to develop major health challenges. What would you do if you knew you had only one year to live? What about one month? Or even only one day? You would live life to the full and enjoy every moment of it knowing it is all a gift from God. You would look at the sky, spend time enjoying the majestic sunrise and sunset, you would stop and smell the roses. Don't wait to be on the verge of death to start enjoying life, do it right now. There is no time better than the present. Have fun with your God, have fun with your spouse, have fun with your children, have fun with your work and remember how blessed you are to have them all.

6. LAUGH

Laughter is proven to increase your immune system response. It increases many glandular, hormonal and organ functions. It decreases stress, depression and anxiety. Norman Cousins wrote a book, *Anatomy of an Illness,* and in it he explained how he healed himself of a chronic degenerative disorder by watching comedies and laughing hours each day. Laughter is healthy and it's fun, so do it every day.

7. VISUAL IMAGERY/DREAM

This is a powerful tool in any mind/body treatment. The bible says, "as a man thinks in his heart so is he." This is visual imagery. It is seeing you and your body as totally healthy or whole all the way from your white blood cell (WBC) activity to your physical performance. Studies have shown if you see your WBC as Pac Man type cells, going around eating all the cancerous cells, this actually boosts your immunity and overall health. Another study took two groups of high school basketball players. One group spent an allotted amount of time each day practicing their free throw shot whereas the second group took the same amount of time to visualize their shots going into the basket without additional practice. The results showed a greater improvement in the visualizing group over the practicing group. See yourself in your mind managing your time, organized, having a lot of time extra time for your spiritual communication with God through meditation/prayer, for your spouse, your family and simply having fun. Visualize yourself doing the best at your work in the least amount of time. As you keep seeing yourself a certain way, this is the way you become.

8. JUST LET GO

In the course of my wife's healing, God gave her a very clear vision: she was holding on to a piece of baggage. He reached out His hand to grab hers, but before she could fully hold on to Him, she had to let go of the baggage she was carrying. The baggage represented all the things in life that we hold on to; some good, some not so good. Things like comfort, security, past hurts, anger, bitterness, unforgiveness. They were all in the baggage. In life, we have to just let go of the things that bind us or hold us back. Sometimes this includes leaving our comfort zone to be stretched to greater heights. We must let go of all the things that hurt us in the past; all the anger, frustration, bitterness, all of it. It does nothing but become a weight that we carry that prevents us from flying high above the clouds of life on "wings of eagles." In life, is it better to always be right, or to be at peace? How much effort and energy are you going to expend to prove you are right? Sometimes it's better to just let go and fly. You must pray to know when to hold on and when to let go, but I think a lot more people would live healthier, happier lives if they would learn to let go more and enjoy the moment. If you knew you only had one month to live, what things in your life would really matter? Money? A job? Always being right? All the annoyance and frustrations that present themselves to drain your joy and peace? I think not. If you knew you had one month to live, you would let go of everything except the highest priorities in your life:

1) God, and 2) Family.

You would start to see the preciousness and beauty of every day that God made and would take time to smell the roses, to see the sun rise and set. You would enjoy the blue sky and white clouds. You would begin to truly live. So I ask you: why do we wait until we know we are going to die before we start to really live? Let's live every day like it is our last. Let's spend some time in quiet meditation with God, being renewed and refreshed each and every day with revelations from Him. Let's enjoy our family, not trying always to be right, but always trying to live in love, joy, and peace. When we learn to let go, we can receive all that we truly desire.

9. PROPER DIET, EXERCISE AND DETOXIFICATION

This will be covered in detail in the chapters to come, but it is important to know you *are* what you eat and think. If I eat cooked, dead, devitalized low nutrient content or high sugar and fat content food, I will cause anything from brain fog or cloudiness, to hyperactivity, to attention problems to various other mental/emotional symptoms like depression, anxiety, gs, tenseness and nervousness. Also, improper diet and exercise ⎰ toxic build up from chemical residue in food can cause the brain ⸎⸎ ⸎ ⸎ oxygen and nutrients which definitely will negatively impact our mental/emotional health by decreasing the amount of energy available for thinking, healing and metabolizing.

How Your Dreams Become Reality

God made us creative spirits because He is a creative Spirit and we were made in His image. Every invention, every innovation, every thing that made this world what it is started as a desire, a dream. How do dreams come true? It starts with knowing that God gives us the desires of our hearts. This is awesome. If we use the process below our dreams can become reality. God made many laws both spiritual and physical that operate and govern the world. Spiritually, the law of sowing and reaping, the law of giving and receiving, the law of faith are a few. Physically, some of the laws include the law of gravity and the law of thermodynamics. What is a law? It means an expected outcome is always produced when the principles are applied. If we jump off a building we will always fall down to the ground. When we plant corn, corn will always grow. When God says He will give you the desires of your heart, He will. His word always is true and more constant than any law. Let us apply these principles to make your dreams become reality.

1) **Desire**

   Desire comes from deep in your heart. It is what you want and how much you want it that determines your desire.

2) **Envision**

   This is the process of painting the picture created with your desire on the canvass of your mind. This is seeing your desire already accomplished. Living as if it already was reality and enjoying it. Enjoying it means feeling the enjoyment in your heart as if it was already done. How would it feel if you really accomplished your dream? In this step you must see it, feel it and enjoy it no different than if it truly had already occurred. This is the enjoyment of the journey.

3) **Pray**

   In your quiet time before God you present your picture that you created before Him and seek His guidance to refine your picture, to show you the best path to complete the picture. This is crucial to the dream process because God knows all things and led by Him, you will open the right doors along your journey. Without His guidance and input, the dream process becomes hard work instead of great joy.

4) **Speak the Dream**

Speak out the dream as if it were already reality because not only does it strengthen your faith in it, but it also strengthens the faith of those around you who start to see the picture of your dream. Your words give strength to your desire.

5) **Know It**

You live and believe as if your dream has already occurred so much so that when it really does occur your reaction is "no big deal" because you already lived it, experienced it and enjoyed it. The journey was the excitement, the destination is anticlimactic, it just leads you to new desires and the creative process begins again.

CHAPTER 11

NUTRITIONAL HEALTH

The first step of our physical health of our ten steps of *total health = wholeness* is our nutritional health, or what we put into our body. This is part of our chemical health, or what goes in. Chemical health addresses all that goes in, good and bad, including nutrients and toxic chemicals and drugs. But here we are just addressing what we eat and drink to impact our *total health = wholeness.*

To be healthy, the body needs oxygen, water, and bioelectrically charged food that contains: 12 amino acids, 16 vitamins, 60 minerals, 3 fatty acids, complex carbohydrates, enzymes, antioxidants, phytochemicals. If a body takes in these nutrients daily it has all that it needs to grow, repair, and maintain itself. However, these items alone do not guarantee good health, because as you will see later, "getting the good in" is just part of our total physical health. We also need to get the bad out — the chemicals in our air, water and food that find their way into our bodies. We need to regularly remove them with periodic detoxification methods that we will discuss later.

In previous chapters, I have explained the problems with eating the wrong foods. To review: The healthiest diet is one that is vegetarian, completely excluding animal products and as close to 100% raw or living as possible. This is called a living food vegan diet and it is the most health-promoting, most anti-cancer, most anti-heart disease diet and always has been.

Why a Vegan Diet?

A vegan diet is a vegetarian diet exclusive of all animal products. No dairy, no butter, no cheese, no yogurt, no eggs—nothing from animals. Many people might say that they could never eat this way. I said the same once not to many years ago. What caused me to change? It was one (knowledge) of the two most common motivating factors that causes a person to change their diet. They are:

1. Because of knowledge—knowing that the chemicals, toxins, hormones, parasites, bacteria and cholesterol content will eventually destroy one's health.

2. Because of fear—this being once one has contracted either symptoms or the actual disease itself, and the desire not to be sick or die motivates one to change.

If you are driven by the first choice of knowledge, the desire to know and do what is best for your health both now and in the future, then some of the following facts will be important in your decision:

1. 50% of Americans presently die from cardiovascular disease. This drops to less than 4% with a vegan diet.[1]
2. Since 1978 the German Cancer Research Center in Heidleberg has shown that the immune system is twice as strong in a vegan as opposed to an animal product consumer.[2]
3. Nine out of 10 Americans (88%) will die from either cardiovascular disease or cancer and of this between 60-90% could be prevented with diet (vegan) and lifestyle changes.[3]
4. Dr. Harold Foster studied 200 cancer patients that were healed without any conventional medical treatment. The highest common denominator between them all was 87% of them changed their diet to vegan.[4]
5. In Dr. Dean Ornish's program for reversing coronary heart disease, along with daily exercise and relaxation techniques, a vegetarian diet was adopted to reduce coronary blockages as severe as 90% preventing these patients from needing bypass surgery.[5]
6. The University of Oslo and the National Hospital is Oslo, Norway found that arthritis pain was substantially reduced in patients who adopted a vegan diet. No pain reduction was seen when animal products were consumed.[6]
7. Countries with the highest consumption of meat and animal fat have the highest rate of breast cancer. In Thailand, the animal fat intake is $\frac{1}{10}$ that of the U.S. and breast cancer is $\frac{1}{20}$ the rate.[7]
8. The risk of dying of prostate cancer is 3.6 times higher in men who eat animal products versus those who are vegan.[8]
9. The risk of dying from ovarian cancer is three times higher in women who eat animal products versus those who are vegan.[9]
10. The average bone loss in meat eating women age 65 was 35%, whereas the vegan female age 65 was only 18%.[10]
11. Lessons from the animal kingdom. The animals that live the longest are vegan (tortoises). The animals that are the biggest and strongest (elephants) are vegan. Elephants do not drink milk and do not eat

meat, yet they are one of the strongest animals on the planet. They are never protein deficient or calcium deficient with their diet of leaves and grasses. Gorillas are three times the weight of a man and 30 times as strong. Not bad for a fruit and vegetable diet. So much for the myth that you have to eat meat to be strong. Triathalon athlete Dave Scott has won the Iron Man competition (the most physically demanding of all competitions) more than anyone else, and he

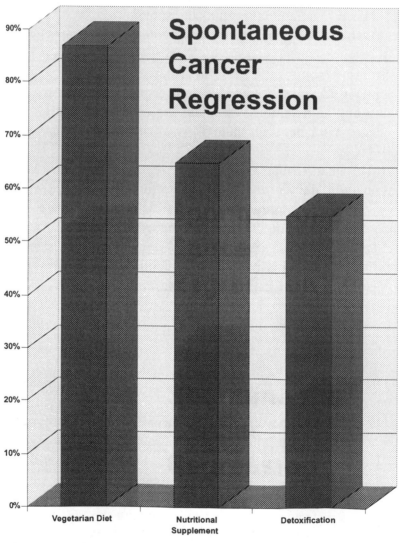

Source: Foster HD, Int J Biosocial Res, 10, 1, 17, 1988

is a vegetarian. The world bench press holder, Stan Price, is also a vegetarian.[11]

12.The length of the digestive tract in animals who eat vegan diets is 8-12 times the length of their torso. This allows for digestion and absorption of the nutrients from the plant material. The length of the digestive tract of meat eating carnivores is 3 times the length of the torso so as to move the quickly putrefying meat out of their system. Mans digestive tract is the length of a plant eater, not meat eater.

13. The saliva of meat eating carnivores is acidic to predigest proteins. The vegetable eating herbivores has alkaline saliva for carbohydrate digestion. Man has alkaline saliva.

14. One of the most convincing of all the facts was the China Project, which proved that the greatest cause of disease came from two diet sources: cholesterol and animal protein, not plant protein. The lowest incidence of disease was when these two were excluded from the diet. This is the vegan diet.

The China Project [12]

In 1983, a cooperative effort began among Cornell University, Oxford University, the Chinese Academy of Preventative Medicine and the Chinese Academy of Medical Sciences.

Answers were sought to why some men in one province in China died of esophageal cancer 435 times more often than men in another part, or why women in one part had breast cancer 20 times as often as women in another part. The reason China was picked was because many families tend to spend their whole lives in the same area eating the same locally grown food. So one can see how diet would affect health and disease.

Some facts related to the project were:

1. Only four in 100,000 males under 65 die of heart disease each year in China while 67 die in United States.

2. The American death rate for breast cancer is five times the rate in China.

Some of the conclusions from the project were:

• High blood cholesterol was consistently associated with many cancers

• Even small intakes of animal products were associated with a significant increases in chronic degenerative diseases

- The greater the plant food in the diet the less chance of getting these diseases
- Chinese eat almost no dairy products and low levels of calcium-rich food, yet get osteoporosis less than those in the United States
- High protein diets cause calcium loss from bones
- Chinese eat about 270 more calories a day than Americans yet have much less obesity. This is thought to come from the fact that when a very low-fat, high plant diet is consumed a slightly higher percentage of calories is burned off as heat rather than being stored as body fat.
- Antioxidants that protect against free radical damage and aging that can then lead to cellular death and the formation of cancer and heart disease were an important part of the diet when they were eaten in whole foods and may not be helpful at all when taken in supplement form. The reason is that the plant foods have phytochemicals that are cofactor components that all work together causing the protective effect of the antioxidant; without all the necessary cofactors as God created them then the missing links will render the antioxidant ineffective. This can be seen in the Swedish study in which supplement beta carotene was given and a higher rate of some cancers was seen. It was not at all seen when the beta carotene comes from orange and green vegetables which reduces cancer rate. God's way is always better than man's way.
- Fat and animal protein causes cholesterol to rise, while plant based foods cause them to decrease.
- Metabolic studies in humans show that animal protein raises blood cholesterol more than saturated fat. This means that lean meat may be just as damaging to your cholesterol levels as a fatty piece of bacon.
- The highest rate of breast cancer is in countries where people eat the most meat.
- Changing our diet to one low in animal products and high in plant products can largely control the playing out of our genetic tendency toward disease.
- Death from breast cancer is associated with high levels of
  - dietary fat
  - blood cholesterol
  - estrogen

- testosterone
- age of first menstruation

All these are associated with diets that are high in animal products.

In a series of experiments, a diet high in animal protein was fed to animals with liver cancer. Their tumors grew rapidly. The tumor stopped growing when animal protein was replaced with plant protein.

- Protein should make up only 8-10 percent of our diet (America is 11-22%)

Final words by Dr. Dean Ornish, director of the Preventative Medicine Research Institute at University of California: "We have to go beyond the (US Dietary) guidelines to a low fat vegetarian diet." Animal products are the main culprit in what is killing us. We can absolutely live better lives without them.[13]

Neal Barnard, M.D. says that ⅔ of Americans alive today will die of cancer or heart disease, most of it diet related.[14] More recently the figure has risen to 88 percent, according to Joel Furlman M.D. That means nine out of ten people will die of diseases that can be cured 60 to 90 percent of the time with diet and lifestyle changes. Scientist estimate that if the people of the world would eat mostly a plant-based diet, cut out tobacco and alcohol and sanitation measures were used by developing countries to reduce the spread of infectious diseases, premature death from all disease could be reduced by 80 to 90 percent.[15]

A health-promoting diet is made of predominantly live food — or food that has enzymes. "Live food" means that the life God put into those foods in the form of enzymes is still there. For example, if you take a raw sunflower seed and plant it in the ground, a sunflower will grow because the seed had active enzymes and was alive. But if you dry-roast that sunflower seed and plant it in the ground, nothing happens, because the enzymes were destroyed by the heat, and the wonderful life-giving properties of the food are gone. Now you can still eat the dry-roasted seeds, but all you get is some carbohydrates, fat, and some fiber — but little to no vitamins, no enzymes, no phytochemicals.

When we regularly eat dead food, we can sustain life for a period of time, but we cannot properly repair, rebuild and regenerate our health once it has declined.

Life promotes life. If one eats live food he will sustain life in his body. If one eats dead food he will deplete the life from his body.

There is a big difference between *feeling* healthy and truly *being* healthy. I have had patients who live on a predominantly dead-food diet, eating donuts and coffee for breakfast each morning, and say they feel great. But these feelings can be deceptive, because God made our bodies to live, and the spirit He breathed into us will do whatever it can to keep us healthy, so some people abuse themselves and *appear* to maintain good health. It's like the story of The Prodigal Son (Luke 15:11-32), who took half of his father's inheritance and left for a distant land. If that boy would have properly invested that money, he would have been set for life. But he spent it on a partying lifestyle, and one day woke up to the horror of having no more money in his account. After that, he could hardly find work, and almost starved to death.

Our nutritional "bank account" is very important — like my patient who feels great while eating donuts and coffee and dead food. It's just a matter of time until he uses up all his resources for good health and wakes up to the horror, finding out he has cancer or some other major health challenge. Remember, how you feel is just the tip of the iceberg of health; it is not an indication that everything is great. This can be seen when one has their blood pressure taken. If it records $^{200}/_{150}$ this person is on the verge of a heart attack or stroke, whether they feel good or not.

LEVEL	**VIBRANT HEALTH** (BODY IS RECEIVING WHAT IT NEEDS)
	APPARENT HEALTH (NO SYMPTOMS, BUT BODY BEING DEPLETED/TOXIC)
OF	**NOT WELL** (SYMPTOMS, SUBCLINICAL FINDINGS)
	DECLINING HEALTH (SYMPTOMS, CLINICAL FINDINGS)
HEALTH	**DISEASE** (SYMPTOMS, MAJOR CLINICAL FINDINGS)

The healthiest diet is made up of raw fruits and vegetables and their juices, sprouts, whole grains, seeds, nuts and legume's — as much as possible.

Now, I do not say to every one of my patients, "You have to become a vegan today or you will get cancer." We all need to make the right choices in life and be comfortable with those choices. This can be seen in my life. I did not become a vegan because of some health problem or because I did not feel well. I felt quite well. But as I learned about what is in meat, chicken, fish and dairy products — hormones, drugs, chemicals, parasites and bacteria — I decided these things were not really appealing anymore. And although I liked the taste of these things, I made a willful choice to help my future health instead of hurting it.

This choice was not made out of fear; I was not sick. But many people change their diets out of fear, instead of by choice. I say, better to make changes now out of choice now rather later out of fear.

Remember that oil filter commercial where the man says, "You can pay me now or pay me later?" "Pay me now" was for an oil filter, while "pay me later" was for a new engine. I chose to pay now rather than let my body pass from excellent, vibrant health to apparent health, to subclinical symptoms, to clinical symptoms, to disease. I would rather pay now. The cost? Things like changing my taste-bud preferences from spaghetti in meat sauce with meatballs to quinoa(the most health promoting grain in the world) in marinara sauce with tofu meatballs. And if you ever tasted my wife's cooking, the switch was not difficult.

It's the same way when I counsel people to lose weight. I would rather not see a patient deprive themselves of their favorite unhealthy food for six months and lose 50 pounds, only to eventually break down, lose their discipline and regain those 50 pounds. I would much rather see a patient change their thinking by choosing a more live, raw food diet, losing maybe just a couple of pounds a month, but learning to eat that way and enjoy it the rest of their life. The quick-weight-loss diets are not only hard on the body, they are hard on the mind. Let's just get healthy, and the weight will take care of itself.

I will discuss this in more detail later, but suffice to say for now that the best plan is to eat live food rich in enzymes, to eat food in the right combinations, and to eat food you are not sensitive or allergic to. All three helps keep you healthy. And when you eat this way, you cannot possibly be overweight, unless you have a glandular problem.

One study on enzyme research showed that when pigs were fed cooked potatoes, they gained lots of weight — just like all good farm pigs should before they're sold at market. But when the pigs ate raw potatoes, filled with God's life-giving enzymes, the pigs did not gain any weight.[16] Great for the pigs, not so great for the farmers, but great news for you. Raw food does not and never will promote unwanted weight gain.

Another study of raw-food consumption tracked three types of people — overweight, underweight and normal weight. When eating raw, enzyme-rich food, the overweight people lost weight and became normal weight, the normal weight people stayed normal, and the underweight people gained weight and became normal weight.[17]

What can we conclude? That if we eat predominantly raw uncooked food, filled with enzymes, vitamins, minerals, phytochemicals and antioxidants, our bodies will go to our ideal weight. And our health will become ideal and vibrant, not apparent or subclinical.

And as I have said, it's better to willfully make this choice rather than be forced to out of fear. Because I did not wait to get sick before choosing, I could comfortably make the changes gradually. You can start by eating less meat, chicken, fish, and dairy, and then start substituting tofu meatballs for regular ones, soy hot-dogs and hamburgers for meat ones. Yes, there will be some taste-bud adjustments, but if you keep working with it, you can learn some delicious non-meat recipes. It is a progression of *choice* — if you are not presently sick.

I am eating healthier today than I have ever been, but I am not yet where I want to be. All my food is not raw and alive, but more and more it is. It is a joy to eat food that you know is giving health and life to your body. You no longer feel the guilt and condemnation of eating unhealthy food that someday might make you sick.

The health-food industry is exploding. They are making more and more vegetarian products that taste good. So get started. It will not be as bad as you think.

FOOD

It is important here to understand the importance of the food we eat in our *total health = wholeness*. Just as what you say and what you think has the power to bring life or death to you, so to does your food. What we put in our mouth can and is either making us more vital, more full of life or it is making us less vital and slowly bringing on death.

This is a fact many would like to deny because of the pleasure food brings to us. So much of our life revolves around food, it is the center of our social structure, all holidays, gatherings, parties and social meetings revolve predominantly around food. This is great if the food brings life into the body; it is not great is the food brings slow death into the body.

Why do I say slow death? Because what you put into your mouth today does not have an immediate negative effect on your health by bringing death, but a progressive weakening of your body and eventual death. The seeds you planted yesterday are bearing fruit today with ill health, but the seeds you plant today of proper diet, nervous system balance, proper thoughts, etc. will bear fruit tomorrow of vibrant health. With 88 percent of people in this country dying from either heart disease or cancer and of those almost 9 out of 10 people, 60-90 percent of them could be made well if they would only change their diet and lifestyle. It shows us how much health is our own responsibility, not putting the blame of our sickness on anyone or anything else.

The problem is the flesh — the part of our bodies that says "feed me" and "I just want to indulge in what makes me feel good for the moment." These attitudes are killing us. If we just look around, 80 percent of the U.S. population is overweight and 30 percent obese. This is the largest percentage of any population in the entire history of the world. Now it is understandable that a certain small percentage has physiological problems affecting glands and organs that cause weight gain and those people are not always to blame for their weight problems.

The largest percentage, however, is people who have grown up on poor food choices due to incorrect food instruction, poor eating habits and seeking pleasure in life from an area that was never meant to bring pleasure, just to sustain health.

1. Poor Food Choices

From the time we were born, we were taught to eat. So many mothers weaned their children off the best food source on the planet for infants (mothers' milk), and switched them to a very poor substitute — cooked refined cereals and other cooked processed foods. The results: and early onset of immune system weakening and the development of food sensitivities and allergies. If this was not bad enough, as we grow we are indoctrinated into the classic "four food group" concept in which two of them have contributed greatly to the declining health of our nation. (Dairy, Meats), Breads/Grain and Fruits and Vegetables.

If you could only understand how milk and all dairy products, meats and all animal products in general are slowly destroying your gift of vibrant health. If you could only get the revelation that we are what we eat and if we eat death (animal food) we will bring slow death to our bodies, but if we eat live plant base foods of vegetables, sprouts, whole grains, legumes, seeds, nuts and fruits, we will bring more vibrant life. Remember, dead food makes dead people, live food makes living vibrant people.

I discussed all this in the section on "Why a Vegan Diet?", but let me just restate a few reasons to support this view. The China Project was a huge study done in China to research sickness and disease. It found that the two greatest causes of ill health were cholesterol (an animal product) and animal protein (even lean meat like chicken and fish). So by eliminating animal products from one's diet, one would greatly and positively impact one's health. How great? Well, with the average American who consumes animal products, his /her chances of dying of a heart attack are at least 50 percent. By contrast, the chance of having a heart attack for a person who consumes a total Vegan Diet (the removal of all animal food from the diet) drops down to less than four percent.

We need to rethink our food choices and rethink why we eat and what we eat. Don't just do it because it's always been done that way. Instead, seek and explore and you will discover what food choices really are the best.

2. Poor Eating Habits

This is everything from eating too quickly to not chewing your food at least 25 times per bite to eating too much at one time, to eating too many different types of food at one time, to eating at the wrong times. These will all be covered later, but each one of these can make a big difference in your total health.

3. Seeking pleasure where pleasure was not meant to come from.

So many people eat for all the wrong reasons. They eat because it is one of the few things in life that gives them pleasure or makes them happy. They eat because they are depressed, they eat because it's the right thing to do socially. God made food to sustain our bodies so they would last at least 120 years. And what food did he mean us to originally eat? In Genesis 1:28-29 we see that green food or plants were meant to sustain us. It is no wonder that in all the studies in cancer treatment and diet that the single greatest common factor was green vegetables — just what God said back in Genesis 1:28-29. The intent of this book is not to solve everyone's deep psychological issues, but to keep it simple. Our greatest pleasure in life comes from a personal intimate relationship with the God who created us, after that comes the pleasure of an intimate relationship between husband and wife, then comes family, then comes friends. Food is not included and never was meant to be. Also it's important to know that if you struggle with food as an addiction or bondage, God can set you free if you just turn this area of your life over to Him. Self-discipline is good in life but it almost always fails when it comes to eating because it is based on your own abil-ity and strength. Self-control, the spiritual gift, on the other hand always succeeds because it comes from God and is His strength placed inside of your weakness. With God all things are possible. So do not give up, just seek your pleasure in life from the right source and know that you EAT TO LIVE, NOT LIVE TO EAT.

What is the ideal diet?

Let's look at the average American diet. It consists of the following:

    50% of calories from animal products

    42-45% of calories from processed food

    5-8% of calories from fruits and vegetables, legume's, seeds and nuts

Up to 95 percent of what we eat is deteriorating our health. What should we be eating? Instead of five to eight percent fruits and vegetables, legume's, seeds and nuts, it should be 100 percent. This is a vegan diet or completely animal free diet. In addition, 75 to 100 percent of it should be raw, living, uncooked food. (see Digestive Health chapter)

    60% vegetables, sprouts, sprouted grains and their juices

    15% legume's, seeds and nuts

    15% fruit

    10% healthy health food store items

If people are in a diseased state, the percentages change to:

95% raw vegetables, sprouts and their juices

15% percent sprouted raw legume's, seed and nuts

If a person is trying to regain their health, the diet should be 100 percent uncooked and all sugars, even fruit, should be eliminated because of its weakening affects on the immune system. Live, uncooked vegetables, sprouts and their juices have the highest concentrations of enzymes, oxygen, bioelectricity, phytochemicals, vitamins and minerals. When food is cooked above 110 degrees Fahrenheit, it loses all the enzymes, oxygen content, bio-electric charge and many of the phytochemicals and vitamins.

The Ideal Diet from a biochemical aspect is the following:

High Water	Bioelectrically Charged
High Oxygen	High Enzymes
High pH(alkaline)	High Phytochemicals
Low Sugar	
Low Fat	High Vitamins (from food)
Low Protein	High Minerals (organic plant bound)

The most important nutrient to put into your body is oxygen. It is the most vital and must be efficiently transported to every cell of the body. The highest oxygen containing foods are living green plants ie sprouts (wheat grass, buckwheat sprouts and sunflower sprouts), next comes other chlorophyll containing plants from land and sea like raw green vegetables, chlorella and spirulina. Sugar and oxygen content are inversely proportional in the body, as the sugar content goes up in the blood, the oxygen content decreases. Fat of all types in the blood causes a 20% decrease in blood flow for up to 8 hours after a meal thus a reduced amount of oxygen transported into the cells and a reduced amount of waste products moved out of the cells. Why is oxygen content in the body so crucial? Because healthy cells thrive in an oxygenated (aerobic) environment. Unhealthy cells like cancer thrive in a low oxygen (anaerobic) environment. Other factors that affect this ideal diet are:

- Lower sugar in the body causes higher oxygen in the blood
- Lower sugar in the body causes a higher pH or more alkaline environment
- Lower the fat intake the more oxygen can circulate to the cells, the more waste products can be removed
- Lower protein in the diet has less a negative impact on the body's normal alkaline pH
- High protein makes the body more acidic or lowers the normal alkaline pH
- Fat intake increases the cancer rates of certain types of cancers

The ideal diet for growing cancer cells is one that has low oxygen (anaerobic), acidic (lower pH), higher protein, higher fat and higher sugar intake. The average American diet unfortunately.

VITAMINS

The purpose of this chapter is not to go over every vitamin and tell you what it's for and how much to take. There are volumes of books that do that already.

My approach is different. I would like as many vitamins and minerals as possible to come from whole-food sources and live food. As I have noted, there are 16 vitamins, 60 minerals, 3 essential fatty acids, and 12 amino acids necessary for good health. All of these should come from our food as much as possible.

I want to explain the difference between a vitamin pill and a whole-food source of vitamins. There are three questions one must ask when comparing vitamin-mineral supplements:

1) Is each vitamin complete, having all the necessary cofactors, enzymes, and phytochemicals to allow maximum utilization in the body?

2) What is the source of the vitamins and minerals?

3) Are the vitamins and minerals maximally absorbed so they can be maximally utilized by the cells of your body?

Did you know that all vitamin supplements are commercially processed with various chemicals, additives, preservatives, fillers and are synthesized in a laboratory? They are man-made, not God-made. They are only minimally absorbed into the body and only under very deficient states. Children in Africa who are starving and losing their sight when given synthetic vitamin A will regain their sight because God made our bodies to MAKE a way and will use anything to prevent diseased state. Most people in the U.S. are not this deficient, so synthetic vitamins have minimal benefit, if any, along with all the added chemicals. Man-made vitamins are not balanced, and therefore cannot be maximally utilized in the body.

Let me explain the difference between organic food and synthetic sources for our vitamins. In a Swedish study, two groups of silver foxes were fed identical diets, except the first group was given synthetic B vitamins while the second group was given brewer's yeast and other natural foods, which is very high in naturally occurring B vitamins. The foxes in the first group, given synthetic vitamins, failed to grow, had extremely poor fur and developed many diseases. The second group, given the whole-food form of vitamin, grew normally, had beautiful fur and maintained good health.[18]

Dr. A.J. Carlson of Chicago University said, "On the whole, we can trust nature further than the chemist and his synthetic vitamins."[19] Paavo Airola, Ph.D., further states, "We must keep in mind that in nature vitamins are never isolated. They are always present in the form of vitamin complexes. There are 24 known factors in Vitamin C-complex. There are 22 known B-vitamin factors. When you take natural vitamins — like in the form of rose hips, brewer's yeast or vegetable oil — you are getting all the vitamins and vitamin-like factors that naturally occur in these foods. That is, you're getting all those vitamins that are already discovered as well as those that are not yet discovered."[20]

Vitamins; Help Or Hindrance?

The Finnish study published in the New England Journal of Medicine in the spring of 1994 and the Agnes Faye Morgan experiments at the University if California at Berkeley in the 1940s, proved that taking synthetic vitamins is worse than starvation. The synthetic vitamins will kill you quicker. The concept is that most all vitamins are synthetic and made in a laboratory unless they are found in foods. Synthetic vitamins are chemicals and as such cause chemical reactions in the body. They have to be broken down and metabolized by the liver, filtered through the kidneys and excreted. In the Finnish study, people that took synthetic vitamin A and beta-carotene actually had a significant loss of protection from lung cancer, stroke and other forms of death. Remember how it was stated before that vitamins have to have many natural cofactors to be utilized properly in the body and without these cofactors the vitamin becomes ineffective. To add to this argument, Dr. Royal Lee, founder of Standard Process Vitamin Company showed in the 1930's that although synthetic vitamins have the same molecular structure, they are in fact a mirror image of the natural vitamin. This means that they look identical in every way but are really the exact opposite of the natural vitamin, which accounts for the minimal absorption and utilization by the body.

The question arises "Well, I feel much better when I take my (synthetic) vitamins. How can this be? Very simple, if synthetic vitamins are chemicals, they can have reactions in your body similar to chemicals and drugs. For example, people say they feel more awake in the morning after their two cups of coffee. Is coffee a natural food source with natural occurring vitamins, minerals, phytochemicals, cofactors and enzymes? Or is it just the chemical, caffeine, in the coffee that is artificially stimulating the body to feel energetic, but in fact is causing a slow decline of one's *total health = wholeness.*

I studied at one of the premiere health institutes in the United States that had tremendous results in improving health and eliminating disease of all types. Upon acceptance to the institute, one is instructed to leave all their vitamins at home. The director of the institute remarked that some people start to regain their health just by not taking their vitamins, which can act like chemicals or toxins when they build up in the body. This build up causes the liver to have to work harder increasing the toxic load on the whole system.

PHYTOCHEMICALS

Phytochemicals are plant-bound chemicals that maintain healthy plant life. New research shows that phytochemicals could also be a major key in human health. Scientists estimate that a single tomato can include more than 6,000 different phytochemicals.

The function of phytochemicals varies from being strong antioxidants (helping the cells live longer), to strengthening the immune system, to inhibiting cancer cell growth and changing precancerous cells back to normal cells, to destroying already-formed cancer cells.

Some phytochemical families include: allyl sulfides, found in garlic and onions; indoles, found in broccoli, cabbage, kale and cauliflower; isoflavones, found in soybeans; and phenolic acids, found in tomatoes, citrus fruits and carrots.

Why so much about vitamins and phytochemicals? Because you need to see that there's no comparison between organic whole food and whole food supplements like SupremeFood— loaded with vitamins and all their cofactors, minerals, trace minerals, enzymes, and phytochemicals to make a complete vitamin mineral food supplement — and synthetic vitamins, which have little to no cofactors, no enzymes, and no phytochemicals, but instead have added chemicals, preservatives, and fillers.

The next question in evaluating vitamins and minerals is, "Where do they come from?" All vitamins and minerals were not created equal. Let's look at where vitamins and minerals come from, if they are not totally synthetic.

According to the United States Pharmacopoeia (U.S.P.), if two products look similar in analysis, then they are identical, regardless of what they are made of. Take salicylic acid, for instance. It is considered the same product whether it comes from wintergreen leaves or from boiling coal in carbolic and sulfuric acids. Similarly, glycerin, according to the U.S.P., is the same whether it comes from fresh vegetables or from boiled-down animal bones and joints with toxic minerals.

You can see now that labels can be deceiving, because you cannot always know what you are really buying and consuming.

But you *can* know what you are consuming with products like SupremeFood.

For instance, most so-called "natural" vitamin supplements are made out of some not-so-nice substances. All "natural" Vitamin B-12 is made from either cow's liver (which is toxic) or from activated sewage sludge.

That's not the case with SupremeFood, where the Vitamin B-12 comes from Hawaiian blue-green algae — spirulina. Most other "natural" B vitamins come from coal tar and petro-chemicals, whereas in SupremeFood it comes from non-active nutritional yeast.

The choice is yours: God-made? Or toxic pseudo-natural or synthetic?

Minerals are much the same story. When you take multi-mineral supplements, you are usually taking ground-up rocks, shells and metals. These are great for plant fertilizer, but not for human consumption.

Here's the best way to get the minerals we need: God created plants to draw inorganic mineral (rocks and metals) out of the soil and assimilate them for health and strength. In turn, God designed man to eat plants that have already converted these inorganic minerals into organic plant-bound minerals, which are nearly 100 percent absorbable in the human body. This is why one can take horse-pill-sized calcium supplements for 30 years and still end up with osteoporosis. Your body simply was not designed to absorb inorganic minerals from the earth (which most commercial minerals are.)

But your body was designed to absorb organic plant-bound minerals from eating fruit and vegetables. This is why the calcium from broccoli and kale is much better than from horse-pill-sized calcium supplements. Not only does the plant form of calcium absorb at the highest possible percentage, it also has all the other health-promoting cofactors' vitamins, enzymes and phytochemicals.

Another point to consider: Many synthetic supplements pass through the stomach, intestinal tract and down into the toilet, virtually undigested. An owner of a portable toilet service said that he saw so many vitamin pills in the toilets that he could build a mound out of them. He also said he could even read the brand name on many of the pills. How is that for absorption?

Remember, if what you put into your mouth is not being assimilated into the cells of your body, then you are just flushing your money down the toilet — and all the while becoming more and more vitamin- and mineral-deficient.

To close this comparison of synthetic vs. toxic pseudo-natural vs. complete balanced organic food vitamin-mineral supplements, remember that we still do not know — and may never know — how all these complexes, cofactors, enzymes and phytochemicals work together to maintain the life and function of the cells of our bodies. But God knows, and that's why he told man to eat plants for food and use them for medicine. Whom do you trust with your health? The knowledge of man or the infinite wisdom of God?

Is this to say you should never take a vitamin pill? No, I just mean it's better to get all the essential nutrients from our food, rather than compromising with an unhealthy lifestyle — or trying to salvage your health by taking a handful of vitamins.

God's food is always balanced. He made it that way so when you eat, not only do you get an ideal balance of vitamins and minerals necessary for good health, you also get phytochemicals and enzymes that you do not get in a vitamin pill.

Phytochemicals are the myriad of chemical components in a plant that are a part of the perfect food for good health. Reports show that phytochemicals are essential in fighting cancer and other life-threatening diseases.

There are many health components of raw fruits and vegetables that have not even been discovered yet, but God knew *all* the health benefits when He made the food.

The food industry tries to show us that processed food has the same vitamin and mineral content as non-processed. But let's look closer by comparing whole grain bread with white bread that's "fortified" and "enriched." These words simply mean that they have been stripped of the God-made vitamins, minerals, enzymes and phytochemicals, only to have synthetic man-made vitamins replace them. So, the label *implies* that this bread has 100 percent of the required daily allowance of everything — everything, that is, but the ability to keep a person healthy. It's nothing more than empty calories.

So remember, the best choice is whole food in the raw, live state. The second choice is, if you have to cook food, at least make sure it's in its natural state before cooking. So, I encourage you to eat as much raw food as possible.

Juicing

One great way to get your daily allotments of vegetables, without spending all day eating, is by drinking raw fresh vegetable juices. Fruit because of its high sugar content should be eaten and not juiced. The beauty of juices is that they are high in vitamins, minerals, enzymes and phytochemicals. As long as they are consumed within 15 minutes of juicing, they are one of the most power-packed foods available. Juicing is similar to a blood transfusion — you get all those needed nutrients directly into your body without the stress of a lot of digestion. This is why many natural-healing cancer treatments include all-day juicing. This process infuses the nutrients into the body without stressing it by putting a digestive load on it, or without risking incomplete digestion due to food sensitivities or improper food combining.

One great thing about juicing is that you can mix four or more vegetables and get the daily recommended number of servings along with a wide array of phytochemicals, as well as loads of enzymes, vitamins and minerals. In his book Live Food Juices, H.E. Kirschner, M.D. comments that we assimilate 1-35% of the nutrients by eating raw food depending on our level of health, but by juicing we assimilate up to 92% of the nutrients. The most health promoting juices are the green juices: wheat grass, barley grass, sunflower and buckwheat greens, kale, collard greens, broccoli and dandelion greens.

Juice Fasting

One of the most powerful therapies for restoring or maintaining health is fasting. Fasting has the following benefits:
1. Detoxifies the body
2. Strengthens the immune system
3. Increases lifespan
4. Increases energy store
5. Increases enzyme bank account which tremendously improves total health and vitality
6. Promotes spiritual growth

The fasting I usually recommend is juice fasting with fresh organic juice consumed within 15 minutes of juicing to ensure enzymes activity (alive.) Water fasting can be beneficial also but needs much more physician supervision so I usually do not recommend it.

1. Detoxification

One of the simplest and easiest ways to start a detoxification program for your body is to stop eating and start juicing. This can be illustrated as a smoke-filled room with a fire place and air filter. If the fireplace is no longer being used then no more smoke will enter the room. This allows the air filter to clean the air more quickly of the smoke. Once all the smoke is gone, the air is increasingly purified from dust allergens, pollens, mold, etc. The air becomes more pure the more times it runs through the filter.

When we fast with organic juices we shut off any outside sources of chemicals from our food and water and allow our bodies to "catch up on cleaning the house," just like the air filter makes the room air more and more pure.

2. Strengthens the Immune System

When we do not eat, we do not waste our precious white blood cells' (WBC) time by making them eat our food. As I have stated and will continue to state, non digested or partially digested food particles that enter our blood stream from maldigestion and malabsorption (i.e., leaky gut syndrome), cause our WBCs to attack it as if it were a bacteria or virus and digest it. The problem is if your WBCs are constantly eating your breakfast, lunch and dinner every day, there is little time for them to eat bacteria, viruses, parasites, candida and cancer cells. This can lead to a drastic weakening of the immune system. Now you can see that the most important thing to do when you want to boast your immune system is to stop eating and start juicing organic produce, especially vegetables and sprouts. Fruit is sweet and great eaten as a snack, but because of the high sugar content it should not be juiced when trying to strengthen the immune system.

3. Increases Lifespan

Studies done at Brown University showed the importance of overeating versus starvation. One group of animals was overfed each day while the other group was just maintained on a starvation diet. The results were very eye opening. The starvation group live on average about 40 percent longer than the overfed group.[21] Another study was done in which two groups of rats were used. One was fed every two hours, the other only once a day. The rats that ate once a day lived 17 percent longer and had higher enzyme levels and activity.[22] The people that live the longest typically eat a low calorie diet of raw fruits and vegetables, sprouts, whole grains, seeds, beans and nuts. They drink pure water, breathe clean air, work physically (like farming) 10-12 hours per day and are separated from the stress of the world. Even fruit flies exceed their lifespan many times over when they are fasted and just given essential nutrients.[23]

4. Increases Energy

Anyone who juice fasts regularly will tell you how great they feel and how much energy they have and rightly so because eating and digestion is a tremendous energy drain. This is if we are eating properly, not consuming foods we are sensitive to, not over-eating, not drinking with our meals to dilute the digestive enzymes, and not improperly combining our meals. All these lead to increased intestinal permeability (leaky gut syndrome) which causes toxins and large undigested food particles to enter our bloodstream. This causes us to become toxic, and have weakened immune systems. The number one symptom of toxicity is fatigue and sluggishness. Juice fasting will restore your energy level.

5. Increased Enzyme Store Bank Account Which Tremendously Increases Total Health and Vitality

When you juice fast you do not waste your enzymes on digestion. So the 50-60 percent of the body's enzymes that were being wasted on digesting dead, cooked enzymeless food can now be used to strengthen the immune system, heal the body, and allow the body to function at greater levels of *total health = wholeness*. Just think of the enzyme content in your body like a bank account. The more raw, live, uncooked food you eat, the more deposits you are making in your *total health = wholeness*. The more dead, cooked food you consume, the more you have to withdrawal from your body's own enzymes causing depletion of the enzymes needed to maintain vital health or *total health = wholeness*. This type of eating makes heavy withdrawals from your enzyme bank account. Once you are enzyme bankrupt, disease begins.

If instead of eating dead, cooked enzymeless food which drains your body of enzymes and energy, you were to drink live, uncooked enzymes, vitamins, minerals and phytochemical rich juice,you would not only stop the degeneration dysfunction and death of your cells, tissues, glands and organs by not eating and having to digest food, but you would add enzymes from the raw juice to your enzyme store (bank account), promoting *total health = wholeness*. The higher your enzyme levels, the lower the risk of diseases. It's a simple fact of life. This is why you could eat anything and do anything and stay up all night when you were young and you never got sick. The younger you are, the higher your enzyme store (bank account) balance was, because you had not made as many withdrawals yet.

6. Promotes Spiritual Growth

Fasting is a powerful method to enable one to live and walk in the Spirit of God rather than in the flesh. As mentioned previously, the flesh is not just a sin nature that wants to live independently from God; flesh is also what you do in your own strength and ability as opposed to doing in God's strength. When you start to fast immediately your flesh cries out "feed me" and those who are very weak in the flesh give in and let their flesh have whatever it wants, i.e.: food, drink, sex, entertainment, etc. So in order to tame the flesh, we must learn to live and walk not in our weakness but in HIS strength. What this means is as the Apostle Paul said so wonderfully when I am weak then I am strong (2 Cor. 12:10.) When I get to the end of myself that's when Jesus can then carry me in His strength. This is living and walking in the Spirit of God. Just as Jesus walked in the Spirit and did not give in to the temptations of the devil while he fasted for 40 days in the wilderness, we also can walk in the Spirit drawing on the Spirit's power to strengthen us in our weakness. This is truly glorious because when we start embracing weakness, so all the more His strength manifests and then God will get the glory for bringing us through the circumstance and we will grow spiritually learning how to live in the strength of the Spirit rather than the strength of the flesh. Another benefit to fasting is more clearly hearing the voice of God. When we put ourselves in flesh weakening situation like fasting, we start to experience the awesome presence of His Spirit strengthening and empowering us to do what we knew we could not do by ourselves, or in our own ability. As we experience more and more of this walking in the Spirit of God and not in the flesh, the flesh and the worldly system have less and less a hold on us. The first time I fasted for one day I thought I was going to die. I was starving — by 1:00 PM and decided to compromise by fasting only until sundown rather than 24 hours. This was my flesh crying out and I giving it what it wanted. But as I learned to walk in the strength of the Spirit, I actually started to embrace the hunger pangs because I knew I was reaching the end of my strength and will power and that is when God's strength would manifest to carry me through. So embrace the weakness and pain of fasting because you will experience the presence and glory of God's Spirit carrying you through.

Lastly I would like to clarify the purpose of fasting. Fasting does not move God in anyway. It does not impress Him or get Him to hear you more because of it. Fasting changes YOU. It opens you more to experience and live in the Spirit of God, and as you do this, His voice will be heard more clearly by you. Remember that God loves you no matter what you do because God is love. His love is not dependent on what you do, but on who He is. So do not fast too legalistically, trying to move God on your behalf, but instead fast to experience the presence, wisdom and power of God as He manifests, and you will mature in Him and walk in the strength of His Spirit.

To close, fasting should be a way of life. Everyone should fast somehow in their life, whether a one day juice fast per week or three day juice fast per month or a seven day juice fast four times per year (season changes) or even all of the above. Whenever you are ill, stop eating and start juicing, you will get better a lot quicker. Also, when juicing try to stick with pre-dominantly vegetable juices (as opposed to fruit juice) and go green whenever possible. The green vegetables, grain grasses, and sprouts are the most health promoting of the juices. Fasting will greatly add to your healthy body, healthy mind and healthy spirit, promoting *total health = wholeness*.

The first time I juice-fasted for seven days, I was concerned I would lose energy and become very tired and weak. On the contrary, not only did I have loads of energy, I also was able to stay up later, get less sleep and still feel great. It also enabled me to hear the voice of God much more clearly.

SPROUTING

Sprouted grains, seeds, beans and nuts have the highest life giving elements of any other food source on the planet. They contain the highest top three necessary components for vibrant health:

1. Oxygen
2. Enzymes
3. Bioelectricity

They also have the highest concentrations of phytochemicals, vitamins and minerals. To put it simply, sprouts are the healthiest food choice available and are the health food of the future. The chart on page 217 shows how the vitamin B_2 content is 13 times higher in sprouted oats compared to raw oats and 100 times higher in sprouted oats compared to cooked oats.

To see how complete these sprouts are, we can take an example of a sprouted mung bean. It has the following contents:

—vitamin A content of a lemon
—thiamin content of an avocado
—riboflavin content of an apple
—niacin content of a banana
—vitamin C content of a pineapple
—calcium content of a plum
—potassium content of a papaya
—iron content of a loganberry

Because sprouts are growing, living food, they are predigested and have a higher biological efficiency than raw or cooked foods. Biological efficiency is the ability to get to the cells of the body what you initially put into your mouth when you ate. The higher the value, the more easily the food is digested and assimilated by the body. Remember, it's not what you eat that counts, but what gets into each of the cells of your body.

Sprouts tremendous regenerating effects on the body are attributed to their superior:

1. Oxygen content
2. Enzyme content
3. Bioelectricity
4. Phytochemical content
5. Vitamin content
6. Vitamin cofactor content
7. Mineral content

They also have high RNA and DNA nucleic acid amounts, which are necessary for all living cells to function and are only found in living cells. Synthetic vitamins are not living food with all these necessary components.

Sprouts are the health food of the future because they are

- cost effective, much more than organic produce
- easy to grow
- can be grown anywhere, in any season with the help of a plant grow light

Since sprouting is so vital to one's health, one can either sprout with:

1. *Sprouting Jars*- Most economical but limited to the variety of sprouts you can sprout (no wheat grass, barley grass, sunflower greens or buckwheat greens). Also, you must rinse the sprouts three times per day every day so you must be close to the house throughout the day. All in all this sprouting is easy, and a great way to add living food into your diet every day.

2. *Sprouting Trays*- This is done by putting soil on trays and planting the seeds in the soil, watering them 1 time per day, and keeping them under a plant grow light. This method works well with wheat grass, barley grass, sunflower and buckwheat greens.

So, let's look at our diet:

1. We are trying to eat mostly raw, living food and no animal products — high in enzymes, high in phytochemicals, high in bioelectricity.

2. We want to eat foods that contain the balance of the 90-plus essential nutrients, 60 minerals, 12 amino acids, 16 vitamins and 3 essential fatty acids.

3. We supplement with SupremeFood, trace minerals, and digestive enzymes to make sure we get our 90 essential nutrients, and that we do not deplete our enzyme store and ensure a wide range of phytochemicals.

Let's talk about what I recommend everyone on the planet take in the form of supplements to their raw live food diets.

Number One: **SupremeFood**

SupremeFood is a perfectly balanced blend of foods and herbs specially formulated to supply you with organic, natural food source vitamins, minerals, amino acids, and essential trace nutrients. These are all God-made nutrients, not man-made synthetic vitamins. The ingredients are from the richest whole food sources available, and all the ingredients are organic.

SupremeFood includes healing herbs, which are simply concentrated foods. Some herbs can be referred to as superfoods because of their great healing and nourishing abilities. These are God's food, not synthetic chemicals made in a laboratory. All of the ingredients are from the richest whole-food sources on the planet. This formula has NO fat, and will give you quick energy because it nourishes the cells of your body; healthy cells produce an abundance of energy and vitality.

I recommend that SupremeFood become one of the foundations of your health-building program, along with an abundance of fresh, live, whole food.

SupremeFood contains the following:

Spirulina — Blue-Green Algae

Spirulina is the most nutrient-rich food source on the planet. It also is the highest natural source of complete protein at 70 percent (compared to beef's 22 percent and soybeans' 34 percent). Spirulina is also the world's highest natural source of Vitamin B_{12}, and one of the few plant sources of this vitamin. One teaspoon of spirulina contains 2½ times the RDA of B_{12} and over twice the amount found in an equal portion of liver. Spirulina is also rich in beta carotene, Vitamins B_1, B_2, B_6, D, E, K, chlorophyll, enzymes, all necessary minerals and trace minerals (the sea is rich in these), RNA, DNA nucleic acids, iron and GLA essential fatty acids. Spirulina also contains phycocyanin, the blue pigment found only in blue-

green algae, which has been shown to increase the survival
with liver cancer. Other studies have shown that when spirulina wa
to patients with mouth cancer, 45 percent of them saw their cancer disap
pear. Spirulina has also been shown to increase red blood cell volume and
oxygen-carrying capability in anemic people within 30 days.[24] It has also
been able to cure all symptoms of gastric ulcers, and more than 70 percent
of duodenal ulcers in clinical trials.[25]

Probably one of the most exciting benefits of taking spirulina is its ability to help with weight loss. By supplying the perfect nutrition when the
body is deficient in essential nutrients, the "hunger signals" usually sent
are no longer necessary. Spirulina's super-nutrients enter the blood stream
in 15 minutes, causing cravings and hunger pangs to leave. Most people
who regularly take spirulina notice decreased appetite, weight loss,
improved energy levels, and increased mental alertness and clarity.

Chlorella — Green Micro Algae

Similar in its nutrient content and health benefits to spirulina, our
chlorella has had its cell wall broken mechanically, unlike other processed
chlorellas which have been chemically broken. This process makes the
nutrients more available to be digested. Chlorella is very rich in the
carotenoids and in magnesium, along with being a powerful blood detoxifier due to its content of chlorophyll, which can inhibit cancer in all human
organs.

The high carotenoid content in chlorella and spirulina has turned precancerous cells back to normal.[26] Carotenoids also protect against heart disease. Cholesterol does not cause artery blockage until it is oxidized;
Vitamin C and carotenoids play a big role in preventing this reactive
change.

Chlorella is also high in magnesium, crucial for heart function, immune
function, blood-sugar balance, muscle strength and relaxation. According
to the USDA, 80 percent of Americans are magnesium-deficient. With
heart disease being the No. 1 killer in the U.S., magnesium deficiencies
become a significant factor.

Chlorella also has been helpful in eliminating toxic metals like cadmium and uranium.

Purple Dulce Seaweed

Seaweeds are one the richest sources of assimilable minerals and trace
minerals found anywhere. Dulce is especially high in chlorophyll,

:nzymes, Vitamins A and B, protein and iron. Dulce has 33 percent more total fiber and 16 percent more soluble fiber than oat bran. A single 7-gram serving supplies 42 percent of the RDA of Vitamin B-6, 23 percent of Vitamin B-12, and 243 percent of iodine. With thyroid dysfunction and disease prevalent in the U.S. today, dulce is one of the best naturally assimilable sources of iodine. Seaweeds also helps protect against the toxicity of heavy metals.

Grasses are the most nutrient-rich phase of grains, usually without any of the allergic or gluten-containing side effects. They are all enzyme-, vitamin-, mineral- and chlorophyll-rich.

Alfalfa

One of the richest mineral and trace mineral foods found on land because its roots can grow up to 130 feet deep. Alfalfa also has a cholesterol-lowering and anti-atherosclerotic effect. Alfalfa is also known to help in allergies because of its alkalizing effect on the blood. Alfalfa is a very good choice for arthritic sufferers because they are frequently mineral-deficient.

Barley Grass

Not only is barley grass mineral- and enzyme-rich, it also contains good amounts of calcium, iron, all the essential amino acids, and Vitamin C with bioflavonoids. Barley grass has been helpful in healing stomach and duodenal disorders, along with pancreatitis. It is also an ideal anti-inflammatory plant. The chlorophyll in barley and wheat grass may also protect against aging and cancer.

Wheat Grass

It has been said that one pound of fresh wheat grass is equal in nutritional value to 25 pounds of the choicest vegetables.[27] It has been shown that wheat grass therapy, along with eating live food, has cured cancerous growths and has greatly improved many other health disorders, including mental-health problems.[28] Because of its high chlorophyll content, wheat grass has long been known as a blood builder and detoxifier. Anemic animals have their blood counts return to normal after five days of ingesting chlorophyll-rich foods like wheat grass.[29] Because of its high chlorophyll content, as well as beta carotene and Vitamin C, wheat grass is an excellent immune system stimulant.

Beet Root

Beets are powerful blood builders as well as a lymph gland stimulant. Beets are a good source of minerals and trace minerals, as are all root vegetables, which change inorganic, non-assimilable minerals to organic, very-assimilable minerals. They also contain high amounts of iron, calcium, sulfur, magnesium, potassium, chloride, beta carotene and Vitamin C. Research has shown that when test animals with malignant tumors drank beet juice regularly, they became cancer-free and lived an average 20 percent longer than the non-cancer control animals.[30]

Spinach

Spinach is another great blood builder, since it's one of the highest sources of assimilable iron. It's also a very good source of calcium, beta carotene and Vitamin C. Spinach has more protein than any other leafy vegetable. Spinach cleanses and regenerates the intestinal tract, as well as stimulating the liver, blood circulation and lymph glands.

Rose Hips and Orange Peel

These are the best sources available for a balanced Vitamin C complex. They contain bioflavonoids, hesperidin, rutin, calcium, and all the necessary trace elements needed to assimilate Vitamin C. Studies have shown that if Vitamin C isn't given with bioflavonoids (like hesperidin and rutin), the vitamin either does not work or its results are significantly decreased.

Rose hips and orange peel are also very strong immune system stimulators, helping to fight all types of infections, bladder and urinary tract problems, and for wound healing. Citrus peels are also one of the highest sources of pectin, which removes heavy metals like lead and mercury.

Nettles

Some top herbalists call Nettles "natures most perfect superfood." Nettles contain extraordinarily high amounts of minerals, vitamins and chlorophyll, and 3.5% high quality protein. Very commonly used in treatment of allergies, respiratory problems and as a liver tonic for ridding the body of numerous internal as well as external toxins.

Astragalus

Used as an immune system tonic it has proven to elevate the white blood cell count in fighting off sickness and disease. Astragalus seems to be very preventative and healing for viral infections and is being used with HIV patients. It also strengthens digestion and raises metabolism.

Astragalus, unlike echinacea, can be taken daily as an immune system boost without fear of over stimulating or depleting the immune system in any way.

Non-Active Saccharomyces Cerevisiae Nutritional Yeast

Nutritional yeast is the highest available source of the B vitamins (except B_{12}). It also contains 16 amino acids, 17 vitamins and 14 or more minerals, including chromium, a glucose tolerance factor that regulates blood sugar. Nutritional yeast is ideal for people who have hypoglycemia, or who have regular problems with fatigue. Nutritional yeast is great for nervous system disorders of all types because of its high B vitamin content. It can also boost the immune system and is a very important nutrient during cancer therapy. Other benefits of nutritional yeast: increased mental clarity, alertness, increased physical energy and effectiveness.

Probably the two most important functions of nutritional yeast are the reduction of fatigue and stress, the top two complaints of the average American. This nutritional yeast is totally safe for people who have candida or are on yeast-free diets, because it has been heated high enough to destroy all yeast activity, but not high enough to decrease the Vitamin B content.

Remember, it's not how many milligrams of each vitamin and mineral you consume that counts, but how much you assimilate or get into the cells of your body. A synthetic vitamin pill, man-made in a laboratory, might have 100 percent of all the necessary vitamins and minerals, but your body might assimilate less than 10 percent.

Also, find the source of these man-made vitamins. For example, does the Vitamin B_{12} come from beef liver (which is toxic), or from activated sewage sludge? Or does it come from spirulina, blue-green algae? What about that mineral supplement? Does it come from ground-up rocks, bones, shells and metal, or from ocean seaweeds?

The choice is yours: Man-made or God-made? It's up to you.

Just two tablespoons of **SupremeFood** added to your favorite raw juice gives you a complete blend of vitamins, minerals, antioxidants and phytochemicals. You can assimilate these foods so easily; the nutrients are going to work in your bloodstream within 15 minutes. If you are feeling run down or your level of health has dipped into the subclinical symptoms stage, then you can take two tablespoons in the morning and two tablespoons again in the evening.

SupremeFood can be combined with juice fasting to help in the treatment of all major diseases including cancer, and heart disease. A general rule is take **SupremeFood** once a day to maintain health, and two times a day to restore health, or if you have a very demanding or stressful schedule.

Since taking **SupremeFood**, I am amazed at my increased energy and ability to push myself and not get sick. Not that I recommend this, but one can tell one's level of health by how one's body handles extremes. Someone on the verge of getting sick cannot go without sleep, or eat junk food, or become severely mentally stressed without contracting some virus or bacteria or other sickness. But a body nourished with what it needs can handle these stresses and stay healthy, even when short-term unhealthy habits are engaged in.

Again, let's look at our bank account analogy. When we eat raw, live vegan food, rich in enzymes, vitamins, minerals, phytochemicals and bio-electricity, we are making deposits on our health bank account. When we drink raw vegetable juice, consumed within 15 minutes of being juiced, we make another deposit on our health bank account. When we eat cooked dead food, devoid of enzymes, most vitamins and minerals, we make a withdrawal on our health account. When we eat refined processed food, like white bread, white sugar and white pasta, we make a bigger withdrawal from our health account. When we eat fried foods, filled with trans-fatty acid; when we eat foods with long shelf lives, soaked in preservatives and hydrogenated oil and/or sugars and salt, we make even larger withdrawals on our health account.

Remember our Total Health continuum:
VIBRANT HEALTH (BODY IS RECEIVING WHAT IT NEEDS)
APPARENT HEALTH (NO SYMPTOMS, BUT BODY BEING DEPLETED/TOXIC)
NOT WELL (SYMPTOMS, SUBCLINICAL FINDINGS)
DECLINING HEALTH (SYMPTOMS, CLINICAL FINDINGS)
DISEASE (SYMPTOMS, MAJOR CLINICAL FINDINGS)

Most people are born with vibrant health, and from that point on, we make deposits and withdrawals. The person who does the most depositing and least withdrawing is the one who has the best chance to live in vibrant health the longest. Also note that deposits and withdrawals are not made just of what we eat (the nutritional health part of our wholeness), but deposits and withdrawals are made in all areas of our *total health = wholeness*:

1) nutritional health
2) digestive health
3) assimilative health
4) eliminative health
5) circulative health
6) immune health
7) oxidative health
8) structural/energetic/organ/gland health
9) mental health
10) spiritual health

Remember, even if you eat totally raw food, take SupremeFood and juice daily, you cannot experience *total health = wholeness* if you are spiritually lost, not having an intimate personal relationship with the Living God who fills you with His love, joy and peace. This spiritual stress flows over into your mental health and causes you to live ever seeking, but never finding, the love, joy and peace that you were created to live in. A spiritually lost person may have made a nice deposit in the nutritional health part of his wholeness, but he has made the greatest withdrawals he could make by not knowing that the Spirit gives life. The most important part of wholeness is spiritual, then comes mental, then all others follow. If you are making withdrawals in these two, not all the deposits in all the other areas will be able to keep you in vibrant health.

Number Two

Digestive Enzymes. I have already spoken on the importance of enzymes from raw, live, uncooked food. Now I want to explain the importance of taking digestive enzymes with all your cooked meals. According to the enzyme theory, most diseases have two causes: 1) enzyme deficiency and under nutrition, and 2) irritating factors like carcinogens, toxins, chemicals, virus, parasites and bacteria. The enzyme theory states that the second cause of disease can only bring out disease if the first is present. Which means, if you have been eating live, raw enzyme-rich vegan food and have been taking the right digestive enzymes, then you have satisfied half of the first requirement. The second half of that first requirement means making sure you daily get your 90-plus essential nutrients, 60 minerals, 16 vitamins, 12 amino acids, and 3 EFAs and complex carbohydrates. If both parts of the first requirement are fulfilled, your body tolerates much longer the stresses of No. 2 (toxins, chemicals, and carcinogens, etc.) before slipping into disease.

The food enzyme concept, as stated in *Enzyme Nutrition* by Dr. Howell, says "When we eat enzymes in raw, live food or take them in the supplemental form, this causes the food we are eating to be more thoroughly digested."[31] This decreases the withdrawals on the enzyme bank account, remembering that cooking kills all the enzymes in the food. This causes major withdrawals from our enzyme account, causing enzymes to be used for digestion instead of their regular purpose: for every cellular, glandular and organ function, and in order to stay healthy and fight disease. An interesting fact from Dr. Howell's Enzyme Nutrition: Although the body makes less than two dozen digestive enzymes, it uses up more of its enzyme potential supplying these than it uses to make the hundreds of metabolic enzymes needed to keep all of the organs and tissues functioning with their diversified activities.[32]

Wow, that means we are wasting more than 50 percent of our enzymes needed to keep us healthy, just trying to digest our food. I will talk more about this in our digestive health chapter.

When God made Adam and Eve, all they ate was live, raw, enzyme-rich food. They made tremendous deposits to their enzyme bank account, allowing them to use all their enzymes to keep them healthy, instead of wasting more than half of their enzymes on incomplete digestion. Research it: The people, who live the longest primarily eat raw, live food. So if enzymes are a possible major key to our health, all we have to do is make sure we eat lots of raw food and juices ... and when we do not, we should supplement with digestive enzymes.

The product I recommend is Total Health Institutes Enzymes because they are hypoallergenic, vegetarian and they contain the same formula recommended by Dr. Howell, one of the world's premier enzyme experts. This product is made completely from vegetable sources. Most other enzymes on the market are made from cow, ox and pig pancreas and liver, which can be toxic. Dr. Howell also stated that these animal enzymes would be destroyed by the hydrochloric acid in the stomach and rendered inactive whereas the plant-based formula was stable in the low pH of the stomach. This vegetarian based enzyme would also still be active in the small intestine where it needed to digest the food eaten.

Number Three

Plant Bound Organic Minerals

The following is an excerpt from The United States Senate Document Number 264, which explains the importance of minerals in our diet: "Do you know that most of us today are suffering from certain dangerous diet deficiencies which cannot be remedied until the depleted soils from which our foods come are brought into proper mineral balance? The alarming fact is that foods — fruits, vegetables and grains — are being raised on millions of acres of land that no longer contain enough of certain necessary minerals. These foods are starving us — no matter how much of them we eat! No man today can eat enough fruits and vegetables to take in enough mineral salts required for perfect health, because his stomach isn't big enough to hold them!"

The amazing thing about this statement is that it was made more than 60 years ago, in 1936. If our soils were depleted then, with deficiencies leading to disease, imagine what they're like now! Improper farming methods, erosion and weather have contributed to a loss of ⅔ of our topsoil. And what's left of the soil is mineral deficient, resulting in plants that vitamin and mineral deficient, and thus weaker and more susceptible to disease.

Thousands of years ago, much of the earth's soil contained most, if not all, of the more than 100 minerals present on Earth. After years of farming, today's average soil contains 17 to 22 minerals. As a result, carrots have a beta carotene content as low as 70 IUs, when the count should be some 18,500 IUs. A Rutgers University study compared organic produce to conventional (non-organic) produce, finding that on average, non-organic produce was 87 percent deficient in mineral and trace mineral content. The mineral content difference was sometimes staggering; for instance, organic spinach had 86 percent more iron than non-organic spinach. So, to get as much iron out of the non-organic spinach as you would out of the organic, you'd have to eat twice as many servings!

Much of our soil's mineral deficiency has come in recent years. You'd have to eat 75 servings of spinach today to get the same amount of iron you would have received from one serving of spinach 50 years ago. That's why Senate Document 264 says we can't eat enough to get the required minerals in our body.

According to Gary Price Todd, M.D., the human body requires at least 50 minerals for optimal health — to go along with the 12 essential amino acids, 16 vitamins and 3 essential fatty acids. The problem is obvious: We need 50 minerals, but today's soil has only 22. And most of today's mineral supplements contain no more than 15 minerals — and they come from ground-up rock, clay or sea beds.

I liken this problem to the building of a toy structure. We've got plenty of the yellow building blocks, but we're missing the purple connector pieces. So we can't finish the building. It's the same with your heath. If you repeatedly don't get enough of the enzymes, minerals, vitamins, amino acids, essential fatty acids and complex carbohydrates into your body, the living miracle machine will start to break down. You'll regress from vibrant health to apparent health, to subclinical symptoms, to clinical symptoms, to diseases.

You need all 90-plus types of pieces to build and maintain this structure. So getting only a maximum of 22 minerals from a conventional (nonorganic) vegetarian diet is not enough. We need to eat organic produce or sprouts; the Rutgers Study shows that organic soil tends to be much richer in minerals than commercial chemically-treated soil.

Another problem is non-uniformity of soil. The mineral selenium is high in the soils in South Dakota, but low in the Midwestern and Southern states.

Minerals are also important for vitamins to do their jobs. Minerals act as co-enzymes and cofactors for both vitamins and enzymes. This means that vitamins and enzymes can't do their job properly without the proper minerals — the purple connector pieces that enable us to finish the structure.

If God's creative plan for the earth called for more than 100 minerals, we obviously need more than the 12-13 that the U.S. Government says are necessary for health. I tend to agree with Dr. Todd, who says we need 50 minerals — and even this might be a conservative estimate. All of the 90-plus minerals in the world today can be found in human tissue; at least 50 of them have various metabolic functions in maintaining health.

Obviously, minerals are vital to our health. But what type?

Three types of minerals will help us erase our deficiency and maintain *total health* = *wholeness*. They are metallic, chelated, and organic plant bound.

Metallic minerals are the worst of the three, because they are hard to digest and assimilate. Only 5-8 percent of metallic minerals are actually assimilated into the body; if you take 500 mg of metallic calcium, a maximum of 40 mg will actually be used. And that's only if they're fully digested, which can take 15-21 hours. Unfortunately, metallic minerals are the most commonly-used types in supplements sold. They are also less expensive than the other types.

Chelated minerals are metallic minerals that are bound to, or surrounded by, amino acids, which actually tricks the body into accepting the metallic minerals, making them easier to assimilate. Chelated minerals are assimilated at a rate of 40-50 percent, much higher than the 5-8 percent of metallic minerals. Unfortunately, metallic and chelated metallic minerals are hydrophobic, or less water-soluble.

Plant-derived, minerals are far superior than the other types for *total health = wholeness*, because they are almost 100 percent assimilated into the body. These minerals come from plants which have absorbed the metallic mineral through its root system and the synthesis of plant growth and life. Plants convert large hydrophobic metallic minerals into microscopic hydrophilic (very water-soluble) colloidal minerals, which absorb directly into the blood stream without going through the 15-to-21-hour digestion period. Colloidal minerals are up to a thousand times smaller than the smallest metallic mineral — and about .001 or $\frac{1}{6000}$ the size of a red blood cell.

In a typical day, you take in 1.5 grams of minerals and about 500 grams of all other nutrients. So, minerals make up about .3 percent of your total daily nutrient intake. But without minerals, you wouldn't be able to utilize the other 99 percent of the food you eat.

The best form of plant bound minerals are from living sprouts, sprouted seeds and from raw vegetables especially root and sea vegetables.

Let me tell you a short story about the value of plant-derived minerals. My wife, Laurie, started to experience chronic, severe leg cramps. She had been taking chelated metallic minerals for years, and didn't know why she was having these apparent mineral-deficient leg cramps. She increased her chelated mineral to twice the recommended amount, and nothing happened. This kept up for six months. Finally, she started consuming plant bound organic minerals in the form of sprouted seed milk , and a day later, her leg cramps were completely gone. Needless to say, we were impressed.

Now, let's move on to the 12 amino acids. Of these 12, nine are essential — which means your body doesn't make them and must get them from your diet. Where do we get them? There are quite a few possibilities.

First, your morning intake of **SupremeFood** gives you all the essential amino acids. **SupremeFood** is a complete protein, and over 55 percent of it is protein. As I've said, we don't need as much protein as originally thought; in fact, too much protein leads to osteoporosis, kidney disease, tiredness, weight loss and often toxic blood, due to a putrefaction of undigested protein. Your body can only assimilate about 25 grams of protein in any one meal, so anything beyond that is wasted. The average American female only needs 25-50 grams of protein per day, which can be attained in one meal, preferably lunch. Why lunch? Because food is digested better further from the time you go to sleep.

Ideally, you should have raw green vegetable juice blended with **SupremeFood** for breakfast. This starts the day with everything you need, and it's a high-energy meal, easy to digest.

It's all right to have a heavier meal with protein for lunch, because you will digest your food better. You're also giving yourself 12 hours to digest that meal and its protein.

The best vegetarian sources of complete protein come from spirulina and chlorella, next from live sprouts and sprouted grasses, next from sprouted seed spread and seed milk, and then from quinoa, which has been called the "supergrain" because it is the only grain that is a complete protein as well as a complex carbohydrate. Also complete proteins can be made by combining either any legume or bean with any grain, nut or seed. This will cover all 12 amino acids. Some examples:

legume/bean		grain/seed/nut
black bean	with	rice
pinto beans	with	corn
soy beans	with	rice
chick peas	with	sesame seed

It was once thought that these combinations had to be eaten in the same meal. Now it is known that it's all right to get them in the same day. For instance, it's OK to eat grains for breakfast and beans for dinner.

Essential Fatty Acids (EFA's)

The three essential fatty acids (EFAs) can be found in a combination of flax seed (highest in linolenic acid), sunflower, pumpkin and sesame seeds added to your diet. EFA's are also present in SupremeFood. In his book, *Fats That Heal and Fats that Kill,* Udo Erasamus stresses the importance of having good fat in your diet and keeping bad fat out. Our nervous system and brain need EFAs to function properly.

THE WHOLENESS DIET

The SAD (Standard American Diet) is truly out, and rightly so. It contributes little to total health.

But the Wholeness Diet (optimal health-promoting diet) is a diet with as much raw vegetables and sprouts as possible (including raw vegetable juices consumed within 15 minutes of preparation), plus whole grains, seeds, nuts, legume's and beans. This is ideal and will promote total health.

Remember, health is a decision, and YOU ARE TOMORROW WHAT YOU BELIEVE TODAY. So don't feel guilty because you don't eat only organic vegetarian food. I want you to think of "diet" as a journey. After reading this book, I pray you will be much more knowledgeable about *total health = wholeness*, and that you would like to make some changes for the better, for your total health. This is where the journey begins: Wanting to make a change. The end of the journey might be a totally organic, raw, living vegan diet, or it might be just eating more raw food and getting away from fast and junk food. Whatever, it is your journey and you have to make decisions today that will affect your tomorrows.

If you had asked me many years ago if I thought I would become a vegan having no animal products in my diet, I would have laughed and said you were crazy. But the more I learned about what's in the animal products we eat — chemicals, hormones, antibiotics, drugs, bacteria, viruses, parasites — the more I willfully decided I wanted to live a life of *total health = wholeness*. I decided I didn't want to put these things in my body anymore. And now I feel great — much better than I used to — due to my vegan diet and my **SupremeFood** breakfasts. I made the choice to change; no one forced me. This is how you should transition into a healthier diet: by having the facts (they're all in this book) and making your own decisions.

I am reminded of the Scripture, "My children perish from lack of knowledge" (Hosea 4:6). Always learn, always grow, always live your life in *total health = wholeness*. Remember the small steps of a dietary lifestyle. Changes are to be celebrated, like a baby's first step. The baby doesn't run until he learns how to walk first. So go for it at your pace, but go for it.

There is only one exception to this rule, and that is if you have dropped into the clinical symptoms or disease categories. Once you are there, you have no choice but to do all that it takes to repair and restore your health. This is critical, because if you don't get the 90-plus nutrients in, along with enzymes, antioxidants and phytochemicals, and get the toxins out, you will continue to worsen. Don't wait until then; start now and make gradual changes. You won't regret it, when the plague of the this century hits — toxicity. Toxicity leads to many conditions, but most importantly a weak immune system which opens the door to cancer, bacterial, viral, fungal and parasitic infections.

I purposefully did not spend a lot of time in making a new diet that promises health and weight loss, because God already created such a diet. As I said, the closer our diet resembles Adam and Eve's diet, the healthier we'll be, and the less weight problems we'll have.

Remember the pigs that ate raw potatoes and didn't gain any weight? And remember the study where eating a raw-food diet caused overweight people to become normal weight, underweight people to become normal weight, and normal weight people to remain normal. What else can be said? Eat as much raw as possible, and cook as little as possible.

WHOLENESS DIET

Upon Rising -   Drink 3 glasses of distilled water, wait 30 minutes, then drink 8 oz of freshly juiced green vegetable juice (Sunflower sprouts, kale, collards, broccoli and dandelion greens) with two tablespoons of SupremeFood blended. Remember, breakfast means breaking a fast and ideally only water and juices should be consumed in the morning

Mid-Morning -   If you are hungry eat some raw vegetables (red peppers yams, carrots, cucumber) or drink 8 oz of fresh vegetable juice

Lunch -   Large mixed sprouts/greens and vegetable salad with a very small amount of organic flax seed oil or extra virgin olive oil and fresh squeezed lemon or raw organic apple cider vinegar (if not yeast sensitive.) Have sprouted seeds/nuts ground up into a spread with this meal. With major health challenges oil should be kept to a minimum or avoided because it slows the blood flow and oxygen and nutrient exchange into the cells

Afternoon -   If you are hungry, eat some raw vegetables (red peppers, yams, carrots, cucumbers) or drink 8 oz of fresh vegetable juice

Dinner -   Mixed green/sprout and vegetable salad like the one you had for lunch, with either quinoa, millet, wild rice or baked yam (if not sugar sensitive i.e. candida, cancer, chronic fatigue, diabetes or weakened immune system); eat all raw if you have **ANY** major health challenges.

Evening-   Seed milk shake (sprouted sesame, sunflower, pumpkin, flax blended with distilled water). You can add a banana if you are not sugar sensitive or immune depressed. This drink can be blended in the morning with SupremeFood instead.

If you presently need to change your health you should eat 80-100% raw, live food — not cooked. Also, you should drink at least 24 oz. of fresh, raw vegetable juice each day (8 oz three times per day.)

If you are in transition in your diet, then you can eat whole grains and have cooked food at lunch and dinner if necessary (i.e,: baked yam, millet, quinoa, wild or brown rice and beans.)

Combine vegetables with proteins (nuts or seeds) for one meal.

Combine vegetables with starches (grains, rice, yam) for the other meal. Never eat starch with protein in the same meal. Fruit is always eaten separately as a meal itself or in between meal snack.

Drink one quart (32 oz) of distilled water per 50 pounds of body weight per day: upon rising, between breakfast and lunch and between lunch and dinner. Water should be consumed no later than 30 minutes before a meal and at least one and a half hours after a meal so as not to disturb digestion of your meals.

Take vegetable enzymes with all cooked meals if maintaining health and with every meal if regaining health.

Beverages	Wholeness Diet	Transition Diet
	Fresh extracted vegetable juices, herbal teas, distilled water	Organic bottled juices, cereal coffees

	Wholeness Diet	Transition Diet
Dairy	None	Non-dairy cheese, milk i.e.: rice or soy
Meat/Fish	None	None
Fruit	Fresh (limited)	Unsulfered, dried Frozen (limited)
Grains	Sprouted raw quinoa, millet	Whole grains cereal Stick with millet and quinoa if you have not been food tested
Nuts/Seeds	Raw,sprouted unsalted almonds, sunflower, sesame, pumpkin, flax	Other nuts and seeds Avoid peanuts and cashews
Oil	Raw flax seed oil Extra virgin olive oil (limited)	Cold pressed canola, sunflower and cold pressed non-dairy, mayonnaise
Vegetables	All raw	Cooked fresh, baked yams
Soup	Raw, cold	Cooked homemade
Seasonings	Herbs - fresh garlic onion, parsley	Herbs - bottled
Sweets	Raw fresh fruit (limited) Stevia (herb)	Stevia, (herb) rice milk, unsulfered molasses, raw unfiltered honey organic maple syrup (limited)

Now let me address some questions you may have about this type of diet:

What if I'm already very thin? Will I be in danger of losing too much weight?

Not according to the study where underweight people became normal weight when eating raw food. If you're concerned, add more good vegetable fat to your diet — like avocados (no more than 3 per week), soaked, sprouted nuts (especially almonds) and seeds. Sunflower, pumpkin, sesame, flax seeds are great blended into seed milk. Peanuts and cashews should be avoided because they contain potential cancer causing toxins and residues. Also, you can add a little more cold-pressed organic oils like flax, sunflower, sesame, canola, and extra virgin olive oil (too much oil will burden the liver and slow the blood flow.) If you eat nuts and seeds, make sure you chew them thoroughly to baby-food consistency. This greatly aids in digestion and helps prevent intestinal problems. Remember when you lose fat you should reshape your body with resistance exercises like weight training and rebounding. Muscle weighs more than fat.

Will I get enough calcium in my diet if I cut out milk?

Where does a cow get it's calcium from? Green plants—and so should you.

There is quite a bit of calcium in dark-green vegetables like broccoli, kale, collards, dandelion and spinach. Unhulled sesame seeds are also high in calcium. And remember, it's not how much you eat, but how much you assimilate that counts. Calcium in vegetables is organic and almost 100 percent assimilable. Seed milk shakes made with sesame, sunflower, pumpkin and flax are calcium powerhouses.

In one study, a low amount of calcium was ingested in a vegetarian diet. The body compensated by assimilating more calcium to balance the deficiency. God designed us perfectly, and the body is designed to do whatever needs to be done to keep you in total health. Also know that whenever calcium is heated like in pasteurized milk, it changes from organic absorbable to non organic, non absorbable.

Will I get enough protein without meat?

Where does and elephant get it's protein from? Green plants—and so can you.

We discussed the value of spirulina, chlorella, quinoa, and sprouted seeds and nuts as protein sources, and also how to combine a legume or bean with rice, grains, seeds or nuts. Most Americans eat 2-3 times as much protein as necessary, which leads to fatigue, kidney problems, osteoporosis, and improper weight loss, toxicity and a cancer friendly acidic environment. You only need 25-50 grams of protein per day, depending on your size.

I know I should cut out meat and dairy, but I have a hard time saying no to these foods.

Three points were previously addressed: 1) knowledge, 2) will, and 3) self-control versus self-discipline.

Knowledge. I once talked to a man who worked at a chicken plant, where they processed the chicken all the way through from the killing to packaging the final product. He simply said, "If you saw what I saw, you would not eat chicken. The tumors, the pus and bacteria, just to name a few.

And to know only one in every 20 chickens is inspected curbs your appetite." I remember a similar talk with someone who worked at a hot-dog factory, who told me that all the parts of the animals are used — and I mean all the parts. Knowledge is, if you knew what they knew, you wouldn't eat them either. This is why I changed my diet to an animal free vegan one. When I found out all the drugs, antibiotics, hormones, parasites, bacteria and viruses that can be transmitted to us when we eat meat, chicken, fish, or dairy products, I made a choice to eat as much health-promoting food as I could. I wasn't forced to make this choice, because my health was good. But I chose to do it because our second son was starting to eat food and my wife, Laurie, felt God speak to her heart that our son wasn't supposed to eat animal products. So we all became progressively more and more vegetarian or vegan.

Knowledge is more than just knowing facts. It also comes from God speaking to us through His Spirit. When our family decided not to eat meat anymore, we based this decision on factual knowledge as well as from asking God to reveal what was best for us. There is nothing as powerful as hearing God speak clearly to your heart on something, because once He does, you know, even if you don't fully understand.

Will. Your will is your choice. God did not make us robots in His image. He made us living spirits with a free will to choose whatever we think is best. Our will is what gives us eternal life, because the Word said "choose life" (Deut.30:19) so in Christ "you and your children might live." Moses told us to choose between life and death, blessings and curses. When we willfully make a choice, we choose between two options: following the flesh, or following the Spirit. The flesh is the part of us that wants to live independently of God, satisfying itself. The flesh is made up of the body and the unrenewed mind. The unrenewed mind is programmed with the things of the world, not things of the Spirit. It is a mind that puts "self" on the throne of one's life, and wants to satisfy all the cravings of the body and unrenewed mind. Think of it this way: your flesh tells you what to do rather than you telling your flesh what to do. Your flesh tells you to eat things that aren't health-promoting but health declining. This kind of choice comes out of the weakness of the flesh rather than the strength of the spirit. Most people live their whole lives being led by their flesh that tells them what to eat, what to watch, what to do. There is a better way: to be led by the Spirit of God.

Self-control versus Self-discipline. Self-control is one of the nine fruits of the Spirit, a part of the very nature of God. True self-control is of

God and empowered by God. True self-control says, "I cannot do it, but in Christ's strength I can do it, for when I am weak, that is when I am strong." This is key to spiritual health — to walk totally God-dependent, led by His Spirit rather than living independently or self-dependent, led by your flesh.

Self-dependence is self-discipline, which says "I will not do it. I will not, I will not, I will not do it." This is where all diets fail. They fail when self-discipline fails. And it always fails, sooner or later, because it depends on you. God didn't create you to depend on yourself; He created you to depend on Him. Self-control in your diet — or any area of your life — is a glorious wonder because it comes from God, from seeking Him in prayer and saying, "Father, I know I can't stop eating these sweets. Lord, give me strength to have victory in this area of my life."

When we live this way — not in our weakness, but in God's strength — we suddenly start having victories where we always had defeats. The victories keep coming as we learn to walk in His strength, led by His Spirit.

So to recap the question: We have to have knowledge — both head knowledge from the facts, and heart knowledge from God's Spirit — before we make a decision. Then we have to make a willful choice to choose life (*total health = wholeness*) rather than death, health rather than sickness. Then we have to be empowered by the Holy Spirit to give us self-control when temptation comes, or when we feel weak, because in our weakness, all the strength of God lives inside us to meet our every need.

To summarize this chapter, here's my recommendation for nutritional health: A predominantly raw, living-food vegan diet rich in enzymes, vitamins, minerals, antioxidants, bioelectricity and phytochemicals. You should be eating:

1) 75% complex carbohydrates, 15% proteins, 10%fat.
2) More plant food and much less animal food.
3) More raw uncooked vegetables, fruits, seeds, nuts, sprouts and less cooked food.
4) More organic food and less conventional (non-organic) food.
5) SupremeFood, 2 tablespoons, 1-2 times per day.
6) Digestive enzymes whenever eating dead or cooked food, 4-6 capsules per meal.
7) Plant bound organic minerals, in the form of seed milks and raw fresh vegetables and their juices.

CHAPTER 12
DIGESTIVE HEALTH

Digestion is the action of taking the food we eat and breaking it down into its component parts, parts which will be assimilated by the body and used to maintain *total health = wholeness*. Thorough digestion is a great step toward assimilation into the blood stream.

In this chapter, we discuss five categories of digestion:
1) mastication (chewing)
2) HCl production in the stomach
3) bile production in the gall bladder
4) enzyme production in the pancreas/enzyme content in living food
5) food combining

Mastication

Mastication is the act of chewing. The more thoroughly you chew, the better it is for your *total health = wholeness*. When you chew food thoroughly, it is mixed with saliva, which includes the enzyme amylase, which digests starches. Completely-chewed food is broken down into a much larger surface area, meaning more digestive enzymes can work to break down proteins, fats and starches into their components parts — the building blocks for all your cells.

Here's what it looks like.

Imagine a head of cabbage, with 20 layers of leaves, sitting in your stomach. Enzymes can only attach to the outer surface of food, like the outside of the outer layer of the cabbage. To fully digest it, we would need to pull all the leaves apart and break them into small pieces, like running it through a food processor, exposing much more of the surface area of the cabbage for the enzymes to attach to. The enzymes then go to work, attacking all sides of the pieces, breaking down the food into its usable components for the assimilation phase.

OK, I know you cannot swallow a whole head of cabbage, but you get the point: That's comparable to people who only chew their food a few times before swallowing. Little chewing produces little surface area for digestion, meaning fewer nutrients are pulled out of the food.

Bottom line: The more we chew, the more we break up our food into tiny pieces, giving our enzymes more surface area to work with, improving the whole digestion process many times. When this is done, enzymes digest even more food, helping to get more valuable nutrients — vitamins, minerals, enzymes, antioxidants and phytochemicals — into our blood for *total health = wholeness*.

How many times should you chew your food? Until it is the consistency of baby food, usually 25-40 times per bite of food.

When I first started chewing my food thoroughly, I realized that I had been swallowing my food after 8-10 chews. I had to work hard to train myself not to swallow so soon. It took time, but I have learned, the more I chew, the more nutrients enter my body.

Another benefit of thorough chewing is that it "predigests" starches in your food. An enzyme secreted in your saliva digests starches by at least 50 percent before they even hit the hydrochloric acid of the stomach, and then amylase produced in the pancreas finishes the job thoroughly digesting starches and carbohydrates.

Poor chewing habits, meanwhile, can cause maldigestion syndrome, which leads to increased intestinal permeability ("leaky gut" syndrome), which leads to toxicity in the blood — the precursor to sickness. I discuss this more in the next chapter. This is what happens: Your food is made up of starches (carbohydrates), fats, and proteins. If your food is not thoroughly chewed, sufficient surface area is not produced to completely digest all the components of the food. What happens next is a progression of steps that lead to ill health. The carbohydrates start to ferment, the proteins start to putrefy, and the fats start to oxidize, and all become free radicals (which are the most destructive compounds in the body causing rapid destruction of the cells) which are cancer producing. Just imagine putting what you had for dinner last night all mixed together in the oven on very low heat just high enough to keep it warm, then let it stay like that for days, weeks, months, even years. Can you imagine the stench, the bacteria, and the toxic mess you would have? That is exactly what is going on in your digestive tract when your food is not properly chewed and digested. Some of it irritates our bowels and we pass bowel movements with terrible odor, some of it gets pushed into the diverticuli (pockets) in the bowel, where it remains for months to years or until some bowel cleansing program is initiated to remove this toxic mess. All this can occur from NOT CHEWING YOUR FOOD 25-40 TIMES PER BITE. So, relax and enjoy your food, take more

The Importance of Thoroughly Chewing Your Food

If we swallow a piece of food the size of a 2cm cube without chewing it, the available surface area for digestive enzymes to act on is 2cm x 2 cm x 6 sides = 24 square cm.

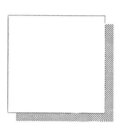

Now imagine this same piece of food is cut into 1mm slices. This would increase the surface area for digestion to 2cm x 2cm x 2 sides x 20 slices = 160 square cm.

If those slices were run through a food processor, the surface area available to digestive enzymes would be increased tremendously.

The surface area available for digestion goes up 666% when we go from a cube to a slice. When we go from a slice to finely chewed food of baby food consistency, the surface area available for digestion goes up by even higher percentages. So chew your food thoroughly at least 25 times per bite.

time eating your meals, then you will greatly add to your *total health = wholeness*.

HCl Production

Hydrochloric acid, or HCl, is produced in your stomach and secreted to help break down food, giving it more surface area to improve digestion and assimilation of essential nutrients.

HCl breaks down hard-to-digest protein rich foods, like meat. Meat is a very tough protein to break down in the stomach, so tough that only a super-strong acid — like HCl — can do the job.

The stomach starts secreting HCl as soon as you start chewing and tasting your food. This is why gum chewing does not promote health; it prepares the body for food it never gets. This causes the unnecessary release of acid and other enzymes in the stomach, resulting in excess acid.

The opposite problem occurs when your stomach secretes not enough acid — one result of not chewing your food enough.

When your stomach has either too much acid or not enough, a couple of conditions commonly occur. Excess acid leads to gastric duodenal ulcers, and acid deficiency leads to food allergy and sensitivity — which lead to all kinds of symptoms and diseases (discussed in the next chapter.)

Some of the diagnostic symptoms of low acid secretion are:
> burping, fullness for an extended period of time after eating, bloating, easily upset stomach

Some of the diagnostic symptoms of high acid secretion are:
> stomach pains, stomach pains just before and/or after meals, antacid dependency, stomach pain when emotionally upset, sudden acute indigestion, relief of pain by drinking carbonated drinks or milk.

Bile Secretion

Next along your digestive journey is your gall bladder's secretion of bile from your liver, which is essential in fat digestion and toxin removal. Bile is produced in the liver and stored in the gall bladder, from which it is secreted into the small intestine. In the small intestine, bile emulsifies, or breaks down, fat — like soap does to oil and dirt when we wash our hands — further preparing it for digestion and assimilation. Without bile, fat digestion would be greatly reduced. This can be seen in people who have no gall bladder; when they eat fats, it's not digested, and often results in diarrhea.

You might say, "Well, we do not want to digest fat, do we?" Remember, you need three essential fatty acids in your diet for *total health = wholeness*. Without them, you would have many deficiency symptoms that could lead to disease.

Enzymes

Enzymes are tangible physical substances that contain life itself. They are the keys to life and health. Every breath, even every thought, requires enzymes.

In the last chapter, we stressed the importance of enzymes, which control every function of the body at the cellular level. Here's an analogy: To build a house, we need raw materials like lumber, nails, cement, etc. But we also need the workers. Enzymes are the body's workers. They put the building blocks of proteins, carbohydrates and fats together to form the "building" of your body — your cells and organs.

Enzymes are alive. They promote life. When you plant a seed, it will germinate and grow because enzymes in the seed promote life and growth. If you take that same seed and dry-roast it in the oven, then plant it, it will not grow — because the cooking process destroyed its enzymes. Without the workers, the building will never get built.

You can see the importance of eating raw food. (I am not talking about raw meat, chicken, or fish; those things should always be thoroughly cooked to kill parasites and bacteria, but raw and living plant based food.)

Why raw food? Because raw food — seeds, nuts, vegetables and fruits — is alive, full of living enzymes. If planted, raw food will propagate, because not only does it include the raw materials (proteins, carbohydrates, fats), but it also includes the workmen (enzymes) who can build the building and keep it running in good repair.

One theory says we are born with a certain number of enzymes, and that once we make too many withdrawals without making enough deposits, we are enzyme-bankrupt — and life no longer exists. So clearly the more cooked food (with no enzymes) and the more over eating we do, the more our enzyme supply declines. The only way to slow this decline is to eat much more living and raw food. And when we are not eating living and raw food, we should add vegetable-source digestive enzymes to our diets.

Just think of your enzyme health as a bank account. You start your life with a tremendous inheritance of enzyme health. As life goes on, you are spending more and more enzymes in digestion, in over eating, in metabolic function. So you need to implement an "investment program" to keep your inheritance, to keep your account healthy. Otherwise, the price will one day have to be paid in the form of ill health and sickness.

The best way to make deposits on this account is by eating as much living and raw food as you can. Don't over eat at any one meal, but eat smaller meals more frequently throughout the day.

Raw vegetables include their own enzymes which help digest your food, saving your body's own enzymes for other metabolic functions.

Your body includes three classes of enzymes: 1) enzymes from raw and living food, 2) metabolic enzymes made by your body, and 3) digestive enzymes your body makes. Let's take a closer look at each.

1. Enzymes from raw foods are vital in your diet.

The Differences between Raw and Cooked Food

In 1946, Dr. Francis Pottenger conducted a research project to see the differences on health benefits from raw food versus cooked food. In this study he took 900 cats, half were given raw food the other half were given the same food except it was cooked. The cats that ate the raw food were healthy and produced healthy kittens with no premature deaths. The cats that ate the cooked food did not fare so well. They developed all the diseases common to mankind: heart disease, cancer, pneumonia, thyroid disease, kidney disease, paralysis, arthritis, liver disease, osteoporosis, decreased sexual interest and diarrhea. The first generation of kittens from the cats that were fed cooked food were sick and abnormal, the second generation were diseased or dead, and by the third generation the mothers were sterile.[1]

From the book Goldot by Lewis E. Cook, Jr., a three-part experiment was done in which three groups of rats were tested:

Group 1

A group of rats were fed a raw diet consisting of vegetables, fruits, nuts and whole grains. These rats grew very healthy and never suffered from any disease, never became fat, mated regularly, were gentle, affectionate and lived in harmony with each other. After reaching an equivalent of 80 human years they were put to death and their organs, glands and tissues were found to be in perfect condition with no signs of aging or deterioration.

Group 2

The next group of rats was fed a diet of cooked food, white bread, meat, milk, salt, soft drinks, candies, cakes, vitamins, minerals and medicines for any ailment. This group from early on in life contracted colds, fevers, pneumonia, heart disease, cancer, arthritis, poor vision and cataracts. Most of this group died prematurely and became very antisocial, fighting, stealing, each other's food, and trying to kill each other. This caused them to have to be separated to avoid total destruction of the group. Epidemics of sickness affected the group and as they died, they were autopsied and found to be in advanced degeneration in all their organs, glands and tissues. Their offspring were all sick and had the same problems their parents had.

Group 3

In this group the rats were fed the same diet as Group 2, the average American diet, and had all the same diseases and behaviors that were exhibited in Group 2. Extreme sickness, antisocial behavior and early death were all seen. Some of this group were put to death at an equivalent human age of 40 years and were autopsied and found to have extensive degeneration of all parts of their bodies.

In the next part of the Group 3 experiment the rats after 40 human years were put on a strict fast with only water to drink for several days, after eating the typical American diet for the equivalent of 40 years. Then when food was reintroduced into their diet it was only the raw food that Group 1 received. This diet was alternated with times of fasting and within one month the behavior was completely different now being very docile, playful, living together in harmony with each other. Then once again at the age of 80 human years equivalent these rats were autopsied and found to have no signs of aging or disease just as in Group 1.[2]

A study of baby cows produced similar results. Cows that were fed pasteurized (heated) milk — instead of raw milk — died within 30 days.[2]

In another study, pigs that ate cooked potatoes gained lots of weight, whereas pigs that ate raw potatoes gained no weight.[3]

And I've already mentioned the study about humans — some under-weight, some over weight, and some normal weight — eating a diet of raw food. All three groups went to a normal weight.[4]

Adam and Eve ate raw food. God designed it that way: Our body's enzymes are meant to be used mostly on metabolic functions, and little to none on digestion. But today, we use up to 60 percent of our enzyme bank on digestion, causing depletion of organs, gland and tissues, which leads to ill health.[5] If God wanted us to eat cooked food, we would not suffer enzyme depletions for doing so. People who do not cook their food main-tain optimal enzyme levels.

The same goes for the animal kingdom, as noted in the above studies with cats, cows and pigs. There is not much disease in the animal kingdom. Animals in the wild do not contract cancer, heart disease, diabetes, and arthritis like we do because they eat raw, live food. We humans are the only creatures on the planet that primarily eat dead, cooked, enzyme-less food — and our disease rate shows it.

Let me tell you about Luigi Cornaro, a 15th-century nobleman from Venice, Italy. In his youth, Luigi over-indulged in every way. Then he decided to change his ways by living a life of moderation. He set a goal to live 100 years — in an era when the average life span was about 35 years. Luigi lived to 103, his mental capacity sharp to the end. What was the key? Starting at the age of 37, he lived the rest of his life on a diet of fruits and vegetables totaling about 1500 calories per day.[6]

Dr. P.R. Burkholder of Yale University found the following increases in B vitamin content in sprouted oats as compared to dry oats. Then he com-pared the dry raw oats to the average 87 percent loss in vitamin content after cooking. *(See "Living Sprouts" on next page.)*

The Miracle of Living Food

What accounts for the over 1500% increase of vitamin content in raw versus sprouted oats (and probably all food)? It is truly a miracle as we see sprouted food produce higher vitamin content with the addition of only water and light. These foods truly are alive and able to produce higher vita-min and nutrient (enzyme/phytochemicals/bioelectricity) contents as they prepare to grow. This is very important in our maintaining *total health = wholeness.*

Recent research studies have shown that broccoli sprouts contain up to 50 times the amount of anti-cancer properties that mature broccoli plants

Living Sprouts vs. Raw vs. Cooked

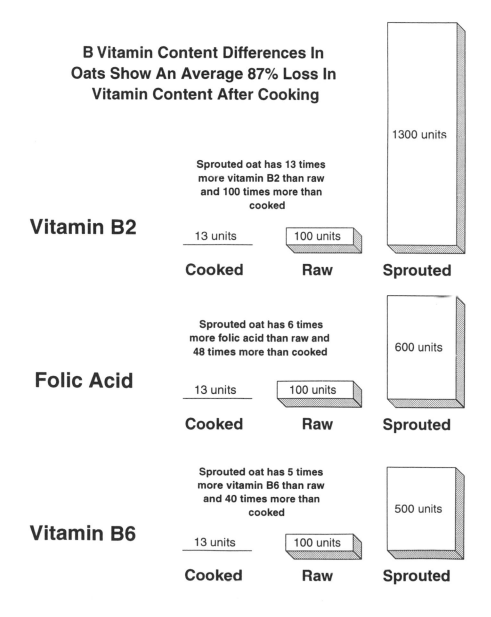

B Vitamin Content Differences In Oats Show An Average 87% Loss In Vitamin Content After Cooking

1300 units

Sprouted oat has 13 times more vitamin B2 than raw and 100 times more than cooked

Vitamin B2

13 units   100 units

Cooked   Raw   Sprouted

Sprouted oat has 6 times more folic acid than raw and 48 times more than cooked

600 units

Folic Acid

13 units   100 units

Cooked   Raw   Sprouted

Sprouted oat has 5 times more vitamin B6 than raw and 40 times more than cooked

500 units

Vitamin B6

13 units   100 units

Cooked   Raw   Sprouted

have. The same holds true for us as human beings. When is our body the most vital, enzyme rich and most impervious to poor diet, lifestyle, chemicals, toxins and stress? When we are children. This is linked to our enzyme bank concept that says if we do not take in much live enzyme-rich food then our enzyme account decreases making us more susceptible to all disease. Remember when you were 18 you could eat junk food (burgers, fries, and pizza) drink soda, stay up all night and feel fine the next day? Not so when you turned 30. If you can keep a high proportion of your diet living foods, sprouted, oxygen, enzyme, vitamin/mineral, phytochemical and bioelectrically rich foods, our cell tissues, organs and glands would have the necessary components to maintain, repair and flourish. So when it comes to the healthiest diet choices they include in order of their importance:

1.   Sprouts and their juices
2.   Green vegetables and their juices
3.   Vegetables and their juices

So, remember that sprouts have up to 13 times the vitamin content of the unsprouted grain and up to 100 times the vitamin content to the cooked grain.

2.) Metabolic enzymes

These make up the bulk of your enzymes. They cause every reaction of every cell, tissue and organ. They are the sparks that light the fire that makes everything work; without them, you would die immediately. When your supply of metabolic enzymes dwindles — due to them being used in digestion — you see a gradual decline in health.

White blood cells are loaded with enzymes. When you eat a cooked meal, or simply eat too much, your WBC count elevates to bring extra enzymes to digest your food — and taking WBCs away from their primary job of fighting bacteria, viruses, parasites, fungi and cancer cells. Your immune system suffers. Cancer will soon be the No. 1 killer in the United States. AIDS and other viral diseases are on the rise. Antibiotics are not stopping more and more bacterial infections. The key is a strong, healthy immune system. You get this by eating raw food, which keeps the WBC count normal.

3.) Digestive enzymes

These are vital for digestion, the process of breaking down food into its component parts — fats into fatty acids, proteins into amino acids, carbohydrates into simple sugars. There are four types of digestive enzymes:

1) lipase, which breaks down fat
2) protease, which breaks down protein
3) amylase, which breaks down starch
4) cellulase, which breaks down plant cellulose.

The pancreas secretes these concentrated enzymes to thoroughly digest your food. This is why we never want to drink with our meals; the liquid dilutes the digestive enzymes, which then causes maldigestion and leaky gut. So if you drink with your meals make sure it is just enough to keep your mouth moist and only water. You can drink your liquids 30 minutes before a meal or one and one half-hour after to ensure proper digestion.

Why is it important to break down fats, proteins and starches into their component parts? For the same reason that a building cannot be built without all of its component parts. We need thorough digestion for good health.

Here's an example: When someone drinks milk and lacks enough lactase, the enzyme which breaks down lactose into its component simple sugar, the lactose starts to ferment, causing gas, irritable bowels, possible diarrhea, aggravated candida problems, and the potential for increased intestinal permeability ("leaky gut").

The same is true with the milk protein casein. Most people lose the enzyme to digest casein at around age 4.[7] As a result, casein becomes a sticky glue-like substance that interferes with intestinal assimilation. It also coats the respiratory tract with mucus, bad news for allergy, asthma or sinus sufferers.

Another good reason for breaking down food into its component parts is to avoid immune stimulation complexes. These complexes can trigger many allergic reactions. If you eat a food that you are sensitive and it is totally digested into its component amino acids and fatty acids, there is no allergy provoking component to any basic building block of food or else your body would have an allergic reaction to every meal you eat. This means that even if one is sensitive to tomatoes he is not allergic to its simple amino acids or fatty acids because all component parts are neutral or non-allergenic. A persons severe allergic reactions are triggered by larger protein molecules which consist of multiple amino acids connected together. This is why complete digestion of these larger protein molecules can help to reduce the allergic reaction to foods.

If digestion is incomplete, larger food particles can enter the bloodstream via "leaky gut" — trigger problems such as allergies, asthma, joint pain, arthritis, inflammatory bowel conditions, neurological symptoms, etc.

In one study, a cooked-food diet — devoid of enzymes — led to enlargement of the pancreas, an organ that secretes digestive enzymes, and eventually exhaustion and degeneration of pancreatic tissue. Man is the only animal with a cooked-food diet. The following chart shows the result: Our pancreas makes up a much bigger percentage of body weight than it does for other animals, indicating how overworked our digestive glands really are.[8]

	Body Weight (Grams)	Pancreas Weight (% of Body Weight)
Sheep	38,505	0.0490
Cattle	455,265	0.0680
Horse	543,600	0.0603
Man	63,420	0.1400

Enlargement of the pancreas is a possible cause in the development of diabetes, blood sugar problems, pancreatitis (inflammation of the pancreas) and pancreatic tumors. In one study, 86 percent of the diabetics examined were deficient in amylase, the enzyme that converts starch to sugar. After adding amylase to the diet in oral digestive enzyme form, 50 percent of the diabetics who used insulin could now control their blood sugar without insulin.[9]

In a study at George Washington University Hospital, patients were fed 50 grams of raw starch. The average rise in blood sugar was 1 milligram per 100 cc in one half-hour, with a decrease of 1.2 mg after one hour and a decrease of 3 mg in two hours. Patients fed 50 grams of cooked starch saw an increase in blood sugar of 56 mg at half an hour, 51 mg at one hour, and down to 11 mg after two hours. Fatigue and anxiety accompanied this great swing in blood sugar.[10]

The importance of a high enzyme diet cannot be stressed enough. Enzymes are the key to all life and in order to live a full life as God meant us to live we must take in enough enzymes to keep our enzyme bank account high. If not as stated we will become enzyme bankrupt and disease will begin. There are only two ways to keep the enzyme store adequate for *total health* = *wholeness:*

1) Eat a total raw food diet which consists of uncooked fruits, vegetables and their fresh raw juices, seeds, nuts, sprouted grains and their sprouted grasses.

2) Add vegetable based digestive enzymes to your diet whenever you eat cooked food. This is not as good as the total raw food diets but becomes more practical for most people. Simply take 4-6 capsules with each meal to ensure complete digestion of the food. This not only prevents leaky gut syndrome along with a long list of health disorders linked to low enzyme stores but also helps to preserve your present enzyme account, ensuring many years of vibrant health.

Some of the many disorders that have been shown to be either directly or indirectly attributed to by low enzyme levels in the body are:
- immune system weakening, impairment and disorders
- obesity and weight related disorders
- circulatory disorders
- neurological and mental disorders
- cancer
- cardiovascular disease
- allergies
- child illness (including hyperactivity and A.D.D.)
- gastrointestinal disorders
- hormonal disorders
- decreased life span

This is to name just a few of the disorders and diseases that are caused by low enzyme levels. It is not the scope of this book to describe the details of each of these that a low enzyme level will bring on, but enough to say that having a steady high level of enzymes in your body, whether from raw foods or from vegetable digestive enzymes taken with meals, is one of the most important keys to your total physical health if not the most important. So make sure your enzyme bank account is large so your dividends of *total health* = *wholeness* never cease.

Vegetable vs. animal based digestive enzymes

Animal based enzymes are produced from the stomachs and pancreas of pigs, cows, ox, etc. These are not recommended because:

1.) Animal enzymes work in an alkaline environment (pH above 7). These enzymes cannot survive and do their job of digestion in the acid pH of the stomach. So when you take these supplemental enzymes you are getting little to no therapeutic effect because they must pass through the stomach which they were never intended to do. In his book *Enzyme Nutrition,* Dr. Howell explains how vegetable based enzymes from aspergilli can tolerate acid from the stomach and predigest food so as to minimize the amount of enzymes being secreted (and used up) by your body.[11] This is why I recommend this type of enzyme (see appendix).

2.) Animal glands are toxic, laden with chemicals, drugs, and possibly even viruses and parasites. For the same reasons I have previously discussed not eating animal products, also applies to taking animal based enzymes.

Food Combining

Food combining dates back to the early part of this century, when research was done to evaluate different digestion times of foods and how certain foods digest better in the presence of other foods. Research also evaluated how certain food combinations caused maldigestion, inflammation of the digestive tract, "leaky gut" syndrome and toxicity.

Food combining really works if you stick to it properly. Let's take a look at our food-combining chart.

The food combining concept is based on digestion rates for all food, how long it takes to digest each food in your digestive tract— fruit (two hours), fresh squeezed juice (15 minutes), and meat (12 hours), starch (5 hours). *See Below*

Now the rule is in the wheel: You can only cross one dashed line and you can never cross any solid line in combining meals. For example, fruit should be eaten alone and between meals, because fruit digests quickly (in about two hours). If you eat a fruit dessert after a steak dinner, it will not digest well. It will just ferment in your intestinal tract, causing bloating, stomachache, abdominal gas, gas pain, foul gas, cramping, diarrhea, or bowel movements with a bad odor. It also causes "leaky gut," and is the primary cause for toxins entering the body and a weakened immune system. So fruit should be eaten alone, or as a between-meals snack.

Food Combining

You can only cross
one dashed line and no solid lines

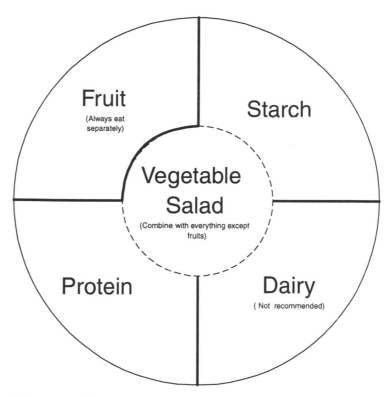

Vegetables and salads can be eaten with starches (rice, grains, potatoes, etc., or proteins (nuts, seeds, beans, meats). Proteins and starches should not be eaten together. Fruit is always eaten separately or in between meal snack. Dairy is not recommended at all, but if you eat it, combine only with vegetables and salads.

If you have a sweet tooth after dinner, should you eat something besides fruit? Yes, but you will want to pick the right combination, depending on what you ate in that meal. If you had a vegetarian stir fry of brown rice and vegetables, you will want to combine the starch of the rice with a starch-like dessert — like mochi, which is baked, brown rice sweetened squares with a cinnamon flavor.

White refined sugar is totally excluded in any health-promoting diet. Even sugar substitutes, like fruit source, organic maple syrup, and sucanant (evaporated sugar juice) should be taken in moderation. Stevia, an herb, can be used for it sweetness without having calories or raising one's blood sugar.

Beans, meanwhile, count as a starch even though they can contain some protein.

Starches should predominantly be made up of complex carbohydrates like wild or brown rice, whole wheat (if you are not sensitive), quinoa, millet, buckwheat, oatmeal, barley, rye, whole grain bread, corn, and the list goes on. Starches with a digestion time of five hours can be combined with vegetables or salad with a digestion time of five hours.

Speaking of salads, the best dressing is just fresh squeezed lemon maybe once in a while with a little organic extra virgin olive oil. Get rid of the French (too much sugar), Thousand Island (too much dairy) and Ranch (too much dairy. And avoid croutons, unless it's a starch/vegetable meal.

A meal of protein with vegetable/salad combination is ideal for lunch, because it is heavier which gives your body more time to digest before you go to sleep.

The custom in many European countries includes a heavy lunch, followed by a two-hour break, or *siesta*, and a light meal for dinner. I agree with this practice — I also like the siesta part!

The body cycles through 3 phases after eating a meal. These are associated with 3 eight-hour periods to make up a 24-hour day.

1. Noon -8 PM Digestion phase
2. 8 PM-4 AM Assimilation phase
3. 4 AM-Noon Elimination phase

This further explains why larger meals should be eaten later in the day and lighter meals eaten earlier in the day.

How do you pick a protein to mix with your salad and vegetable for lunch? Some suggestions are soy products, nuts, and seeds or, if you are not a vegetarian, things like chicken, fish, beef, turkey or eggs. These mix well with our near-neutral foods of vegetables or salad. So review the chart and start combining your food properly.

Digestion Time

The digestion time of various foods is determined by how easy they are to assimilate by the body. Foods that are easily digested are often referred to as "mild foods" since they do not require a lot of work and energy to digest. The following are approximate timetables for digestion:

Green vegetables (non-starch) -	5 hours
Raw Juices -	15 minutes
Fat -	12 hours
Protein (meat) -	12 hours
Protein (fat) -	12 hours
Protein (starch) -	12 hours
Starch -	5 hours
Mild Starch -	5 hours
Fruit, sweet/dried -	3 hours
Fruit (acid) -	2 hours
Fruit (sub-acid) -	2 hours
Fruit, sweet/fresh -	3 hours
Melon -	2 hours
Syrup, sugar -	2 hours
Milk -	12 hours

Alkaline/Acid Foods

Now a word about alkaline/acid foods. Our body functions in an alkaline pH. This means that there is a greater concentration of hydroxyl ions (OH-) as compared to hydrogen ions (H+). The hydroxyl ions are in greater concentration in plant origin food whereas the hydrogen ions are in greater concentration in animal origin food. To maintain the absolute necessary 7.4 body pH (7 is neutral) which is slightly alkaline we need to ingest enough plant origin food. A diet that is largely animal products (meat, chicken, fish, milk, and eggs) is very acid forming and stressful to the normal homeostasis or balance of the body. This increases the chances of all diseases like cancer, heart disease, osteoporosis, arthritis etc. So it makes sense that the more alkaline our food is the better it is for our health. Similarly, the more acidic our food is, the worse it is for our health. For the most part fruits and vegetables are alkaline-forming, grains are slightly acid forming (except quinoa, millet and amaranth), and animal products are more acid forming.

The following charts display the alkaline and acid properties of certain foods. They can be used to determine not only what foods are alkaline and acid forming but also to what extent, for example raw spinach is rated at +556 (+ meaning alkaline) and is 100 times more alkalizing on the body than blueberries rated at +5. Blueberries however are 45 times more alkalizing than scallops rated at -226 (- meaning acidic.) So eat as much alkaline forming food as possible and when you have a choice, pick those foods that are the most alkalizing.

Alkaline Ash Foods

Foods are listed in order of their positive affect in replacing alkaline reserve, i.e., raw spinach at +556 is approximately 100 times more effective than green peas at +5.

Raw spinach*	4 c	+556
Beet greens	1c	+478
Molasses	1Tsp	+360
Celery	5 stalk	+341
Dried figs	5	+297
Carrots	3	+282
Dried beans	½ c	+282
Chard leaves	1½ c	+214
Water cress	2½ c	+192
Sauerkraut	⅔ c	+176
Lettuce	½ head	+170
Green limas	⅔ c	+142
Dried limas	⅔ c	+123
Rhubarb**	1 c	+117
Cabbage	1⅓ c	+111
Broccoli	1 c	+101
Beets	⅔ c	+98
Brussels sprouts	6	+95
Green soy beans	⅔ c	+85
Cucumber	10 sl	+71
Parsnip	½ lg	+67

Radishes	7	+64
Rutabagas	¾	+62
Dried peas	½c	+57
Mushrooms	7	+50
Cauliflower	1 c	+50
Pineapple	1 c	+44
Avocado	½	+44
Raisins	½ c	+42
Dried dates	7	+40
Green beans	1 c	+39
Muskmelon	¼	+38
Limes	½ c	+33
Sour cherries	18	+30
Tangerines	2	+29
Strawberries	12	+28
White potato	1	+26
Sweet potato	1	+26
Grapefruit	½ c	+25
Apricot	2	+25
Lemon	½ c	+24
Blackberries	1 c	+22
Orange	½ c	+22
Tomato	1	+21
Peach	1 lg	+21
Raspberries	1 c	+19
Banana	1 sm	+18
Onion	1 sm	+14
Grapes	½ c	+10
Pear	1	+10
Blueberries	⅔ c	+5
Apple	1	+5
Watermelon	½ sl	+5
Green peas	¾ c	+5

*   best eaten raw
**   not recommended

Acid Ash Foods

Not all foods listed are recommended but are listed for your information.

Foods are listed according to their ability to decrease the alkaline reserve of your body. the higher the number the more depletion of the alkaline reserve and the more harmful it is to you.

Scallops	½ cup	-226
Oysters	5	-209
Dried lentils	½ cup	-171
Sausage	6 links	-160
Sardines	8	-160
Oatmeal	1 c	-95
Corned beef	¼ lb.	-80
Lobster	¼ lb.	-78
Peanuts	? lb.	-78
Haddock	¼ lb.	-78
Soda crackers	8	-52
Codfish	¼ lb.	-51
Macaroni, spaghetti	⅞ c	-50
Peanut butter	3 Tsp	-49
Chicken	¼ lb.	-43
Pike	¼ lb.	-39
Wheat germ	1T	-38
Brown rice	⅝ c	-29
Whole wheat flour	⅝ c	-26
White flour	⅝ c	-26
Salmon	1 c	-26
Beef steak	¼ lb.	-24
Turkey	¼ lb.	-23
Barley	⅝ c	-21
Veal chops	1	-21
Lamb	¼ lb.	-17
White bread	2 slices	-15
Wheat bran	1 Tsp	-10
English walnuts	10	-10
Lamb chop	1	-10
Bacon	2 sl	-10

Eggs	2	-9
Whole wheat bread	2 sl	-8
Pork chop	1	-6
Honey	4T	-4
Shrimp	¼ lb.	-4
Fresh corn	½ c	-2
Sugar		0
Corn oil		0
Olive oil		0
Corn syrup		0

Questions

It seems impossible to eat this way. How important is it, really?

First, nothing is impossible when we are in Christ Jesus (Matthew 17:20.) Go back and review my discussion on diet, and how it takes: 1) knowledge from the world and from the Spirit, 2) will (or decision), and 3) self-control (from the fruit of the Spirit), not self-discipline when times get tough. How important is it? Let me say that the greater your total health is, the less important it is to eat the right combinations at every meal. If you want to stay in total health you need to properly combine your foods or else a leaky gut will form and toxicity and a weakened immune system will eventually develop. The weaker your *total health* is, the more important it is to eat this way at every meal.

A healthy 6-year-old has a much more forgiving digestive tract than a toxic 35-year-old who has dropped into the clinical symptom stage of health. We've got a 5-10 percent margin of error in our diet for making wrong choices if our health hasn't hit the subclinical symptom stage or below. It's not what you do between Christmas and New Year's Day that counts, but what you do between New Year's Day and the next Christmas. Unless you're sick, then *everything* you put in your mouth has to promote health.

If I feel great, do I have to eat the combination diet way?

For the same reason you change your car's oil every 3,000 miles, instead of waiting till the red engine light flashes on. Then it's too late. It's always better to make a healthy lifestyle change or diet change when you have the choice to choose life. Too many wait until sickness knocks on the door to start making changes, driven by fear and panic. It's better to build a house on solid rock rather than on sinking sand (Matthew 7:24-27). This is how I see many choices we have in our *total health = wholeness*: We either pay now or we pay later. Paying now is taking the time, energy and effort to make positive changes that will help you for your entire life. Paying later is waiting until you are sick and grasping at anything you can for your needed miracle.

Start small by eating fruit separate from other foods, having your heavier meal at lunch and lighter one at dinner, and starting to cut out dairy and sugar. These small steps eventually end up as one grand step for your *total health = wholeness*.

Where does a cheeseburger fit in?

It doesn't. A cheeseburger breaks all the rules, because meat shouldn't be eaten with starch. You should eat only one or the other, with vegetables or salad. And the cheese is a dairy product, and dairy is always out because it is the number one food allergen, so get used to it. (See the chapter 6 "You Are What You Eat.")

Aren't we free from the dietary laws of the Old Testament?

Good question. What you are free from is any law that says you must do it to become righteous in God's eyes, because in Jesus we are the righteousness of God. "God made him who knew no sin to become sin for us, so we might become the righteousness of God" (2 Corinthians 5:21). Paul said, "Everything is permissible, but not everything is beneficial" (1 Corinthians 10:23.) What he meant is, "I am free in Christ to do what I want, but not everything I could do will be good for me."

So, the Levitical law of dietary guidelines no longer applies to us for attaining righteousness. But it does stand for good health. Why do you think God said not to eat pork? Because pigs are filthy animals that will eat their own dung, and they're filled with parasites. Why do you think God told us not to eat fish that eat off of the bottom of the lake, or beasts that feed off of dead and decomposed animals? Because these creatures are more toxic and more laden with bacteria, virus and parasites than others. So if someone suggests a better way to eat and digest your food more thoroughly, don't throw it back at him and say, "I am free from that law."

To summarize food combining:

- fruit is eaten alone because it digests in two hours
- starches can be eaten with either vegetables or salads or both, but not with proteins
- proteins can be eaten with either vegetables or salads or both but not with starches
- dairy products should be avoided at all times
- fruit 2 hours after a meal (between meal snack) if you are not sugar sensitive (having candida, chronic fatigue, cancer, diabetes, or any weakened immune disorder.)
- protein and vegetables and salad are best for lunch
- starch and vegetables and salad are best for dinner
- poor food combinations can cause poor digestion, "leaky gut" and toxicity, along with putrefaction of proteins, fermentation of sugars and oxidation of fats, which lead to free-radical formation and these structures are highly carcinogen producing
- don't drink but a few ounces of water with your meals, it will dilute your digestive enzymes

To summarize digestion:

- proper mastication (chewing) is a must 25 times per bite
- HCl secretion is needed for proper digestion of protein
- enzymes are a key to health and life
- vegetable-based enzymes should be taken with all cooked meals
- a raw-food diet is vital for its enzymes, vitamins and mineral, phyto-chemicals, oxygen and bioelectricity
- start proper food combining, slowly if you're healthy, always making just a few changes until you feel comfortable combining as a lifestyle

CHAPTER 13

ASSIMILATIVE HEALTH

To assimilate means to take in or absorb all the way into the individual cells. Food and nutrients are no good if you eat and drink them, but do not assimilate them. Assimilation is vital in our *total health = wholeness*.

A lack of assimilation can result in inflammatory bowel conditions like severe colitis or Crohn's disease. In these conditions, when food reaches the inflamed bowel, it simply passes through, with no nutritional benefit to the body whatsoever, ultimately coming out as diarrhea. The body is like your bank account; it's not how much money you make that counts, but rather how much you keep. Likewise, it's not how much or what you eat that counts, but what you assimilate.

Many factors affect how much food we assimilate, including:
1) Increased intestinal permeability (leaky gut syndrome)
2) Food allergy/sensitivity
3) Intestinal parasites
4) Maldigested food
5) Inherited bowel disease
6) Bacteria or viral infections
7) Candida/parasite

Leaky gut (also known as "increased intestinal permeability") and food sensitivity is covered in this chapter. Maldigestion was covered in Chapter 12; bacteria/virus and candida/parasites are covered in Chapter 16.

LEAKY GUT

Leaky gut is exactly what it sounds like. The intestinal tract is like a fine screen or mesh, which only lets nutrients of a certain size through. The nutrients then pass into the hepatic portal blood vessels, which bring nutrients to the liver, your chemical detoxification plant.

In a leaky gut condition, the intestinal tract becomes inflamed and the selective permeability (letting only digested food particles through) breaks down. This allows the passage of not only normal digested nutrient building blocks (amino acids, fatty acids and simple sugars from carbohydrates), but also the passage of larger food particles, like larger chain proteins, fats and carbohydrates, and toxins that were never meant to pass through. This can be likened to a window screen. If the screen is functioning properly with no holes in it, air will pass through, but the flies, mosquitoes and other bugs will not. In leaky gut, the intestinal barrier becomes inflamed. Instead of only letting the digested broken down food particles through, the larger food particles and toxins enter causing the immune system to become weakened and over stimulated. This is like the screen that now has tears, making larger holes that allow all types of insects to get through.

This presents a few problems. Larger chain proteins can trigger not only intestinal irritation and inflammation, but also all kinds of allergies, immune and autoimmune problems, and inflammatory joint conditions like rheumatoid arthritis. Too much protein can also cause kidney damage, especially if it is not digested into its amino acid building blocks.

Leaky gut can also result in toxicity, since toxins leak through the "screen" of your intestinal wall (because of the larger holes produced by the inflammation.) These toxins ultimately end up in the liver, your chemical detox plant. Unfortunately, your liver is by then overburdened, and the toxins end up circulating throughout the body, causing havoc wherever they go. If the toxins deposit in the brain, you might have foggy thoughts, possible memory loss and/or confusion, and even the start of neurological disease like multiple sclerosis or Parkinson disease. If the toxins deposit in the joints, you will have arthritic-type pains. If the toxins deposit in organs that produce white blood cells (WBCs), your immune system will be weakened, making you more susceptible to illness, including cancer.

Toxicity is the primary cause of cancer because toxicity is the primary cause of a weakened immune system. Cancer cells form in your body daily, but your WBCs normally destroys them. But when toxicity weakens your immune system, your WBCs can't do their job, giving cancer cells the opportunity to grow. They eventually form a little colony called a tumor, which WBCs have more trouble destroying. So do not let your defenses down.

What would happen if two armies came to fight, and one side laid down all its weapons? That army would be quickly destroyed. That's why our immune system is to be highly regarded and guarded at all costs.

(See page 235 for a visual conception of leaky gut.)

What causes leaky gut? At least seventeen things:[1, 2, 3]

1) Food allergy/sensitivity is probably the largest daily cause of leaky gut in America. I will discuss this in more detail later in the chapter.

2) Parasites can be found in all of us, especially intestinal parasites. They come mainly from beef, chicken, fish, and pork, but they are everywhere. Parasites feed off of you and excrete their toxic waste inside you. That's why "parasite programs" should be regularly taken, to rid you of these unwanted guests. (Read more about parasites in Chapter 16.)

3) Virus, often in the form of intestinal flu. The most common symptom is diarrhea, causing you to assimilate none of your food.

4) Bacteria like salmonella yield much the same result as a virus, making assimilation nearly impossible.

5) Poor diet, usually manifested in improper food combining, or eating food that is highly processed or preserved, or high in fat or sugar content.

6) Stress causes lack of blood flow into the organs, including the bowel, which can result in leaky gut.

7) Toxic heavy metals—like metallic lead, mercury or cadmium—cause irritation to the intestinal lining.

8) Ethanol, or alcohol, kills tissue and sets off an inflammation reaction, which causes increased intestinal permeability.

9) Drugs have many side effects that can result in poor assimilation. Drugs kill the normal flora of bacterial growth in the bowel, allowing pathogenic bacteria to grow back in a greater proportion. Candida, or yeast, also overgrows the bowel, causing leaky gut. Other drug side effects are corrosion to the gastrointestinal tract, causing inflammation and leaky gut.

10) Candida is a normal pathogen present in the intestinal tract. But when the beneficial or good bacteria in your intestinal tract is killed off because of antibiotic use, the candida overgrow and cause a wide variety of symptoms leading to poor health.

11) Eating or Drinking Toxic Food containing Chemicals and/or Toxins.

When we eat or drink food containing chemicals or toxins this directly causes intestinal lining irritation and inflammation which leads to a leaky gut. Many people would say that their diet doesn't contain any of these, but in truth, practically all food consumed today by Americans is toxic and/or loaded with chemicals. These come from the drugs and chemicals stored in the animal flesh, from the pesticides sprayed on the fruits and vegetables, the preservatives put in food to increase shelf life, the additives like stabi-

Increased Intestinal Permeability (Leaky Gut)

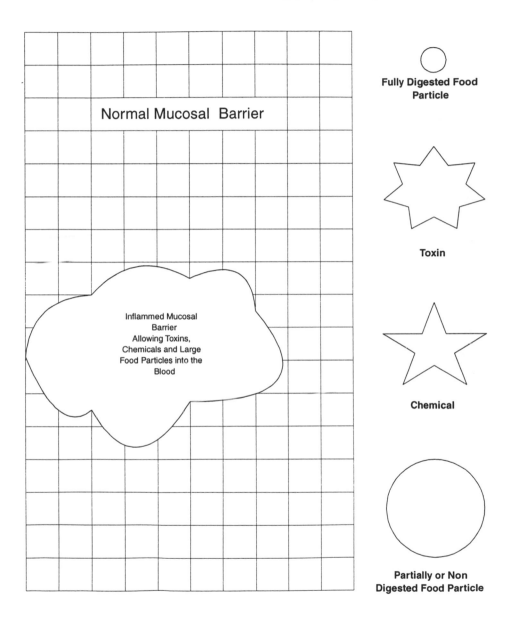

Normal Mucosal Barrier

Inflammed Mucosal Barrier Allowing Toxins, Chemicals and Large Food Particles into the Blood

Fully Digested Food Particle

Toxin

Chemical

Partially or Non Digested Food Particle

lizers, thickeners and other food processing chemicals. The only people who don't eat toxic/chemical laden food are those who eat only organic food and make all their own meals from scratch.

12) Improper food combining causes intestinal irritation and inflammation and will be discussed later in the chapter.

13) Eating acid pH forming food causes stress on the digestive tract and on your total health. This was discussed in the last chapter and will be mentioned later in this chapter.

14) Not chewing your food enough will also cause a leaky gut. Each bite needs to be chewed a minimum of 25 times.

15) Eating too much at one time is a tremendous drain on your digestive ability and if the food is not completely digested (which it cannot be when you over eat) it causes intestinal irritation and inflammation.

Remember each time I mention leaky gut and the causing of intestinal irritation and inflammation, usually it is asymptomatic (cause no symptoms) in ⅔ of the American population. This is why 95% of Americans have a leaky gut and only about 30% perceive that they have any digestive problems.

16) Drinking with meals causes a dilution of your digestive enzymes, which causes maldigestion and leaky gut. This is why only water should be consumed with meals and only enough to keep your mouth moist (no more than 4-6 ounces). Water should be consumed a half-hour prior to, or one and a half-hour after meals.

17) Eating dead or deficient food causes very poor digestion because once you cook the food, the enzyme content of the food is destroyed (unless you add supplemental vegetable based digestive enzymes). This not only causes leaky gut but also greatly reduces ones *total health = wholeness* because of the significant enzyme withdrawal (your enzymes are used instead of the natural occurring enzymes in the raw food to digest the food) instead of deposit to your enzyme health bank account. (See diagram page 238)

The terms "leaky gut" and "toxic buildup" are hardly new. In 1910, Elie Metchnikoff, director of the Pasteur Institute in Paris, wrote a book called *The Prolongation of Life.*[4]

He states, "The natural death of human beings cannot be regarded as due to exhaustion from reproduction. It is more likely due to an autointoxication of the organism." Metchnikoff also said the inherited "structure of the human large intestine and the customary diet of civilized man is especially favorable to the multiplication of toxic microbes that cause intoxication." Very prophetic words from the man who discovered the phagocyte, a type of WBC that eats bacteria, virus, molds and cancer.

Metchnikoff also wrote, "If it be true that precocious old age is due to poisoning of the tissues, it is clear that agents which arrest intestinal putrefaction must at the same time postpone and ameliorate the conditions of old age."

So, the concepts of bowel health and toxicity have been around for centuries; we only seem to have forgotten them in the last 50 years or so.

Leaky gut is probably the greatest cause of sickness and disease. In my practice, I see patients of all ages. It is amazing to see that even in young, healthy children, the first system to show negative physiological changes is the digestive system. The pattern begins: As a person ages, problems gradually spread from the digestive tract to other elimination organs (liver and kidneys), then systematically throughout the body. This causes physiological changes in other organs and systems. The immune system weakens. Toxins deposit in the neuromusculoskeletal system, causing pain and arthritis. Deposits in the neurological system cause brain fog, memory loss, and possibly neurological diseases such as multiple sclerosis or Parkinson's disease. Toxic buildup eventually affects every organ, gland, tissue and cell.

So, how important is a healthy digestive tract? It is the mirror of your total physical health. People with regular constipation, loose bowels or other bowel complaints will likely have significant health problems in the future.

FOOD ALLERGY/SENSITIVITY

It has been said that up to 60 percent of all human illness involves food sensitivities/allergies (or intolerance).[5]

A food sensitivity or allergy is your body's mild or severe reaction to a substance. When a person with sensitivity is exposed to an allergen, his body starts making antibodies. Allergens and antibodies attach to each other, releasing chemicals like histamine into the body. Histamines cause blood vessels to dilate and allow fluid to leak out of the vessels and into body tissues. Some of the results include swollen nasal passages, itching and tearing eyes, hives on the skin, diarrhea or leaky gut. Some reactions are life threatening; fluid accumulation in the lungs and larynx can suffocate a person if proper emergency care is not instituted immediately.

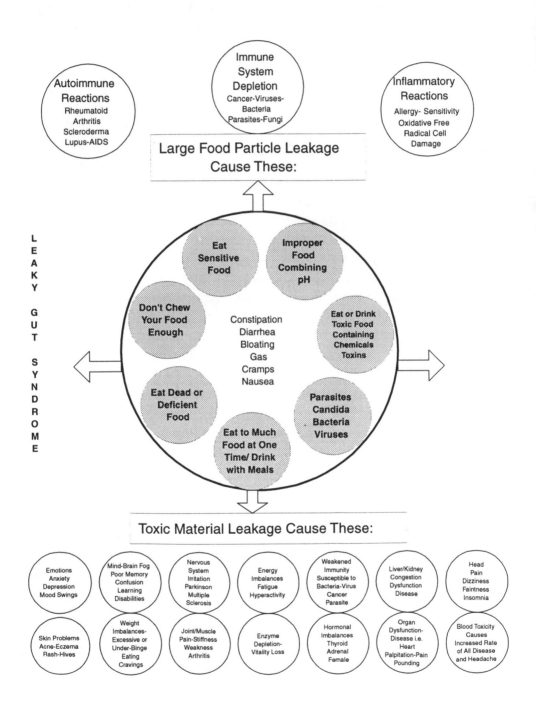

Food Sensitivity

What is food sensitivity and how does it occur? Food sensitivity is an immune system over reaction to a substance you ingest or consume. This reaction causes an increased intestinal permeability or "leaky gut" to develop. A leaky gut allows large food particles to enter the blood stream, thus weakening the immune system even more because it is your white blood cells that have to eat these large food particles instead of eating bacteria, viruses, parasites, candida, and cancer cells.

A leaky gut also lets toxins into the blood which can either throw the immune system into imbalance or deposit in other glands, organs, and tissues, causing the full spectrum of pre-disease symptoms all the way to actual disease itself. What is a possible cause of food sensitivity? Eating enzyme deficient food. When we eat large amounts of cooked, enzyme deficient food, the body sees these heat-altered fats, proteins, and carbohydrates as stressors. The actual cooking process not only changes the chemical structure of the food, but also renders it of little nutritive value. Dr. Burkholder of Yale found that sprouted oats had 13 times more B2 content than raw oats and 100 more B2 content than cooked oats. A diet of high cooked food content can only sustain life but not regain or improve life and health. So how do the allergies occur? We eat the same cooked, enzyme deficient, nutrient deficient food day in and day out. This is why dairy products are the number 1 food allergy. We have consumed cooked (pasteurized) milk daily since we were babies. The solution lies in changing the diet to a high energy, high enzyme, high oxygen, high bioelectricity diet of living, raw foods that are animal product free (vegan). This is vegetables, sprouted grains, seeds, nuts, beans, and legumes. Also, rotating any cooked food in the diet so it is not eaten daily. What about the people that eat a piece of raw spinach and break out in hives? We must realize that not all reactions we experience are allergic in nature. Many times, when we eat raw, living foods and have this kind of reaction, it is nothing more that the enzymes from the food reacting in the body with some toxin or foreign material that has to be expelled. The enzymes in raw and living food actually cleanse and purify the body of unwanted debris and can throw it out through the skin as detoxifying reaction. So when you eat organic, living food and have a reaction, you might just be cleaning and detoxifying your body, so cut back the amounts and build up gradually.

Symptoms of food allergy/sensitivity

Food sensitivity is such a contributing factor in nearly all diseases and causes of ill health that the symptoms are numerous. They range from affecting every system, organ and gland of the body. Some of them are as follows:

Chronic tiredness, sluggishness, fatigue, inability to get up and get going in the morning even after having sufficient sleep. Also a fatigue in the mid to late afternoon. Mental dullness, tenseness, nervousness, restlessness, jitteriness, irritability, depression and anxiety. In children learning disabilities like attention deficit disorder (ADD) and hyperactivity can be traced to food allergies. Authorities feel that 95% of all migraine headaches are do to multiple food sensitivities. Headaches are a common manifestation of food allergy/ sensitivity. Neuromusculoskeletal complaints are common in food sensitivity most commonly back pain, joint pain, and arthritic pain. Skin disorders from eczema, various rashes even acne can be related to food sensitivity. Respiratory complaints are very common, with asthma, upper respiratory tract infections, bronchitis and sinus problems being most prevalent. Gastrointestinal symptoms are believed by some to be the most common manifestation of food allergy. These symptoms include looser bowel movements, bloating, abdominal cramping, increased intestinal gas, bad smelling gas and stools. High blood pressure can also be seen with food allergy

Common Food Allergens

Some of the most common foods people are sensitive to and should be tested for are:

Dairy products	Tomato
Wheat	Egg
Corn	Citrus
Soy	Legumes (peas, beans, peanut)
Seafood	Vinegar
Yeast	Spices

Whenever I am working with patients to restore their health, one of the first things I have done is a food sensitivity test. This way, I am assured that the food they are eating is adding to, not taking away from their health. Remember, if you are sensitive to just one of the above list (and you might have no obvious symptoms) with every meal you are causing a leaky gut to develop and are stressing your total health as well as your immune system. This is why it is so important to be tested, so you can start a plan for *total health* = *wholeness*. This plan begins with what goes into your mouth every meal. As Hippocrates once said, " Let food be your medicine" or as Dr. Victor Rocine said in the 1930's," If we eat wrongly no doctor can cure us, If we eat rightly, no doctor is needed."

What causes food sensitivities? They can be genetic. If one parent has food sensitivity, the child has a 50 percent chance of having it too; the number jumps to 75 percent if both parents have it.

Another cause of food sensitivity is overeating the same food too often. For example, most people drink cows milk daily their whole life. Not coincidentally, dairy products are the single greatest allergen, causing a wide variety of symptoms and diseases. The best way to prevent this kind of allergic response is to totally give the food up for 30 days, then slowly reintroduce it into your diet—starting off only once every two weeks, then progressing to possibly once every four days.

There are four types of testing done to determine or diagnose food sensitivity/allergy:

1. Skin tests in which a small amount of the suspected allergen is injected under the skin and then is checked for a reaction in the skin. According to Dr. Thrash,"Most food sensitivities are skin test negative; in other words, skin tests are not accurate for diagnosis of food sensitivities,"[7]

2. Radioallergosorbent testing (RAST) is designed to pick up the presence of IgE antibodies to each given allergen. "RAST is unreliable for testing for food allergies. It has been shown to produce approximately 20% false positives and 20% false negative results," according to Thrash M.D.[8] Also the RAST test is expensive, being about $12 per allergen tested so 40 allergens can cost up to $480.

3. Blood tests are only up to 25% accurate so are basically considered unreliable by most food allergists.[9]

4. Body reactive testing
        A. Pulse test
        B. Muscle test
        C. Body balancing test
        D. Elimination test

All of these are the simplest yet the most accurate ways of testing for food allergens because they produce a systemic body response to the allergen being tested.

Want to find out if you have got a particular food sensitivity? Then follow this schedule:

For one month, completely avoid a particular food, or anything containing that food. For example, if you want to find out if you are allergic to milk, you must avoid not only milk, but also cream, butter, cheese, yogurt, etc. You must read labels too; even a small amount of a dairy product will trigger the allergic antibody histamine response. After one month of abstinence, you can reintroduce the food and eat or drink it with each meal and see if your body produces any symptoms that it did not have for the time period you abstained from it.

There are two ways to monitor your sensitivity at home. First, you can check for any symptoms of sensitivity, like clearing your throat, mucous in your throat, stuffier nose, closing of nostril or runny nose, any noticeable change in breathing, any tightness in breathing (more difficult to completely inhale), any minor skin reaction or hive, any gastrointestinal problems (looser bowels, increased gas, stomach cramping or colic), headache, brain fog or cloudiness, lack of mental alertness, or any perceivable change that is not present before eating the food.

Another way to monitor sensitivity is with the pulse test, which is a bit more difficult to master. Take your resting pulse before eating the food you are reintroducing. Then eat only the food you are checking for sensitivity. Take your pulse right after eating, then at 20, 40 and 60 minutes. A drop or rise in pulse rate of 20 or more beats is indicative of possible food sensitivity.

There is another testing procedure, but it takes some skill in mastering: the applied kinesiology technique of muscle testing. After eating a single food to be tested, a previously tested strong muscle is tested again right after the food is chewed and put under the tongue. If the strong muscle goes weak, it is an indication of food sensitivity. For example, you could stand and hold your arm straight out in front of you testing the anterior deltoid muscle. After eating the food, the tester applies moderate pressure to your arm, checking to see if the muscle weakens or feels spongy, rather than the firm feeling a normal strong muscle has. The weakness indicates possible body irritation or sensitivity. I discovered another way to test my patients that is very accurate and is not dependent upon the patient's subjective response as in the prior muscle testing. With this technique I test the body for postural balance after each food is placed on the body in the form of an electromagnetically charged small tube that has the same electric nature of the allergen itself. I have tested people who have spent $800 on blood tests to find they apparently have no food allergies, but when I tested them they showed multiple sensitivities, especially to dairy products, wheat, yeast, etc.

At the Institute, we do a food sensitivity test to determine what to limit the diet to. Then 30 days later, we do another one to see what we can reintroduce into the diet. If a person still shows sensitivity to dairy products after 30 days of abstinence, then dairy is and never will be a good food for their total health.

Upon rechecking if you are not showing sensitivity after the first time eating, then you gradually reintroduce the food first after 30 days, then after 14 days, seven days, and then four days. Usually a person can go back to eating the food between once every week to once every four days, but not on a daily basis.

Another way to check for food sensitivities is the elimination diet, which is similar to the procedure described above, but much more rigid. This is for those who have either multiple sensitivities or are just having a difficulty pinpointing the offending food. In this diet, recommended for adults only, you eliminate all food for 3 days, drinking nothing but purified or distilled water. This gives your body a chance to clear itself of all allergens. Then reintroduce only one food only per day and check by one or more of the testing methods described. Keep a record of each food eaten each day, adding one food per day until you find a sensitivity. Make a list of the offending foods, and keep them out of your diet. When you find a food you are sensitive to, wait three days to give your body time to clear the offending food. (Note: If beginning this test with a 3-day fast seems too extreme, you can modify it by eating a food known to not cause symptoms, like brown rice. Once you have eaten just brown rice for five days with no allergic reactions, you can begin reintroducing other foods.

If you find that you have sensitivities to certain foods, you do not necessarily have to completely eliminate them from your diet. You can lessen their damaging impact by going on a rotation diet, in which you eat the "offending" foods only once every four to seven days. Dr. Marshall Mandell thinks a rotation diet done properly will eventually allow a person to eat 50 to 70 percent of foods he is sensitive to.[10] In the rotation diet, list all known food sensitivities and eliminate those from your diet for at least a month. Then write down a 7-day menu, planning only one sensitive food per meal and eating that same sensitive food only every four to seven days. When you plan your meals, avoid foods in the same family—for example, legumes (beans, peanuts, peas, and soy.) In other words, if you have pinto beans for lunch on Day 1, wait 4-7 days before testing another legume, like green beans.

We've used this method in my home. When my son started having very bad headaches, we learned that he was sensitive to soy, which he had been eating two or more times a day. So we kept him off soy for a month and rechecked him; he was no longer sensitive to soy and his headaches were just about gone. So we reintroduced soy once a week, and tested him; he was fine on this schedule. So we gave him more soy after four days and again tested him; he still tested clear, so he was allowed to have soy protein once every four days. A while later, we got a little careless with this, and he started eating soy 2-3 times per week—and soon his headaches were as bad as ever. So this all reinforced to my wife and I that diet and food sensitivity play a big role in our *total health = wholeness*.

The rotation diet is good even if you don't have any known food sensitivities, because it prevents them from occurring. If you've been eating cornflakes for breakfast every day for years, it's time to make a change: Cornflakes one day, oatmeal the next, rice cereal the next, and cream of wheat the next, a four-day cycle. Then start again with the cornflakes. Try to rotate all foods in your diet. This will help prevent food sensitivities/allergies and leaky gut.

To review this chapter:

1) Leaky gut comes from food allergies/sensitivities, parasites, virus, bacteria, poor diet, stress, heavy metals, ethanol and drugs.

2) Leaky gut causes toxicity, which can cause disease processes from cancer to multiple sclerosis, from weakened immune systems to development of cardiovascular disease, from mental dullness to arthritic pain. Toxicity will be the plague of the century and will be the cause of nearly all disease, and leaky gut is the biggest cause of toxicity.

3) Food sensitivity can be tested by increase in symptoms, by the pulse test, by muscle testing or by the body balancing technique.

4) A rotation diet, an elimination diet, or a combination of the two can control food sensitivity.

Questions and Answers

How do I heal a Leaky Gut?

Go step by step through the 17 causes of leaky gut and correct each cause. For example, do not eat food that you are sensitive to, reduce your stress levels, stop drinking alcohol, take only medications that are absolutely necessary, watch your diet for chemicals and toxins, combine your food properly, chew your food at least 25 times per bite, don't eat too much at one meal, don't drink with meals, take dophilus and bifidus bacteria for a healthy digestive tract, to name a few. When every one of the 17 causes of leaky gut is corrected, your chance of having a one is minimal.

Why have I never heard of "Leaky Gut" before, and why hasn't my MD ever mentioned this in my health care?

That is a great question. It has been in the medical literature for many years. To quote a few of their abstract research articles:

- A short review of the relationship between intestinal permeability and inflammatory joint disease (Clinical and Experimental Rheumatology 3:75-83, 1990)
- The Leaky Gut of Alcoholism: Possible Route of Entry For Toxic Compounds (Lancet, Jan 28, 1984)

Even as far back as 1893 an article in the *Journal of the American Medical Association* (JAMA) stated how important bowel health is in overall health and the prevention of disease:

> "The morbid influence of habitual constipation on an organism, otherwise healthy, is an interesting study, but easily understood. The fecal mass having traveled down through the long digestive conduit, finally subsides into the colon and rectum in a complete state of decomposition - a mass of ptomaines to be seized by the active absorbents of these receptacles and thrown back into the general circulation, poisoning tissues where ever they go and defying the liver, kidneys or any other emunctory to cast them out of the system. Congestions, inflammations, abscesses and all the catalogue of pathological complications are liable to ensue. Most likely a large majority of chronic diseases take their origin from this cause...." (*JAMA* 1893:20:559-600.)

Can children get a leaky gut?

Yes, very much so. I have checked young children and found that the intestinal tract is the first body system that starts to break down, this then starts the path to ill health later on in life.

Can children be checked for food sensitivity by these methods you just described?

Yes and no. Yes, if you use wisdom and use what can be done within the child's boundaries. You can do a pulse test, muscle test, or most easily, a body-balancing test. But you cannot have a child fast on just water for 3 days. Principles of the rotation and elimination diet will benefit a child with food sensitivities.

CHAPTER 14
ELIMINATIVE HEALTH

One of the greatest principles of physical health is "GET THE GOOD IN and GET THE BAD OUT."

Up to this point, we have talked about nutritional, digestive, and assimilative health—all means of "getting the good in." The 90-plus nutrients needed for optimal health were discussed, and these chapters talked about all phases of getting the necessary nutrients into the cells that need them.

Now we will address getting rid of toxins in our bodies—"getting the bad out." The bowel is the key to health, and if bowel health is not maintained, then inflammation leads to leaky gut, which leads to toxicity, which eventually leads to declining health and sickness.

In 1994, the colon-rectal cancer was the No. 1 cancer for men and women as a combined group. Why? Some reasons are obvious. Stressful lifestyle. Poor nutritional health. Poor digestive health. Poor assimilative health. Poor eliminatory health. Lack of exercise. Intake of refined sugar, animal fat and processed food. Not enough fiber, and high levels of non-manageable stress. It all adds up to a gastrointestinal health crisis, which leads to a total health crisis.

We've already established leaky gut as a major cause of toxicity and sickness—the opposite of the wholeness which God gave us. One of the most common causes of leaky gut is constipation. Many people don't think they have this problem; they say, "I go every day." But some of the world's most healthy primitive tribes move their bowels 2-3 times a day with no straining or effort. Their bowel matter is loose, easily passed and fully digested. That's quite a difference from the average American, who moves his bowels between once a day to once a week. And for most Americans, there's too much effort used to eliminate this material. After all the energy is put forth, the end result is either a) a very hard mass that appears to be wrapped in cellophane, b) one that resembles multiple pea- and marble-shaped pellets, or c) a solid, low-water content stool which is hard to pass.

What's the difference between the optimal health of primitive tribes and the average American? The tribes have a primarily vegetarian diet, lots of exercise (10-12 hours per day), and much less stress. We have learned that to be normal in bowel health, you should have one bowel movement after every meal, none of them being the slightest bit hard, or wrapped, or marble-like.

Here's a closer look at the bowel:

As food goes down the intestinal tract, nutrients are being absorbed and if a leaky gut is present (see Chapter 13) toxins are also being absorbed. Eventually, the food arrives at the rectum. Then you try to move your bowels, but they don't want to move because of a backup similar to a traffic jam, which results from not moving your bowels with each meal. As pressure and backup build up, fecal material is pushed from inside the lumen into the diverticula, or bowel pockets. Even a person who has 2-3 bowel movements per day may still have a lot of old toxic fecal material stored in these bowel pockets. This same person can go to a gastroenterologist, have a complete enema program before a lower GI series, and hear the doctor say it's all OK—when in fact, they have pounds of old fecal material stuck in them. The average person is walking around with 7-21 pounds of impacted fecal material inside of them and their diverticula, causing resorption of this toxic matter. There have been autopsies of patients who had three bowel movements a day, but still retained 40 pounds of impacted fecal material. This is a result of the narrowing of the bowel lumen and diverticulosis, which causes many bowel movements but narrower, longer, fecal material.

The Merck Manual, the medical standard text for diagnosis and treatment of disease, includes some information about these filled bowel pockets, or saccular herniations, that protrude through the wall of the colon. The incidence of diverticulosis (filled bowel pockets) has been steadily rising over the last 40 years. The manual states that in 1950, 10 percent of adults over age 45 had this disease; in 1955, 15 percent; in 1972, 30 percent; and in 1987, almost 50 percent. The 1996 edition of the manual states that the incidence increases rapidly over the age of 40, and that every adult in this country will have enlarged/filled bowel pockets or diverticulosis. (see chart next page).

To combat this escalating problem, we need to clean, stimulate and tone all the organs of elimination, starting with the bowel. How do you know if you have a bowel problem? Let me say it simply and clearly: You do. The question is how bad is it?

See how do you do on this checklist of optimal bowel health:

Incidence of Diverticulosis
in adults over the age of 45

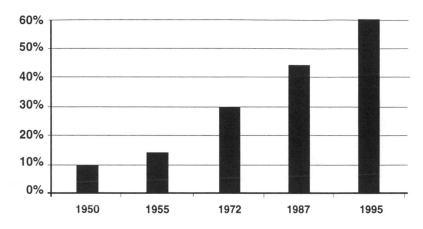

1) I have a bowel movement after every meal, two to three times per day.
2) My bowel movements are normal, soft, formed, and easily passed without effort.
3) I am on the toilet no longer than 5 minutes during bowel movements.
4) My feces are formed and soft. It doesn't discolor the water when flushing. It isn't marble-like or hard, nor does it appear to be wrapped in cellophane.
5) I don't see undigested food and mucous-like material in the toilet bowl.
6) The bathroom does not have a bad odor when I leave it.
7) I don't feel cramped or colic when it is time to have a bowel movement.
8) I have never eaten meat, chicken, fish, or other parasite containing foods.
9) I have had a recent food sensitivity test to know what foods are irritants or inflammatory forming for my intestinal tract, and I have eliminated all these stresses from my diet.
10) I have never been on antibiotic therapy.
11) I do not ever get constipated or diarrhea.
12) I have not had a cold or flu in the last three months.

13) I do not get more than one cold per year.
14) I chew my food 25 times per bite.
15) I take vegetable-based digestive enzymes with each meal.
16) I do regular enema or other bowel cleanse programs at least four times per year.
17) I eat fiber food with every meal vegetables, sprouts, and whole grains.)
18) I don't eat processed, refined food, or starches.

Dr. John Kellogg, at the Battle Creek Sanitarium in the earlier part of this century, said that 90 percent of the diseases of civilization are due to improper functioning of the colon. Dr. Kellogg thought everyone should eliminate the residual contents of a meal 15-18 hours after eating it; if you aren't passing the residual contents within 15-18 hours, you're constipated.

How can you tell if you're constipated? Take the corn test. Eat corn along with a meal, noting the starting time you ate it. Examine each of your bowel movements until corn is visible and write down the time of day. **Don't stop timing yourself until you cannot find any more corn in your fecal material. When this occurs write down the time of the previous bowel movement when corn was seen, this is the finish time. The starting time to the finish time is called your bowel transit time.** This will tell you how long it took to move through your system. If it's more than 18 hours, you're constipated, even if you have three bowel movements per day.

If you eat three times a day but only move your bowels once a day, there will be a backup, causing diverticulosis or bowel pockets. The backup forms pressure, which causes the lining of the bowel to herniate, or push through. If these diverticula are filled with fecal material, they do not pass it because it is not a movement pattern of the normal bowel peristalsis. It's sort of like a creek of running water, with little inlets along the edges of the creek. Leaves and branches flow into the inlets and get stuck there, because they're out of the creek's normal flow pattern.

Once these bowel pockets form and fecal material sit in you for days, weeks, months and years, you have a slow release of toxins, poisons and inflammation of the colon, causing leaky gut.

The longer it takes to have a bowel movement, the worse the problem gets. For example, if one has a bowel movement every two days, that's six or more meals being stored in the colon, causing back pressure, forcing fecal material into the diverticula causing diverticulosis. Eventually this causes overstretching of the bowel muscular lining, damaging muscles and their tone. This can become disastrous, if a person is regularly constipated. In this case, diverticulosis can lead to overstretching of the bowel lining, which can lead to an atonic bowel, or one that no longer has normal muscular peristalsis movement. This results in the inability to ever move the bowel normally without enemas. Needless to say, this person will always be toxic and will struggle greatly with their health.

Just a short note on the "itises" of the bowel, diverticulitis and colitis. The suffix -itis means inflammation, so these are inflammations of the bowel pockets and of the colon in general.

The list of things that cause inflammation is a long one:
- constipation
- poor diet (refined, processed, high protein, high fat, alcohol, coffee)
- food sensitive
- poor food combination
- poor digestion
- lack of proper chewing
- lack of digestive enzymes
- lack of HCl
- diluted digestive (with water) enzymes
- poor assimilation
- bacteria, virus, parasites or candida
- stress
- fear, depression
- anger, worry
- bowel nerve pressure
- structural subluxation of lower back
- lack of exercise
- lack of proper water intake (1 quart per 50 lbs. of body weight per day - not with meals)
- medications

Colitis and diverticulitis cause a leaky gut and toxicity, as well as alternating diarrhea and constipation. We've already discussed some results of constipation; diarrhea, on the other hand, causes malnutrition, because your body never assimilates what it needs to sustain good health—the 90-

plus nutrients needed daily. Without them, your body soon becomes tired and weaker, and sickness can set in.

Colitis, diverticulitis, and constipation can all cause the mucous lining of the bowel to become inflamed and damaged. This causes lack of normal mucous lubrication of the bowel and eventual thickening, which in turn causes more constipation and the possible formation of scar tissue and strictures. These cause permanent narrowing of the normal bowel in particular areas and in turn also leads to further backup and constipation.

I hope and pray you now understand that bowel health is one of the most important aspects of your total physical health picture. An abnormally functioning bowel will always lead to toxicity, which will eventually lead to disease.

If you could only detox one part of your body, it would be the bowel. And if this is all one detoxifies, 60 percent of people would be healed or greatly improved.

A bowel cleanse program will regularly purify your bowel. I recommend bowel cleansing at least every three months for healthy people, and more frequently for those trying to restore their health. Bowel cleansing programs include organic/wildcrafted herbs and possible high enemas. The herb program is easy and very effective, not only in getting rid of constipation, but also in ridding bacteria, yeast, parasites, as well as resorbing the impacted fecal material and its poisons, toxins and even radioactive materials. Bowel cleanse programs also helps tone and heal the bowel. The healing herbs for the bowel include:

HERB	USE
Aloe	Increases bowel peristalsis (increases bowel movements either quantity or frequency)
Cascara Sagrada	Same as above
Senna	Same as above
Garlic	Anti-parasite, fungal, bacterial, viral
Barberry	Liver and bile stimulant
Cayenne	Stimulant to bowel peristalsis, tones bowel, stops bleeding
Ginger	Digestive aid, anti-nausea
Psyllium	Laxitive
Flax	Lubricant, laxative

Activated Willow	
Charcoal	Absorbs chemicals, toxins
Bentonite Clay	removes 40 times its weight
Apple Pectin	Draws out heavy metals and radioactivity
Fennel	Digestive aid, soothing
Slippery Elm	Laxative, stool softener
Marshmallow	Demulcent

Once the bowel is deeply cleansed with the 2 week program, the bowel is maintained with a daily cleansing and maintenance program, capsules taken daily.(see appendix)

People who have inflammatory bowel problems (colitis, diverticulitis, Chron's disease, spastic colon) would only do the second half of our bowel cleanse program, since constipation usually isn't a problem, but diarrhea is. So we have to slow the bowel, heal the linings and resorb toxins, poisons or inflammatory byproducts that are contributing to the condition. I would like to briefly mention what lives in your intestinal tract. There are four main organisms:

1) Beneficial bacteria called bifidus and dophilus bacteria which are extremely important to good bowel health, because they help digest cellulose and produce the following vitamins: B12, thiamin, riboflavin and K.
2) Pathogenic bacteria which if overgrown cause intestinal lining inflammation (leaky gut).
3) Candida, which also can cause leaky gut syndrome if not, held in check by the beneficial bacteria.
4) Parasites, which always present a health hazard if not held in check by a strong immune system. One way to help maintain a healthy bowel is to supplement your diet with bifidus and dophilus bacteria along with fructoligosaccaride (FOS). FOS is a type of sugar that comes from fruits and vegetables that specifically encourages growth of only the beneficial bacteria whereas the pathogenic bacteria and candida cannot exist on it. In her book, The Cure For All Cancers, Dr. Hulda Clark says that parasites are the cause of all cancer. She documents 100 case histories of cancer cures using a program to eliminate parasites from the body. Whether or not parasites are the only

cause of cancer could be debated but it cannot be denied that they do pose a health hazard and should be treated as such. I recommend getting rid of parasites (de-worming) twice a year with an anti- parasite herbal program made up of the following herbs:

1. Garlic -will kill anything that isn't suppose to be in your intestinal tract.
2. Wormwood
3. Black Walnut
4. Pumpkin
5. Lavender flower
6. Grapefruit seed
7. Black Currant
8. Olive leaf
9. Cramp bark

Detoxing the bowel is only one part, but a vital part, of *total health = wholeness*. The best way to correct bowel problems is to correct all areas of total health that we have discussed thus far:

Nutritional Health
- SupremeFood
- 90-plus essential nutrients
- no refined sugar
- low fat
- low protein
- no alcohol, coffee, caffeine
- drink 1 quart of water per 50 lbs. of body weight every day (not with meals)
- eat raw vegetables and sprouts
- high fiber (have to ease into this if you have inflammatory bowel)

Digestive Health
- mastication (chew food 25 times)
- proper HCl amount in stomach
- take digestive vegetable enzymes
- combine food properly

Assimilative Health
- decrease all causes of leaky gut
- do not eat foods you are sensitive to

Eliminative Health
- cleanse bowel four times per year minimum
- structural alignment (spinal manipulation to remove nerve pressure to the bowel)
- maintain normal bowel flora (acidophilus, bifidus, FOS)
- a parasite program twice a year

Mental Health
- address stress, fear, worry, anxiety, depression
- walk in God's love, joy and peace

Spiritual Health
- the Spirit gives life
- remember the flow of wholeness: spirit >mind> body

LIVER/GALL BLADDER

Our next step in "getting the bad out" is liver/gall bladder cleansing.

After the bowel, the liver is the next most important organ to cleanse or detoxify. The liver is truly amazing; it is your body's own detoxifying organ. It daily prevents death by changing every chemical, toxin or drug that circulates through your body into non-toxic byproducts, which are excreted in the bile out into the intestinal tract, enabling you to get the bad out regularly. For example, when you drink a can of diet pop with Nutrasweet, your liver changes the aspartame (the sweetener in Nutrasweet) into a nontoxic chemical to be removed via bile into the small intestinal tract.

The liver does this for everything you breathe, drink, or eat. All chemicals, toxins and medications must be detoxified by the liver, or they would cause you great harm. Air pollution, chemicals like fluoride and chlorine in water, and of course all the toxins in food—all of it has to be broken down by the liver. The problem arises when too many of these chemicals and toxins enter our body. The liver is already working hard enough to keep chemicals and byproducts made inside the body from making the body toxic. When we pour in more chemicals and toxins from the outside, the liver can get overworked.

Chemicals and toxins to be detoxified are either exogenous (from outside the body) or endogenous (by product of cellular metabolism from inside the body.) Adam and Eve's livers just had to deal with endogenous chemicals, because they lived in a pure world. But today, our liver must work double-time, working equally hard on both exogenous and endogenous toxins and chemicals. The end result is toxic buildup in the blood, because the liver simply cannot do it all.

We've illustrated this principle with the image of an air filter in a closed room with a fire in the fireplace. If the flue is partially closed, the air filter can do its job and clear the room of any smoke. But if the flue is closed completely, the air filter can't keep up with the demand, and the room will remain full of smoke. In this illustration, the original smoke in the room represents the regular endogenous cellular byproducts of metabolism that must be purified daily to keep you healthy. The added smoke resulting from the closed flue represents the exogenous toxins and chemicals from this world which cannot be cleared.

So we need our livers to get the bad out, to get rid of the smoke, so to speak. This is the purpose of the liver detoxification program, which essentially opens the door and windows and lets all the smoke out so you can start clean and fresh—this time without adding more smoke to the room.

Remember that your liver was designed to handle the endogenous load, but not the exogenous load of today's environment. Because our environment is toxic, our liver becomes overburdened and toxic. Unfortunately, we can't get rid of all exogenous toxins by modifying our environment, because the air around us is loaded with chemicals and pollutants. But we can choose foods and water that will reduce the toxic overload on our livers. We can choose preservative-free, pesticide-free and herbicide-free organic food. We can choose distilled water or reverse osmosis water, as opposed to tap water. Every bit helps to keep your liver working properly and prevent internal toxicity.

Without your liver, you would die immediately. People with colon/rectal cancer have a better survival rate than people with liver cancer, because you can live without a colon, but not without your liver. Liver cancer prevents the liver from functioning properly, resulting in toxic and chemical overload on your body and, ultimately, death.

Many components are helpful for toxins to be neutralized for excretion.
They are

1) Silymarin (milk thistle), a powerful herb that is very liver protective and is a liver-specific antioxidant, meaning it helps liver cells live longer and break down less due to the oxidizing effect of detoxification, which is very corrosive to the liver.

2) Cruciferous vegetables (broccoli, brussel sprouts, cauliflower, cabbage) contain sulfur, which supports liver detoxification

3) Alpha linolenic acid, which is found in flax seed oil, from the omega three-fatty acid family.

4) Vitamin C and bioflavonoids found in red and green peppers, powerful antioxidants that help protect the liver against oxidative damage.

5) Vitamin E, from whole grains, which improves the liver's oxygen radical detoxification system.

6) Beta-carotene (carrots, yams), which aid the liver's antioxidant properties.

7) Trace minerals, such as zinc, copper and manganese (seeds, nuts).

What can you do to help your liver?

1) Detoxify the liver 2-4 times a year (see liver detox program in appendix).

2) Stay on Liver Maintenance Program (see appendix) which include the following herbs, organic milk thistle, a liver protectant along with other liver
specific herbs: chaparral - a strong detoxifier and antioxidant, dandelion - a liver tonic, barberry, gentian, oregon grape - bile flow stimulants.

3) Eat as many organic vegetables as possible, especially greens like broccoli, dandelion, kale, collards, cauliflower, brussels sprouts, cabbage and carrots.

4) Do not eat foods that are artificial or have preservatives.

5) Drink and cook with distilled or reverse osmosis water only.

6) Have plenty of food-source antioxidants in your diet, like Vitamins E, C and A, all of which are found in SupremeFood. Vitamin E is also found in whole grains, seeds, Vitamin C in green and red peppers and citrus fruit, and Vitamin A in carrots and yams.

7) Don't breathe chemical fumes; keep windows open.

8) Exercise regularly, especially rebounding celular exercise; this circulates and detoxifies the blood quicker.

9) Reduce structural misalignments (via spinal manipulation) which cause nerve pressure to liver and decrease liver function.

10) Reduce mental stress; this flows from spiritual health and stress reduction techniques (Mental Health chapter). When we live in the love of God, it brings us joy and peace.

11) Spiritual health gives you God's love, joy and peace.

After one of my patients went through our bowel and liver detox program for some long-standing health problems, she came into my office amazed, saying, "I can't believe how great I feel. I haven't felt like this in years!"

Her statement says it all. Remember GET THE GOOD IN, GET THE BAD OUT.

KIDNEY/BLADDER DETOXIFICATION

The kidney and bladder area, which also accumulates toxins, must also be cleansed.

Our kidneys are our blood and fluid filters. Kidney function is critical to good health and serve five functions[2]:

1. Regulation of body fluid volume
2. Regulation of electrolyte balance
3. Regulation of acid-base balance
4. Excretion of metabolic products and foreign substances
5. Production and secretion of hormones

More than 150 quarts of fluid, including blood, pass through the kidneys daily. Thankfully, God gave us two kidneys to do the job; one kidney alone could do the job if toxins aren't stored there.

The kidney picks up where the liver leaves off. The liver, as you remember, changes harmful chemicals, toxins and drugs into harmless waste products to be excreted. Some of this nontoxic waste product enters the blood stream and is brought to the kidneys, where it is filtered out of the blood and excreted in the form of urine. Without proper kidney filtration, blood urea levels rise (metabolic byproduct), and toxin and chemical levels rise (foreign substances), eventually becoming lethal.

Think of the illustration of the air filter in the smoke-filled room. If you shut off the filter, smoke would continue pouring into the room—symbolizing regular cellular metabolism byproducts—eventually causing sickness, disease and even death. Another illustration is that of a fish tank. Regularly fed fish regularly excrete waste products, which pollute water with bacteria and chemicals; without a water filter, the fish would eventually die.

People who have kidney failure can still survive with kidney dialysis—a complex machine that filters blood. A person is usually hooked up to this machine three times a week, 6-8 hours at a time. These people are on very restricted diets and are not allowed to drink very much, because they cannot produce and excrete urine.

The biggest threats to your kidneys are:

1) Toxins or poisons (both endogenous and exogenous) circulating in the blood stream, eventually ending up in the kidney. They must be filtered out, or the kidney will eventually stop functioning.

2) Bacterial infections, like Group A Beta Hemolytic strep from sore throats, or skin infection and other general infection.

3) Stone formation, which causes inflammation, ischemia and even cell death. The primary cause of kidney stones is the high-protein diet of average Americans. When digested and metabolized, protein leaves an acid ash residue in the body. This acidic residue leaches calcium out of the bones to help normalize the pH of the body. The calcium circulates and eventually is deposited into the kidney, building up over years until the kidney excretory function is blocked. Then the uric acid level rises, the blood urea nitrogen goes up, and the body becomes very toxic, very quickly. A person in this condition experiences pain ranging from general lower back pain to extremely intense back pain with nausea and vomiting. By the time a person reaches this point, his kidney has probably been malfunctioning for many years.

How do you keep your kidneys healthy?

1) Drink one quart (32oz) of distilled water per 50 lbs. of body weight per day. Distilled water, essential for detoxification, is the purest of water, and pure water is best for washing toxins, chemicals, salts and stone formations out of the body. The more distilled water you drink, the more harmful or potentially harmful toxins, uric acid crystals, phosphates, oxalates, and other debris are washed away.

2) Drink fresh vegetable juices, which are high in potassium and are very detoxifying. Most people who become ill have a high sodium-to-potassium ratio, because their diet includes processed foods and heavily salted foods for flavor and taste. Potassium, on the other hand, is abundant in fresh fruits and vegetables, which the average American eats too little of. Vegetable juices are not only loaded with vitamins, minerals and enzymes, but also potassium, which is very detoxifying and cleansing. In juice fasting, a person can lose a tremendous amount of water weight, because a higher sodium ratio tends to make you retain fluid to try to dilute the sodium. When you balance the potassium-to-sodium ratio, your tissues no longer need to retain fluid for osmotic balance, so they release all the stored water. As a result, blood pressure comes down, weight goes down, and total health increases.

3) Detox your kidneys four times a year for good health, more often if you are ill. The herbs in the kidney detox program are God's medicine: "The fruit shall be your food and the leaf your medicine." (Ezekiel 47:12)These herbs are taken in tea, and tincture form (see appendix for program). Herbs should be organic if possible, and if not, then wildcrafted. "Organic" means no chemicals have been applied to them or their soil for seven years (California Organic Food Act). "Wildcrafted" means the herbs have been collected in natural settings, growing wild away from the chemicals of cities.

The medicinal herbs used and their primary functions are listed below.

HERB NAME	PRIMARY USE
Juniper berries	Diuretic, disinfectant
Corn silk	Diuretic
Uva ursi	Diuretic, mild disinfectant
Horsetail	Diuretic
Burdock root, leaf	Diuretic
Parsley root, leaf	Diuretic, disinfectant

4) Drink pure cranberry juice or take cranberry juice concentrate pills with water. This doesn't mean the cranberry drink or cocktail sold at the grocery store; those are mostly refined sugar in water with very little cranberry juice added. Pure cranberry juice is very strong and is not sweet, but remember, **do we eat to live or live to eat?** Drink this daily if you have had, or are trying to prevent problems of the urinary tract—including kidneys, bladder and urethra. Cranberry juice is the only juice that stays slightly acidic from time of ingestion to time of excretion, thus it helps dissolve stones and crystals. It also decreases bacteria's ability to adhere to and grow inside the bladder and urethra. I have had many patients with bladder infections who were healed—without antibiotics—after taking high dosages of cranberry juice and other immune-stimulating herbs.

5) If you have a fat-malabsorption problem, decrease foods containing oxalate. Some foods containing oxalates are very healthy and should not be avoided, unless you have a problem with fat digestion and absorption. Fat can bind to calcium, which usually binds to oxalate, which can form oxalate crystals and eventually kidney stones.

High oxalate foods include chocolate, eggplant, black tea, spinach, okra, beets, mustard greens, and baked beans with tomato sauce. But remember: Do not avoid spinach, mustard greens, beets, eggplant and okra unless you have a significant problem with fat malabsorption.

BLOOD

Finally, we need to cleanse our blood to keep it from circulating toxins, chemicals and drugs. Your life is in your blood, because without it, no life can exist for more than a few minutes. Blood is the major transportation system of your body, the highway by which all cells are nourished with oxygen, vitamins, minerals, enzymes and phytochemicals. Blood is also the way we get rid of waste products of cellular metabolism (endogenous toxins), and chemicals, drugs and toxins from exogenous sources. Blood carries chemical, toxins, drugs, and other harmful substances to the filtration systems of the liver and kidneys. Blood also transports WBCs, which fight off infections from bacteria, virus, fungi and parasites, and which consume abnormal cancer cells in the body.

Blood is frequently mentioned in Scripture, where it is always equated with life. Blood is the symbol of both the old and new covenants. In the old covenant, animals were sacrificed to show that this covenant was made for life; the shed blood of the animals was meant to be a payment for the sins of the people. In the new covenant, when Jesus Christ shed His blood for us, the blood served two purposes. First, it paid the price for the sin of the world for past, present, and future, because Jesus was the pure, sinless Lamb of God who truly did take away the sin of the world. Second, the shedding of Jesus' blood established the new covenant between God and all of mankind. His shed blood means those who believe can be forgiven of their sins, because "without the shedding of blood, there is no forgiveness." (Hebrews 9:22)

Obviously, life—*both physically and spiritually*—is in the blood.

Unfortunately, many problems can arise in the blood, including:
1) Inability to carry oxygen
2) Inability to circulate oxygen and food to needed areas
3) Inability to fight off bacteria, virus, fungi, parasites, and abnormal cancer cells
4) Inability to clear or purify toxins, chemicals, and drugs

Blood's inability to carry oxygen occurs commonly with certain mineral and vitamin deficiencies, especially iron and Vitamin B_{12}. This causes either abnormal red blood cells (RBCs), which cannot carry oxygen properly, or a lack in production of new RBCs. An RBC's average life span is 90 days. Abnormal RBCs can also result from various diseases, sickle cell anemia and many other anemia disorders.

Blood's inability to circulate oxygen and food to needed areas occurs in certain diseases (like sickle cell anemia) where the RBC becomes sickle-shaped instead of spherical in shape. This causes poor blood circulation through all the small capillaries. The RBCs get caught and cause cellular hypoxia (lack of oxygen) and then cellular death.

High blood cholesterol and fat also commonly cause this. Fat and cholesterol cause coating and narrowing of blood vessels, decreasing movement of red and white blood cells along with all other vital nutrients. If you had to put a fire out, which works better: A fire hose or a garden hose? The fire hose does, because it is at least 15 times the diameter of the garden hose, allowing more water to come out. We want our blood vessels the same way—clean and with the largest diameter possible, so blood cells can move quickly and freely. The more fat we consume, the more sludging or sticking of the red and white blood cells. And the slower RBCs move, the less oxygen, food, vitamins and minerals can get to the needed cells. And the slower WBCs move, the less they can fight infection from bacteria, virus, fungi, parasites, and the less they can patrol to eat cancer cells. So, the lower the fat in the blood, the better the circulation of red and white blood cells.

A meal high in fat content causes clumping of the RBCs which, after several hours, reduces the overall oxygen supply to the body by 20 percent. It takes approximately 12 hours after the meal for blood flow to return to normal[3]. Many people eat fat in all three meals, causing the body to continuously run on only 80 percent of the normal oxygen supply. This can cause major problems, because the ability of RBCs and WBCs to do their job has been reduced by 20 percent.

The greatest threats to blood's vital function are:
1) High animal fat diet
2) Vitamin and mineral deficiencies
3) Toxic buildup of toxins, chemicals, and drugs
4) Diseases of the blood, often triggered by a move away from normal homeostasis (body balance), which is usually a result of toxic buildup

As you can see, good blood circulation is vital to our health. This is why a fever causes the rate of blood flow to increase exponentially. For every degree rise of body temperature, the speed of RBCs and WBCs doubles. So it is not health promoting for someone who is sick to take aspirin, Tylenol, or similar fever-reducing agents, unless the fever becomes uncontrollable with natural healing methods.

What can we do to keep our blood healthy?

1) Change to more of a vegan diet, avoiding as much animal fat as possible. You can have a small amount of quality vegetable oil or fat in only one meal per day (organic extra virgin olive oil). This will protect from constant blood cell sludging and a 20 percent decrease in total body circulation of essential nutrients, red and white blood cells.

2) Get all your essential nutrients for the day, including vitamins, minerals, essential fatty acid and amino acid. These nutrients should come from your food, not from synthetic (and potentially toxic) vitamin and mineral supplements. SupremeFood is ideal for this, because it has the essential nutrients in organic food form. It is not a vitamin or mineral supplement. It is food that God made which contains vitamins, minerals, enzymes, phytochemicals and the other essential nutrients. Take it the way God made it; that's always the best rule. Take your essential nutrients from whole organic food, and take your medicines from the plants and herbs that God created.

3) Reduce the amount of chemicals, toxins, and drugs going into your system, by breathing the purest air as possible. Avoid fumes and exhausts. Drink and cook with pure water, preferably distilled or reverse-osmosis filtered. Eat organic fruits, vegetables, sprouts, whole grains, seeds, nuts and beans. And eat them raw or uncooked and sprouted, to preserve enzymes, vitamins, minerals and phytochemicals, oxygen and bioelectricity. If you can't get organic produce, wash your fruits and vegetables with a non-toxic pesticide remover. Or soak them in organic apple cider vinegar and water. Also, take off the skins, which contain up to 50 percent of the pesticide residue. Avoid processed foods and those containing preservatives—chemicals that will make you more toxic. And remember that whatever touches your skin is absorbed into your blood stream within 30 seconds; you'll look at shampoos, conditioners, and hand-and-body lotions in a whole different way. Read the labels; if you can't eat it, think twice before putting it on your skin or hair.

4) Detoxify your blood 2-4 times per year. Our recommended blood detox program includes these herbs, including their primary functions (see appendix):

HERB	PRIMARY USE
Red clover	Detoxifies, thins the blood
Garlic	Thins, lowers blood pressure, anti-bacterial, antiviral, antifungal
Burdock	Detoxifies, diuretic, cleanses skin
Yellow dock	Detoxifies, iron source
Lobelia	Relaxes body to aid in detoxification
Cayenne	Circulates the blood
Chaparral	Detoxifies, antioxidant

Herbs are God's chosen medicine (Ezekiel 47:12.) So if we use organic wildcrafted herbs in the right combination with the right strengths, the desired effect will be achieved.

Now that we've discussed eliminatory health and the importance of detoxing each system, I would like to stress the importance of doing the detox program in the proper order. Without following the proper order, you risk feeling very ill and potentially hurting yourself.

1) Bowel cleanse

2) Liver/gall bladder cleanse

3) Kidney/bladder cleanse

4) Blood cleanse

Why this order? If you detox the blood before detoxing the liver, all the blood's toxins deposit in the liver, which is overworked and already filled with toxins. This can cause inflammation of the liver, which would reduce its normal functioning capacity, causing you to become more toxic instead of less toxic. The bowel is detoxed first because it is the worst of all areas, and also directly reduces liver overload. When it is cleansed, there are no more leaking bowel pockets to dump poisons into the blood, which goes directly to the liver from the intestinal tract. So keep the proper order of detoxification.

See appendix for more information on detoxification programs and products.

CHAPTER 15

CIRCULATIVE HEALTH

Circulation is movement of blood and lymph throughout the body. The primary organs of circulation are the heart, arteries, veins and lymph channels. With every heartbeat, blood is propelled with tremendous force to move fluid through thousands of miles of blood vessels and lymph vessels. It is truly amazing to know how awesome God created our bodies.

Blood's purpose is to carry essential nutrients, food, vitamins, minerals, phytochemicals and antioxidants to every one of the billions of cells that make up our body, and to get cellular waste products, toxins, chemicals and poisons out of our body.

Think of your blood vessels and lymph channels like highways, railroads and waterways. On our highways, trucks transport food, which includes the nutrients we need to live. Trucks take the food from farmers and bring it to grocery stores throughout the country, and the stores then distribute the food to the people in that area. While the trucks do their job transporting food, trains and barges do their part too in transporting necessary materials.

Now imagine if there was a fuel shortage. Not all grocery stores would receive the food needed for the people in their town. This would be like an iron-deficient anemia, where RBCs are not able to carry enough oxygen to the rest of the body.

Here's another analogy: Suppose there was a nationally imposed speed limit of 20 mph, slowing all traffic. Food and nutrients wouldn't get where needed in time, and the country could not survive. It's the same with poor circulation, which is caused by lack of exercise, out-of-shape heart and blood vessels, poor lymph movement due to improper breathing, lack of rebounding cellular exercise, cardiovascular disease, or high fat diets that cause sludging of the blood.

If the transportation system slows down or breaks down, the RBCs and WBCs cannot reach all points of the body. The WBCs, our soldiers to fight foreign invaders, would not be able to mobilize quickly enough. Waste products would not be removed quickly enough. Imagine local garbage trucks with a 5-mph speed limit: We would have a lot of putrid garbage building up in our neighborhoods, leading to sickness and disease. If our bodies don't remove waste products, toxins and chemicals, homeostasis is no longer maintained. As a result, our level of health will progressively drop—from optimal vital health (total health), to apparent health without symptoms (or suboptimal health), to subclinical with symptoms, to clinical findings with symptoms, to disease.

The Lymphatic System

The lymphatic system consists of lymphatic organs like the thymus gland, spleen, lymph nodes, tonsils, appendix and Peyers patches found in the small intestine.

The lymphatic system's **primary** function is to be the body's defense against bacteria, virus, fungi, parasites and abnormal cells like cancer. The lymphatic system and organs make WBCs called lymphocytes, which stop these invaders from taking over our bodies. Lymphocytes are circulated and stored in lymph nodes around the body, migrating through tissues and seeking to destroy any foreigner. Meanwhile, many WBCs circulate through the blood, constantly seeking to destroy foreigners as well.

The lymphatic system's **second** function is returning tissue fluid into blood vessels. Tissue fluid seeps out when blood goes into capillaries before returning to the veins and the heart. This fluid, known as lymph fluid, collects in lymph channels, which empty into larger and larger lymph vessels until they reach the thoracic duct. The lymph fluid then returns to the circulating blood via the jugular and subclavian vein junction in the neck (which the thoracic duct drains into.)

The **third** function of the lymphatic system is the filtration of bacteria, virus, fungi and parasites in the lymph nodes, which help prevent the spread of infection. The lymph nodes are growth-and-storage areas for WBCs, which consume bacteria or viruses in the lymph fluid, preventing the spread of infections. This explains why when you have a sore throat, your lymph nodes and your neck become enlarged: They are actively killing viruses and bacteria and preventing the spread of infection to other areas of the body. The lymphatic system is also critical in fighting and destroying cancer cells. So, swollen lymph nodes can indicate not only infection in the body, but perhaps even cancer.

The **fourth** function of the lymphatic system is to absorb fats from digestion via the lymph capillaries of the intestinal villa—microscopic finger-shaped absorption tissue.

FUNCTION GONE WRONG

The normal function of the circulation system can be altered by many factors. Here's a list of those factors, starting with the most predominant, in both the circulation of blood and in the circulation of lymph:

Blood
1.   Abnormal heart function
2.   Insufficient cardiovascular exercise
3.   Abnormal tissue/blood osmotic balance
4.   Abnormal vessel opening elasticity
5.   Abnormal RBC production
6.   Abnormal WBC production
7.   High fat diet

Lymph
Same list as above, plus:
8.   Shallow breathing
9.   Lack of rebounding cellular exercise
10.   Lack of cardiovascular exercise

Let's take a closer look at each *(see diagram next page)*:

1. Abnormal heart function is by far the worst cause of less-than-optimal movement of blood nutrients, RBCs, WBCs and lymph. These things just don't get around the body well enough if the heart loses some of its ability to pump blood with significant pressure. This can result from genetically inherited heart defects or birth defects, or acquired defects—like an enlarged heart, and its decreased ability to pump blood properly. Post-heart-attack patients also suffer from abnormal heart function.

2. Insufficient cardiovascular exercise is a problem for many of us. The heart and blood vessels are made of muscle, and muscle must be exercised to stay strong and efficient. The minimal amount of cardiovascular exercise needed for good health is 30 minutes of aerobic exercise (elevated, sustained heart rate), three times per week; daily is preferable for good health. Also, exercise moves blood faster, causing your body's cells to get the oxygen and nutrients they need faster—and to get rid of waste products faster. And since blood is detoxified and filtered through the liver and kidneys, it makes sense to keep your blood moving.

3. Abnormal tissue/blood osmotic balance. A normal balance of sodium-to-potassium affects the amounts of fluid in the blood stream, in tissue

Healthy vs. Diseased Tissue
caused by Excess Fluid Buildup in the Interstitial Spaces between the Cells

---

Blood Capillary

Cell	Cell	Cell	Cell
Cell	Cell	Cell	Cell
Cell	Cell	Cell	Cell
Cell	Cell	Cell	Cell

Cell	Cell	Cell
Interstitial Fluid		
Cell	Cell	Cell
Cell	Cell	Cell

Lymphatic Capillary

Total Cell Health	Tissue Dysfunction/ Disease
No Interstitial Fluid between Cells	Increased Interstitial Fluid between Cells

outside of the blood vessels, and in the cells themselves. This balance can be negatively affected by high sodium (salt) intake, low potassium intake, and the leaking of blood protein into tissues without enough lymphatic drainage back into the bloodstream. High sodium intake causes tissue spaces around cells to fill with fluid, when they should normally have no fluid. This fluid increase causes more blood proteins to enter the tissue spaces, forcing still more fluid there because fluids follow blood protein. If the lymphatic system doesn't move blood proteins and fluid out quickly, tissues remain swollen and cells start to die because the oxygen and nutrients cannot get to the cells. (See Chart)

4. Abnormal vessel opening elasticity. As blood vessels are constantly filled with fat (predominantly bad saturated animal fat), they get coated with cholesterol plaque, a glue-like substance that can kill blood vessels. This is seen in plaque of the abdominal aorta, one of the body's largest blood vessels, which if it is great enough, causes it to explode as an aneurysm, usually resulting in death. Plaque also decreases smooth flow through blood vessels, narrows blood vessels, and causes the normal elasticity of arteries (which move the blood) to greatly decrease. This results in poor circulation and high blood pressure. High blood pressure forces more fluids into tissue spaces, which remain swollen, and cells continue to die.

5. Abnormal red blood cell production. Disease processes that cause abnormal red-blood cell production (like sickle cell anemia) result in poor oxygen circulation. Iron-deficiency anemia or pernicious anemia (lack of organic Vitamin B_{12}) reduces the amount of red blood cells. Anemia reduces circulation, impairing *total health = wholeness.*

6. Abnormal white blood cell production. If the bone marrow, thymus gland, lymph nodes or other lymphoid tissue responsible for WBC production is diseased or damaged, our body's immune system will be impaired. Poor WBC production is caused by deficiencies, such as folic acid (a B vitamin) deficiency. WBC production can also be impaired when a person is highly toxic.

7. High fat diets as discussed earlier cause a sludging of the blood (red and white blood cells) which results in a 20% decrease in circulation.

Circulation of lymph is decreased by:
1. Shallow breathing, or incomplete lung expansion. Deep breathing moves lymphatic fluid more effectively than any other means, even intense exercise. But few people breathe correctly, mostly using less than ⅓ of their lung capacity. According to lymphologist Dr. Jack Shields, deep breathing

drains lymph fluid 10 to 15 times better than any other method. Most people are "chest breathers," never using the lower part of their lungs, which are supposed to supply 80 percent of our body's oxygen.[1] Incomplete lung expansion also causes retention of acid and other waste products that should be expelled in carbon dioxide, when we exhale.

2. Lack of rebounding cellular exercise. Lymph also circulates better during a rebounding activity, like walking or bouncing on a rebounder. Rebounding combined with deep breathing exercise is the greatest lymph circulator of all.

3. Lack of cardiovascular exercise. A person who gets no exercise drains 1-2 milliliters of lymph fluid per minute from tissues. Exercise brings the rate up to 20 mls per minute. More intense, aerobic cardiovascular exercise brings the rate even higher, because of the combination of the deep breathing necessary to sustain the exercise and the increased heart rate.

Now I want to discuss the importance of all lymphoid tissue in maintaining *total health = wholeness*. I wouldn't remove the tonsils or appendix unless absolutely necessary, because they're lymphoid tissues. Losing such tissues causes a reduction of the body's ability to fight off pathogenic bacteria, virus, fungi and parasites. So a tonsillectomy, even in the wake of recurring sore throats, may not be the wisest decision. A better approach would be to naturally boost the immune system with food source vitamin C, plant based organic minerals, echinacea and garlic, and to avoid WBC inhibitors like sugar and food allergens like dairy products. Removing the tonsils removes the first line of defense again pathogens (disease causing agent), because you're removing a filter that prevents these germs from spreading throughout your body. The same is true of the appendix, although it's not removed as freely as tonsils are. Still, using God's medicine of herbs, bowel cleansing, detoxification and proper food choices could save the appendix more frequently. This would minimize the pressure that forces fecal material into diverticuli and into the appendix, causing it to inflame and eventually rupture. I believe everything God gave us has a purpose, and we shouldn't have to remove any parts if we walk in *total health = wholeness*.

What can I do to help my circulative health?

I have nine suggestions:

1. Maintain good heart function. Keep the heart strong and toned with a regular cardiovascular exercise program—preferably daily, but at least three times per week. If you have not exercised regularly, contact your family physician first for him to give you the go ahead. Find an aerobic exercise, which keeps a sustained, elevated heart rate. The easiest and most popular is brisk walking or rebounding cellular exercise. If you're starting from scratch, I recommend starting with one minute per day and adding a minute a day until you hit 30 minutes, then stay at that level. Follow this schedule as long as you're not feeling tired or chest pain, pressure or palpitations. If in doubt, stay at your present level for three days, then increase one minute every three days, if you're able. We don't have to get in cardiovascular shape overnight (or over a month), but we do have to get in shape. Take your time and go at your own pace and follow your doctor's recommendations.

2. Increase potassium and decrease sodium intake. Help your osmotic balance by consuming lots of fresh, raw fruit and vegetables and their fresh juices, using organic whenever possible. These foods and juices include tremendous amounts of potassium, which causes fluid to leave the tissues. Your cells will no longer be waterlogged and dying due to lack of oxygen and essential nutrients. Make a batch of potassium broth (recipe follows), and drink it like tea 1-3 times per day. The broth will flush many toxins, chemicals, poisons and harmful salts and acids from your body, and will replenish vitamins and minerals.

Here's how to make **potassium broth**: Using organic vegetables, fill a large pot with one part potato peelings, one part chopped onions and garlic (50 cloves of garlic), one part celery and dark greens (like spinach), and one part carrot peelings and whole chopped beets. Cover the vegetables with distilled water. You can add hot peppers to spice up the flavor, but never any salt. Simmer for two hours, and let sit overnight. Strain the broth in the morning and put the vegetables in your compost. Refrigerate the broth and it will last about five days.

If you eat lots of raw fruits and vegetables and their juices, drink potassium broth three times a day, and remove sodium from your diet, tremendous amounts of fluid and toxins will leave the tissue spaces, reverting you to a state of total health. Many people who follow this diet lose a lot of water weight, which had resulted from high sodium intake, resulting in osmotic imbalance. Once this imbalance is corrected, life and health returns to cells and tissues. So, start to avoid sodium as much as possible. If you must use some salt in cooking, use only a little of the finest sea salt. And read labels; you'll be surprised to see how much sodium is in many of your favorite foods. Substitute organic spices for salt. Get use to food a little blander or spiced up with alternatives to salt. Stop eating out at restaurants, unless they are extremely health-conscious. Even if you try to completely eliminate sodium from your diet, you'll at best only get rid of 50 percent of it, because it's so hidden in many foods. So, don't worry that you won't get enough sodium. There is enough sodium in all fruits and vegetables and it is in the right ratio of 1 part sodium to 5 parts potassium.

A high sodium intake increases the chance of high blood pressure, which forces more fluid into the tissue spaces, putting a greater demand on the lymphatic system to drain this fluid. So let's all *say no to salt and say yes to uncooked raw fruit and vegetables.*

3. Progressively cut out animal products from your diet. Animal fat is the greatest cause of high cholesterol, which accumulates in blood vessels and narrows their opening. This leads to both ischemia (a lack of blood to tissue) and high blood pressure, which greatly increase the chances of heart attacks and strokes, the number 1 and number 3 killers in the United States. Most people with high cholesterol could be in the normal range in 30 days by eliminating animal products and eating only fresh, raw fruits and vegetables, whole grains, sprouts, sprouted seeds, nuts, beans and legumes. This would drop your cholesterol 100 points, and you would feel so much better.

Sound impossible? Again, *do we eat to live or live to eat?* If you think you live to eat, you're controlled by your body's desires. But self-control, a fruit of the Spirit, combines with your will to become totally healthy. You will be able to control what you eat. There are many excellent meat substitutes available to help you still enjoy eating.

Dr. Dean Ornish, a cardiologist, showed the benefits of such a diet. He put patients destined for heart bypass surgery on a vegetarian diet, had them exercise daily, and meditate or relax daily. As a result, none needed bypass surgery. Impressive, wouldn't you say?

4. Get the proper nutrients in. You need 90-plus essential nutrients, along with complex carbohydrates. The best place to get these vitamins, minerals, enzymes, phytochemicals, oxygen and bioelectricity and all other essential nutrients is with a diet of live, raw food, especially, vegetables, sprouts, whole grains, seeds, nuts and some fruit. The second best placed to get them is SupremeFood, an organic vitamin-, mineral-, enzyme- and phytochemical-rich supplement. It is a balance of whole food that keeps you healthy. (SupremeFood was described in detail in Chapter 11.) For RBCs and WBCs to do their jobs effectively, you need the building blocks to keep producing these blood cells. If you're deficient in just one area, the blood cells won't function properly. It's like a car without an engine; you have all the other necessary parts, but it doesn't work without the one missing part. So eat more vegan (vegetarian with no animal product) organic whenever possible. And take SupremeFood once or twice a day.

5. Take cardiovascular specific herbs

As I have said, herbs are God's medicine (Ezekiel 47:12), so we want to boost our cardiovascular system with God's prescription:

HERB	USE
Hawthorn	Heart protector, healing aid
Motherwort	Heart beat regulator
Red Clover	Detoxifies blood, thins blood
Garlic	Thins blood, lowers cholesterol, regulates blood pressure
Cayenne	Increases circulation
Ginger	Increases circulation
Ginko biloba	Increases circulation to the brain

6. Practice deep breathing. Deep, complete breathing uses your chest and your diaphragm, and it moves lymph fluid through the lymphatic system quicker. This helps prevent blood proteins from accumulating in tissue, a cause of fluid retention and cell death. Deep breathing also circulates WBCs quicker for disease prevention, and it circulates more oxygen through RBCs to all your body's cells.

To practice deep breathing, get in a comfortable chair or on your back. Inhale slowly through your nose to the count of 10, fully expanding the lungs; this may hurt a bit if you aren't used to it. Hold to the count of 2, and then exhale slowly to the count of 10, fully deflating the lungs. During this exercise, hold one hand on your abdomen, right below your breastbone. As this hand moves out away from your body, you're inflating the lower lobes of the lungs, an indication of complete breathing of both chest and diaphragm types. Do this 10 times, and do it three different times throughout the day. It's also wonderful to meditate and have quiet time in communion and communicating with God while doing your breathing exercises.

7. Do rebounding exercises daily. Rebounding exercises are done on a rebounder by gently vibrating up and down (health bounce). This triples the circulating white blood cell count by tripling the movement of the lymphatic fluid. Brisk walking or running in place can also be done (aerobic bounce) for cardiovascular fitness and weight loss. This can be part or all of your recommended 30 minutes per day of cardiovascular exercise (see Item 1 above). If you can exercise at an intense level where you're breathing deeply, you'll receive the benefits of cardiovascular exercise and deep breathing at the same time. Rebounding is also good for people who aren't very physically fit, because one can exercise at their own level and it is the least stress on the joints (see rebounding section.)

8. Castor oil hot packs. Many great natural healers say lymphatic circulation increases when Castor oil is applied with heat. This is ideal for specific areas like the armpit, which is the lymph drainage of the breast. Cotton or flannel cloth is dipped in Castor oil and applied to the area. A hot water bottle or moist heating pad is placed over that, and left on the area for 15-30 minutes per night.

9. Eat low fat meals. This is the vegan diet. The fat from both animal and plant sources causes the red blood cells to clump together and decrease the oxygen getting into the cells. The white blood cells also move slower causing a decrease in immune system response. This reduction of blood flow is up to 20% for up to 12 hours after a meal. The animal fat, however, causes cholesterol build up in the blood vessels. This narrowing causes heart attacks and strokes, whereas the plant fat contains no cholesterol and does not cause blood vessel narrowing.

Apply these nine recommendations to your circulative health and see how your total health improves.

CHAPTER 16

IMMUNE HEALTH

The main function of your immune system is to seek out and destroy foreign invaders to your body, including bacteria, viruses, fungi, parasites, and even cancer cells. These invaders carry antigens, substances that tell your body that they don't belong there. Your body reacts by making antibodies to fight off the invasion. Special WBCs called B cells produce these antibodies, which bind to the invaders and signal other WBCs to come and destroy the invader. (Similarly to putting a flashing light on the head of someone in a crowd to signal others that this is the one.)

The following explanation of WBCs will give you a greater understanding of how your immune system works, so you can really understand this vital system God has blessed us with. The major categories of WBCs are:

1) B cells
2) T cells
3) Granulocytes
   a) Ncutrophil
   b) Basophilic
   c) Eosinophil
4) Phagocytes
   a) Monocytes
   b) Neutrophil
   c) Macrophages
5) Nonspecific effector cells
   a) Macrophage
   b) Neutrophil
   c) NK cell (natural killer)

B cells develop in bone marrow, and move into the spleen and lymph nodes to wait for their call to battle. B cells produce antibodies, which attach to bacteria, fungi and parasites, literally marking these invaders so that, the *phagocytes* — the "eating" WBCs—will know what to devour and destroy.

T cells detect viruses and other pathogens inside the body's cells by reading the genetic code of the invader, which is different from our own.

The T cell then transforms into different T cells, including the killer T cell that actually kills the infected cell. The inflammatory T cells also call the *macrophages* to come and devour the invader. Amazingly, T cells actually "remember" what the invaders "look" like, so they can quickly respond to future invasion attempts by the same invaders.

Neutrophils, in greatest supply in the body, eat bacteria, viruses and fungi that have been tagged with antibody for destruction. (Neutrophils will also eat invaders that haven't been tagged with antibodies.) *Eosinophils* are much like the neutrophils, but more involved with destroying parasite intruders and regulating allergic reactions. *Basophils* are also involved with allergic responses, producing histamine, which is connected to most allergic symptoms.

Monocytes eat bacteria and fungi. They also mature to larger macrophages, which can devour the most bacteria and fungi—even whole RBCs and malarial parasites. Macrophages can eat up to 100 bacteria, five times as much as neutrophils. Macrophages clean up the body's system by eating dead tissue and dead neutrophils, which usually die after eating 5-20 bacteria. Macrophages can live for months, even years, while average neutrophils and other WBCs live only 2-3 days. Some macrophages are stationary, staying in the spleen, lungs and lymph nodes, waiting for invaders to come to them; others roam through the blood tissues of the body, consuming any intruders they find.

NK cells (natural killers) seek and destroy cancer cells and virus-infected cells—without help from other WBCs. Cancer cells constantly form in our bodies, but a strong and healthy immune system can kill them before they multiply and form tumors.

FUNCTION GONE WRONG

The immune system can weaken and falter for the same reasons our general health can decline, including:

1) Deficiency to make enough WBCs
2) Toxins, chemicals, and drugs which weaken, injure, or destroy the WBCs
3) Refined sugar
4) Stress
5) Environmental irritations such as excessive radiation from sun, X-ray, electromagnetic fields, radon, etc.

Let's take a closer look at each:

1. Deficiency. You know about the importance of the 90-plus vitamins, minerals, amino acids, essential fatty acids, carbohydrates, enzymes, phytochemicals, bioelectricity, oxygen and water. These are necessary for the health and life of your body's cells. When your body lacks these vital nutrients, you become more and more deficient, and your body no longer has all the building blocks it needs to produce the quantity and quality of cells it needs. This results in either fewer WBCs or weaker WBCs, meaning your immune system is greatly weakened. And that's the last system in your body you want to be weak or in smaller numbers. The result of nutritional deficiency is sickness, disease and eventual premature death.

2. Toxins, chemicals and drugs all can lead to immune suppression and immune system damage. If you swam in toxic waste, you would eventually get sick and die, because the toxins would eventually enter your body, causing it to malfunction. Same goes for your WBCs and your body's other cells. Toxins, chemicals, and drugs damage your body's homeostasis (balance), all the way down to the cellular level until, normal function is altered and sickness and disease begin. So, again, it's vital to detoxify our bodies on a regular basis. And again, we need to GET THE GOOD IN, AND GET THE BAD OUT.

3. Refined sugar. This weakens the ability of the WBC to eat bacteria, viruses, candida, parasites and cancer cells drastically. Sugar in all refined or processed forms weakens the immune system. These forms include refined sugar; flour, bread, pasta and even store bought juices. It is important to note that in severe illnesses like cancer, diabetes, chronic fatigue syndrome and other immunosuppressive disorders, all sugar should be avoided, including fruit. As stated in Chapter 6, *a study on sugar intake and immune strength was conducted in which three groups of mice were injected with an aggressive malignant mammary tumor. Prior to injection the dietary blood sugar was altered to produce three levels: high blood sugar, normal blood sugar and lowered blood sugar. After 70 days 66% of the high blood sugar mice had died, 33% of the normal blood sugar mice had died and only 5% of the lowered blood sugar group had died.*[1] *(see Sugar Chart next page.)*

4. Stress. There are three types of stress: mental, physical and thermal.

• Mental stress is one of the greatest, if not the greatest, negative factor affecting your health. Stress causes our bodies to secrete hormones that get us ready to fight, ready to run, ready for intensity. If the stress is long-term, the body gets exhausted, burned out and depleted. Mental anguish or

EFFECT OF SUGAR INTAKE ON ABILITY OF WHITE BLOOD CELLS TO DESTROY BACTERIA [2]

Amount of sugar eaten at one time by average adult in teaspoons	Number of bacteria destroyed by each white blood cell	Percentage decrease in ability to destroy bacteria
0	14	0
6	10	25
12	5.5	60
18	2	85
24	1	92
Uncontrolled Diabetic	1	92

THE AMOUNT OF SUGAR IN A 12 OUNCE CAN OF SODA DECREASES THE ABILITY OF THE WHITE BLOOD CELLS TO EAT BACTERIA, VIRUSES, PARASITES AND CANCER CELLS BY 40% FOR UP TO 6 HOURS.

depression actually hurts your immune system. In a study by Dr. Bernard and Margaret Linn at the University of Miami School of Medicine, 49 men were evaluated because of either a recent death or severe illness of a family member. The findings: The men's WBCs were not working up to normal. After the study, Dr. Linn said that people who reacted to stress with less anxiety and fear showed an increase in their immune system response.[3] Mental stress definitely affects your health and immune system. So, in your total health picture, remember that your spiritual health and relationship with the Living God come first, closely followed by your mental health. Your mind does affect your body, for the better or for the worse. So, let's remember Proverbs 17:22, "A merry heart does good like medicine," and Proverbs 23:7, "As a man thinks in his heart so is he."

• Physical stress occurs when we physically push our bodies over their capacity. If this is done for a long time, the system—including the immune system—will start to break down, especially if there's a nutrient deficiency. How far could a horse carry you if you didn't feed it the proper food and gave it little to no sleep? The horse would one day drop dead due to malnutrition and exhaustion. Your body and its cells are the same; they need proper nutrients and rest. Otherwise, you're breaking down more than you're building up, which leads to sickness and disease—the opposite of wholeness.

• Thermal stress involves temperature extremes—heat, cold, or drastic changes from one to the other. A chill from staying out in the cold without a coat is enough to stress and weaken the immune system enough to allow viruses or bacteria to attack and win a short-lived victory—giving your a cold or the flu.

5. Environmental irritations. Ultraviolet rays, X-rays, electromagnetic fields, radon, and other irritants can damage cells and even cause cancer—if you're exposed to them often enough. Occasional exposure, though, isn't necessarily harmful. For example, if I get some sun after working in my yard one day, that's very different from someone who lies in the sun every day to see how tan they can get. Similarly, a complete set of spinal X-rays is a very small amount of radiation compared to multiple upper GI X-ray fluoroscopy studies. It's the difference between one X-ray picture and an entire X-ray videotape equivalent to thousands of pictures. The same principle applies to your diet: It's not what you eat between Christmas and New Year's that counts (seven days) but what you eat between New Year's and Christmas (358 days.)

What can you do to help your immune health?

1.   Eat a predominantly vegan diet of organic, raw vegetables, sprouts, seeds, nuts, and whole grains. Freshly juiced organic vegetables are also excellent sources of vitamins, minerals, enzymes and phytochemical. Avoid food that you're sensitive or allergic to—especially dairy products like milk, cheese, butter, cream and yogurt.

2.   Use SupremeFood to help "get the good in," providing your body with many of the 90-plus essential nutrients, along with enzymes and phytochemical. Without proper nutrients, your cells—including WBCs—cannot live.

3.   Detoxify regularly to help "get the bad out." We've spoken of a four-phase detox program prescribed by God: "The fruit shall be their food and the leaf their medicine" (Ezekiel 47:12.) The proper order for complete detoxification is first bowel, then liver, then kidney, then blood. Organic and wildcrafted herbs, which are chemical-free, are the best medicine to detoxify the body.

4.   Be led and empowered by the Spirit of God. The Spirit is always with us to lead us, guide us and to show us the right choices for our total health. What a better way to approach any part of our *total health = wholeness.*

5.   Let your mind and heart be filled with love, joy and peace. These fruits of the Spirit help your immune system—all your body's systems—to work as God created it to. The opposite of stress is peace, even in the midst of the storm. The Living God said He would never leave nor forsake us, and that we could cast all our cares upon Him because He cares for us.

6.   Exercise daily, preferably 30 minutes of rebounding cellular exercise and aerobic or sustained elevated heart rate exercise. Exercise is one of the best ways to get your body's blood and lymphatic fluid flowing quickly, taking WBCs where they need to be—fighting disease, bacteria, viruses, fungi, parasites, and cancer cells. Deep breathing exercises, described in Chapter 15, also improves lymphatic movement.

7.   Completely avoid sugar and refined flours, breads and pastas. Studies have shown how detrimental refined sugar is to the body, especially the immune system. If you have cancer, chronic fatigue syndrome, diabetes, candida or any immunosuppressive disorder you should also avoid fruit.

Now let's put this in perspective. Cancer will be the No. 1 cause of death in the United States. Cancer results from a weakening of the cancer police patrol WBCs—killer T cells and NK cells whose purpose is to seek out and destroy cancer cells. Eating sugar reduces the ability of your WBCs to do this critical work. Some people regularly eat some form of refined sugar with each meal or between meals, resulting in a weakened immune system to fight off cancer. You can't fight when 50 percent of your immunity is impaired on a regular basis due to refined sugar intake. This gives cancer cells a chance to grow and eventually form a tumor. Once a tumor has developed, it is much more difficult (although it can be done) to stimulate your WBCs to kill this mass of cancer cells. So, cut out the sugar and help protect your body from cancer, bacteria, viruses, fungi, and parasites. The gaining of a few calories from refined sugar is the least of our problems. Certainly, we don't want the added weight, but we really don't want cancer or other illnesses. So, the next time you reach for the sugar, remember that your body is God's temple. It is also important to note that refined breads, pastas and store bought juices all turn into sugar in your system, which weakens the immune system response.

8. Avoid dairy products. Of all the foods I've tested, dairy is by far the most sensitive, most allergenic, most non-health promoting food, outside of refined sugar. Dairy products, which are not digested as an adult, cause mucus formation, coating the respiratory and digestive systems. Dairy products also contain contaminants, pesticides, chemicals, antibiotics and hormones that are likely linked to certain cancers. This is not something you want to put into your body.

9. Eat raw garlic, perhaps the greatest herb of all. It is proven to decrease chances of heart disease. It lowers blood pressure and cholesterol. It is an effective agent in cancer therapy. One third of all medicinal research about garlic is cancer-related. The National Cancer Institute said that garlic reduces the incidence of cancer; this is especially seen in France, Spain and Italy. Garlic has been shown to help protect WBCs in their fight against cancer and their ability to destroy tumors. Garlic boosts the immune system by enhancing NK cells, stopping tumor growth and reducing the pain associated with cancer. Garlic has been proven to reduce the incidence of colorectal cancer and stomach cancer. In one study, stomach cancer patients who ate garlic were 10 times more likely to have a cancer reduction than the non-garlic-eating group.

Garlic also is a very powerful antibiotic, antiviral and antifungal herb. Garlic destroys both gram positive and gram negative bacteria, making it broad spectrum. Garlic destroys streptococcus, staphylococcus, typhoid, diphtheria, cholera, tuberculosis, tetanus, and pneumonia-causing bacteria, to name a few. The biggest difference between garlic and prescription antibiotics is garlic's selectivity in its bacteria destruction. Garlic kills only bacteria that can damage our bodies, leaving normal intestinal flora undisturbed. Prescription antibiotics, meanwhile, kill all bacteria in the body, both bad and good. The death of normal, needed intestinal bacteria is the beginning of bowel lining inflammation due to an overgrowth of candida (yeast) and harmful bacteria. This leads to leaky gut syndrome, which leads to toxicity, which leads to immune dysfunction and eventually disease. See how powerful garlic truly is?

Garlic is also a powerful antiviral. It will help cure the common cold, flu, and upper respiratory infection, as well as destroy the viral infections of measles, mumps, mononucleosis, chicken pox, herpes simplex, herpes zoster (shingles), viral hepatitis, scarlet fever, rabies, and possibly HIV and AIDS. Garlic's antifungal properties are more potent than any antifungal agent (including the prescription Nystatin), and will stop the growth of candida albicans (yeast.)

As you can see, there is nothing more powerful than garlic for boosting your immune health. Garlic truly is God's given medicine, the "leaf" for medicine described in Ezekiel 47:12. When we take what God meant us to take for disease, there are no harmful side effects.

The biggest reason that people don't enjoy all the benefits of garlic is its odor. Garlic capsules and tablets made to be odorless are all right and have some value, but they're nothing like the real thing. The best way to ingest garlic is to take 6-8 large, raw garlic cloves per day. How? Put it through a garlic press and then into some juice in a blender, then liquefy and drink. Or, you can chop the cloves up, put them on a piece of bread and eat as a sandwich. You can also put the cloves in a juicer first with other produce you are juicing. However you do it; get it in. To help with your breath, buy some inexpensive essential oil—like peppermint oil—at your health food store. Just a drop or two every couple of hours will do the trick.

I relate a story about an elderly woman who had a virus, which led to pneumonia and an uncontrollable infection. The hospital sent her home to die because nothing further could be done. The woman started taking more than 200 cloves of garlic per day (not necessarily my recommended dose), and in seven days, she was on her way to total recovery.

10. Take echinacea, a powerful immune stimulant that was used by American Indians for hundreds of years to fight infection and disease. Echinacea can be taken in many forms, including teas, capsules, tinctures and tablets. The most concentrated form is tincture or liquid extract. When echinacea is combined with alcohol, the alcohol draws out all the medicinal value of the herb and stabilizes it indefinitely. So an echinacea tincture can be kept for years without weakening or losing its immune-stimulating ability.

When buying herbs, make sure they are organic or wildcrafted, with no chemicals added. Make sure they're the proper strength to do the job; many commercial herbs have been diluted, and lose their beneficial properties. How can you tell if echinacea is effective? If it makes your tongue temporarily tingle and go numb; if it doesn't, it's too weak to affect a change in your immune system. Echinacea is usually taken for 7-14 days, as an antibiotic would be taken, to boost your immune system in fighting bacteria, viruses, fungi, and parasites. As an immune stimulant, it should not be taken all the time. To illustrate: if I slapped your hand, your body would be stimulated, but if I continued to slap your hand, your body would get irritated. The adult dosage of a strong echinacea tincture is two dropperfuls five times per day, for 7-14 days or until you are well. All parts of the echinacea plant are medicinal, but the root is the most powerful.(See Appendix)

11. Take Vitamin C, in the form of red and green peppers. It is a strong antioxidant, which means it helps your cells—including WBCs—live longer. Nobel Prize winner Dr. Linus Pauling was the biggest promoter of Vitamin C for good health. Studies have shown Vitamin C's value in combating bacterial and viral infections, especially the common cold. Vitamin C is abundant in many fruits, especially citrus, and is highest in green peppers and red peppers.

12. Drink water, which circulates blood and keeps all the tissues healthy. Your body is 75 percent water, and the average American is slightly dehydrated. So, it is important to drink one quart (32 oz) per 50 lbs.of body weight per day of distilled or reverse osmosis, and even more when you're fighting sickness or disease. Entire books have been written about the vital health benefits of drinking water. So drink up.

13. Eat light, especially whenever you feel ill or are fighting off some sickness or disease. Avoid heavy proteins. Stick mainly with fresh, raw vegetables, sprouts and their juices and powerful whole grains like quinoa and millet.

You've heard the question, "Do you starve a cold and feed a fever, or feed a cold and starve a fever?" The answer is, "You starve everything." When animals get sick they stop eating; they just drink water, and they get well much quicker than we humans do. So start juicing organic fresh produce and drink up. It will energize you, packing you full of vitamins, minerals, enzymes, phytochemicals, oxygen and bioelectricity.

In closing this chapter, let me remind you that in the years to come, there are predictions of many virulent, deadly diseases of viral and bacterial origin, AIDS being just one, along with the ever increasing cancer threat. The people who will survive will be the ones who learned how to achieve *total health = wholeness* BEFORE the storm comes. So get in good habits NOW, change your diet NOW, learn how to boost your immune system and how to fight off cancer, sickness and disease NOW. It's much easier now than waiting to hear the news that you are very sick, and out of fear you desperately try to regain your health. Optimum or total health is a gift from God, and should be treasured and taken care of daily.

CHAPTER 17
OXIDATIVE HEALTH

Oxygen is what our bodies need most and can do without for the least amount of time. The average person can go 30 days without food and four days without water, but only two minutes without oxygen.

Oxygen is why we have life on our planet. God made Earth with a self-containing atmosphere that worked like a greenhouse. He then created plants, which produce oxygen. Then God created animals and man, which need oxygen to live. In turn, animals and mankind produce carbon dioxide, which is what plants need to live. So you see God's perfect balance of plants, animals and man; we need each other to live.

Every human cell, tissue, gland and organ must have sufficient oxygen, or it will die. We must get oxygen to every cell efficiently and effectively, because our lives depend on it. Cardiovascular exercise and deep-breathing exercises with rebounding cellular exercise do a great job of getting oxygen to our cells. At the cellular level, oxygen, combined with simple sugars from complex carbohydrate digestion, is used in complex biochemical reactions to produce energy. This energy keeps our bodies warm, our hearts beating, our lungs expanding and contracting, and enables us to do all the bodily functions necessary to sustain life.

What causes our cells to get old, wear out and die? I think it all goes back to the beginning, in the book of Genesis. God created man and woman, perfect in spirit, mind and body. They would have lived forever, just as we will in heaven because we have trusted Jesus Christ as Savior and Lord. But a problem developed in the Garden of Eden. God had made a covenant with man, and all man had to do was obey God. God had given Adam simple instructions—to tend the garden, name the animals, and avoid eating the fruit of the Tree of Knowledge of good and evil. God told Adam if he ate this fruit, he would surely die. We all know how the story went: Adam ate the fruit, and death followed. "Death," for man, doesn't mean "ceasing to exist," but "separation." When we physically die, our soul and spirit separate from our bodies. When Adam and Eve sinned by disobeying God, the covenant was broken. As a result, man died first in the spirit, then in the soul (mind, will and emotions), then finally, 900 years later, in the body.

When man sinned, he was separated from God spiritually. His daily walking and talking with God ended. "Death" meant separation of the soul from God. Man's soul changed from a perfect mind, will and emotion, to a soul that lost love, joy and peace, and experienced fear for the first time. Man's first words after the Fall were, "I was afraid." I believe the moment of the Fall was also the beginning of the second law of thermodynamics, which states that everything goes from a state of order to a state of disorder. That day, everything began to break down and change and eventually die, all the way down to the cellular level.

THE OXYGEN PARADIGM

After the Fall, oxygen not only gave life, but it started a new process called oxidation, which eventually caused death. On the molecular level, oxidation means that molecules lose electrons spontaneously. Nothing external causes this—except, I believe, the Fall. So oxygen not only gives life, but also takes it away.

Oxidation is easily seen. It's the process by which steel rusts, food spoils, and fruit ripens and then becomes rotten. It's the process by which all things break down, including us. Our bodies no longer live forever because since the Fall, from the day we're born, we start to oxidize and thus start to die. Your body is constantly oxidizing, or "rusting." Oxygen is like the match that can start a fire that burns down an entire forest. It's like the wick that, when lighted, causes a bomb to explode.

How can we put the oxidative fires out? By a chemical reaction called redox, which means the reduction or balancing reaction of oxidation. Oxidation causes us to lose electrons, breaking our bodies down. In redox, molecules gain electrons. Unlike oxidation, redox is not spontaneous; it requires energy. This is why fruit won't "unrot" and old milk won't "unspoil."

What causes oxidation? Primarily, the Fall of man and a broken covenant with God. It's also caused by the following:

1) aging
2) toxins, chemicals and drugs
3) allergies/sensitivities
4) stress

Let's look at each:

1) Aging has been causing oxidation since the Fall of man, when death entered the world and aging began. We all age (oxidize) and die, sooner or later. Death may seem sad, but it can be glorious, if we have trusted in

God's provision for breaking the covenant, which is His Son Jesus Christ. Jesus died to pay the price of our sins, to restore us spiritually to communing with God once gain. If we believe this, death is glorious, because to be absent from the body means to be in the presence of the Lord Jesus Christ, our heavenly Father and His Holy Spirit for eternity. So we can actually look forward to death, as did the Apostle Paul, who said, "To live is Christ and to die is gain" (Philippians 1:21.) Many people can't understand that statement, because they see death as the end of everything. But it can be the beginning of an eternity of nothing but love, joy and peace in heaven. Heaven is a place of no pain, no struggles, no temptations, no strife, no fear, no stress, no hate, no selfishness, no jealously, no depression, no anxiety, no worry, no bitterness, no pride, no sickness, no disease, no wanting for anything. For those who trust Christ, there is no fear of death.

2) Toxins and chemicals are the coming plague of this century. They damage cells and cause most sickness and disease. Toxins and chemicals speed up the oxidation rate of cells, hastening their death. During oxidation, toxins can damage the genetic material of cells, causing cells to grow uncontrolled, leading to cancer formation. Toxins can also affect your immune system, with oxidation weakening and shortening the life of WBCs, which are needed to fight off bacteria, virus, fungi, parasite and cancer cells. So, in a nutshell: Toxins hasten oxidation, which hastens cellular death, which leads to the death of tissues, glands and organs, which leads to the death of people.

Two types of toxins affect cells. *Exotoxins* damage cells from the outside to the inside, while *endotoxins* damage cells from the inside out.

Exotoxins are primarily byproducts of pollution, of chemicals in food, water and air. Exotoxins are also byproducts of cellular metabolism which, if not filtered out of the body, become toxic. The toxic waste builds up until it's potentially fatal.

Endotoxins are also byproducts of cellular metabolism. They build up inside the cell and can eventually rupture the cell. This is most commonly seen when viruses attack a healthy cell. The virus injects its own DNA or genetic blueprint into the healthy cell, which actually starts making more and more viruses. These waste products build up in the cell until the cell membrane ruptures, killing the cell and releasing hundreds of viruses into the body to infect other cells.

3) Allergies and sensitivities. Food and environmental allergens set off a chain reaction that cause tissue inflammation, oxidation and cell death. One source states that 60 percent of all sickness is related to food allergy/sensitivity.[1] Food sensitivity especially affects the intestinal lining. Allergens cause intestinal inflammation, which causes increased cellular oxidation and increased cellular pressure. As a result, cells die, weakening the mucosal lining of the intestinal tract, resulting in leaky gut, which we have discussed in detail.

4) Stress, and our response to it, may be the most detrimental factor in our mental and physical health profile. Stress causes the release of adrenaline, which triggers an "oxidative fire" inside our bodies. Over a period of time, this can be quite damaging.

Let me further explain. Adrenaline is called a "driver" hormone because it causes the body to react in a greatly increased capacity. When you're stressed, your body secretes adrenaline, which enables you to react in "hyperdrive." Adrenaline prepares you to handle any physical demand to the limits of human capacity. An adrenaline rush has enabled mothers to lift cars off their children, and perform other unbelievable feats. That might sound great, but such bursts of adrenaline secretion are extremely oxidative. Dr. Majid Ali states in his book, RDA, "Adrenaline is one of the most, if not the most, potent oxidant molecules in the body."[2]

An adrenaline rush creates an "oxidative fire" that creates a tremendous amount of energy and heat, just as if a fire were burning. These oxidative fires are meant for survival, not for everyday living. If we are under continual stress, adrenaline secretion never stops and the oxidative fires never stop burning. This continual adrenaline secretion damages and kills cells, tissues, organs and glands, and uses all the body's antioxidants (reduction agents) to counteract the constant oxidative fire. As a result, antioxidants can longer battle the normal oxidation of cells from normal bodily function, cellular metabolism, aging, toxins, chemicals and allergies. Consequently, cell damage continues until disease sets in. Imagine a fire truck with a limited supply of water stored inside. That amount of water will put out most typical fires (from aging, normal cellular metabolism.) As more fires flare up (from toxins and chemicals), it becomes more difficult to control them. When an enormous, raging fire comes on the scene, we pour all our water (antioxidants) in that direction. We may control the fire, but we can't extinguish it. Meanwhile, the other "normal" fires we'd been fighting all along are now raging out of control. And suddenly, we've used up all our water. This is occurring daily in most Americans, and they're not even aware of it—until their health starts to decline.

These oxidative fires produce a lot of energy and cause a lot of damage. It only takes one match to start a forest fire, but the fire can rage for weeks until it has finally run its destructive course. The forest has been burned to a crisp, leaving little to no life. The same thing happens at the cellular level in the wake of raging oxidative fires.

In his book, *The Butterfly and Life Span Nutrition*, Dr. Majid Ali says adrenaline and related catecholamines act as powerful oxidant molecules. These molecules and other potent oxyradicals poke holes in cell membranes, killing the cells.[3] These cells become oxidative as a result of toxins in food, water and air, allergies and sensitivities, and viral infections.

It also does not matter what causes adrenaline secretion, whether it's stress, anger, hostility, anxiety or panic. The end result is the same: Cellular damage and death.

What Can I Do for My Oxidative Health?

1) **Pray.** In his book, RDA, Dr. Ali says "prayer is the best antioxidant."[4] How does this work? Prayer is communication with God, who speaks to us through the Holy Spirit and His Word, answering every question, problem, trial or test of life. Prayer, and God's response to our prayer, calms our fears and eases stress. And when there's no more stress, there's no more adrenaline production, no more oxidative fires, no more weakened immune system. Jesus said, "Do not worry about your life, what you will eat or drink; or about your body, what you will wear. Is not life more important than food, and the body more important than clothes? Look at the birds of the air; they do not sow or reap or store away in barns, and yet your heavenly Father feeds them. Are you not much more valuable than they? Who of you by worrying can add a single hour to his life?" (Matthew 6:25-27.) We have no reason to worry or fear: "For God did not give us a spirit of fear, but a spirit of power, of love and of a sound mind" (2 Timothy 1:7NKJ.) God's love, joy and peace will keep us from being stressed, and therefore from secreting adrenaline and starting lethal, oxidative fires. Commune with the Living God, and He will give you rest: "Do not be anxious about anything, but in everything, by prayer and petition, with thanksgiving, present your requests to God. And the peace of God, which transcends all under-

standing, will guard your hearts and your minds in Christ Jesus"
(Philippians 4:6-7.)

2) **Consume high oxygen and bioelectrically charged foods**, like
wheat grass, barley grass, spirulina, chlorella, sunflower sprouts and
buckwheat sprouts.

3) **Eat high-antioxidant foods,** predominantly raw, fresh, organic
fruits and vegetables and their fresh juices. The best antioxidant
foods contain Vitamins A, C and E, and selenium, so try to include
them in your diet as much as possible. Vitamin supplement pills are
mostly synthetic, have a poor absorption rate, and can have toxic
side-effects.

Vitamin A is found in dark green and dark organic vegetables, sweet
potatoes, carrots, dried apricots, spinach, kale, collard, mustard greens, and
pumpkin. All are high in beta carotene, which converts to Vitamin A.

Vitamin C is found in red and green bell peppers, citrus fruits, broccoli,
Brussels sprouts, cauliflower, cabbage, strawberries, and spinach.

Vitamin E is found in wheat germ, raw sunflower seeds, soybeans,
almonds, and vegetable oils.

Selenium is found in raw Brazil nuts, raw sunflower seeds, oat bran, and
wheat cereal.

Juicing is a tremendous way to get plenty of antioxidant nutrients into
your body. Yams and carrots are loaded with beta carotene the vitamin A
precursor that is non-toxic. Add some red peppers to the yam or carrot
juice, and you add natural vitamin C.

Remember: Juice should be consumed within 15 minutes of juicing,
because of oxidative loss of the enzymes and vitamins. Remember if you
have cancer, candida, chronic fatigue, diabetes or any immunosuppressive
disorder you should not juice any sugar containing vegetables which
includes sweet potatoes, yams, carrots, beets or parsnips.

4) **Don't eat highly oxidative foods** or foods that quickly become free
radicals. Free radicals are intermediate products of metabolism or
catabolism (a break-down process) that are highly reactive and highly oxidative. Free radicals are like the sparklers you see on the Fourth
of July; sparks fly off of them in every direction, starting oxidative
forest fires. Free radical damage to cells is often a first step to cancer
formation and other disease.

So what foods should you avoid? Many fats, which oxidize into perox-
idases and form free radicals. What kind of fat should you eat? Your body

needs three essential fatty acids, predominantly from the unsaturated fats found in flax seeds, sunflower seeds and sesame seeds. In the right blend, these seeds have all the essential fatty acids necessary for good health. (See Appendix)

But one problem with healthy oils is that, like all oils, they're heat sensitive. Heat changes all kinds of oil into free-radical formers. Flax seed oil is the best oil you can consume, but it should come directly from the seed not from a processed oil. If you must cook with oil, use organic, pure, cold, pressed super canola oil or organic extra virgin olive oil which are somewhat heat stable. But as a rule, oil/fat and heat don't mix.

Animal fat is predominantly saturated fat, and it's very free-radical forming with heat. Animal fat is also dangerous because of its cholesterol, artery-clogging content. Americans eat too much fat, especially animal fat. By the way, did you know that cholesterol is good and necessary to your body? God created your body to make its own cholesterol. But when cholesterol is heated, cooked, oxidized and eaten, it changes into a free radical. Not only that, but it turns into a glue-like substance that sticks to and coats arteries, leading to the No. 1 cause of death in the United States, cardiovascular disease, heart attack (due to coronary artery blockage) and stroke (due to cerebral artery blockage). So when it comes to fat and cholesterol, stay away from the heat. Literally.

The worst fat or oil is the chemically changed variety through a process called hydrogenation (or partial hydrogenation). This is done to keep it more stable for food processing and to extend its shelf life. Hydrogenated fats and oils are almost like plastic in your body, and they're intensely free-radical forming. Try this experiment: Put a pat of margarine between your fingers, and see how long it takes to totally liquefy like water. Then do the same with pure butter. The margarine never completely melts between your fingers because of hydrogenation, but the butter does. So, is butter better? No, neither is better. Both form free radicals when heated. And butter is a problem because it's a dairy product. So, check labels for the words "hydrogenated" or "partially hydrogenated," and stay away from them. And avoid all fat except the essential fatty acids found in the flax seeds, sunflower seeds and also in SupremeFood.

5) **Eat extra vitamin C foods,** known for their antioxidant qualities. If you're not eating enough foods containing Vitamin C—like citrus fruit (if not sugar sensitive), red and green peppers, add more to your diet. Newer research suggests vitamin C reduces artery blockages.

Dr. Linus Pauling, two-time Nobel Prize winner, recommends that adults and children get enough vitamin C daily. The best way to take Vitamin C or any other vitamin is in food, because it's balanced with phytochemcials and other metabolites and cofactors that make God's pharmacy the best.

6) **Detoxify regularly**. The best way to stop oxidant free-radical damage is get the toxins and chemicals out of your body on a regular schedule. I recommend the bowel, liver and blood detox to be done four times per year, and then followed up with a daily bowel and liver strengthening program. (See Chapter 14 for more information on detoxification.)

7) **Avoid food and environmental allergens.** Up to 60 percent of disease may be related to food sensitivity. Here's what happens during an allergic reaction: Food allergens cause an oxidative fire, known as a histamine release, from mast cells. This causes tissue swelling and increased metabolic activity. This results in increased oxidation and decreased cell life, and a depletion of antioxidant molecules which have been used to put out this huge oxidative fire.

Food sensitivity can also cause inflammation in the intestinal tract, resulting in leaky gut syndrome.

If you're interested in finding out what food sensitivities and allergies you might have, review Chapter 13.

Cancer

Many leading experts believe that cancer grows in a predominately low oxygen environment called anaerobic. Most healthy cells thrive in a high oxygen environment called aerobic. If this is true then oxygen can be even more vital to combat disease than we ever realized. To promote vitality or total health in all the cells of our bodies and at the same time prevent cancer cells from forming and spreading, oxygen therapy is extremely important. Oxygen therapy is any method by which we can increase the oxygen levels in the blood. Some of these include:

1) Deep breathing with full, deep inspiration and complete expiration
2) Exercise with rebounding cellular exercise to increase the rate of oxygen exchange into the body and into the cells.
3) Oxygen promoting nutrients like chlorophyll. Chlorophyll is found in high concentrations in green plants especially in chlorella, spirulina, wheat grass, barley grass, sunflower sprouts and buckwheat sprouts.

In summary, oxygen is simultaneously vital to life and an instrument of death. For life, we need to get oxygen to every cell in our bodies, using methods like deep breathing and cardiovascular/ rebounding cellular along with oxygen promoting nutrients. If oxygen is left unhindered, it will oxidize cells and tissues, eventually killing them. So, as Dr. Ali said in his book RDA, "Oxygen ushers life in. It also terminates life. Oxygen is the spark that revs up all engines in living beings. It can also cause instantaneous combustion of all life forms unless it is held in abeyance by cellular carburetors."[5] Thank God for oxygen and the antioxidant molecules that balance it.

CHAPTER 18
ORGAN/GLAND HEALTH

The next part of our *total health* = *wholeness* is the health of our organs and glands, which is affected by four main factors: 1) genetics, 2) structural imbalance, 3) toxicity, and 4) organ/gland specific nutrition.

1) Genetics means inherited strengths and weaknesses. For instance, heart disease runs in some families; for others, it might be cancer or diabetes. But some families seem to have an almost indestructible genetic code. These people can smoke, drink, eat bacon and eggs every day for breakfast, drink milk three times per day, and never look at a vegetable... and yet, for some unknown reason, they can live 100 years or more in good health. That's great, but these days, we can't simply "live off our genes," mainly because we don't know that much about our genetic code. This is evident in families where one generation lives into their 90's, while the next dies by the age of 60. Also, today's toxins and chemicals are stronger, more lethal, more oxidative, more free radical forming and cancer-producing than ever before. Whatever your family's genetic history, thank God for how He made you and how He blesses you and your children with good health. Even if heart disease runs in your family, God's Word says all things are possible for him who believes. So don't spend too much time either worrying or boasting about your genes.

2) Structural imbalance is subluxation (or misalignment) in the spine. Subluxations can put pressure on a spinal nerve that might be the life energy to any organ, gland, or tissue, causing dysfunction. I have treated patients with all areas of their spine subluxated, which produced a variety of organ and gland problems, from hyperactive functioning of glands and organs (causing burnout) to sluggishness of them, (causing decreased function.) Different areas of the spine are correlated with different parts of the body: The neck generally supplies nerves to the eyes, ears, nose, throat, thyroid and head; the upper back to the heart and lungs; the middle back to the stomach, pancreas, liver, gallbladder, spleen; and the lower back to the intestinal tract, kidneys, bladder and reproductive organs.

What causes subluxations? Many things (see the list below) but two of the main things are: Traumatic occurrences, like a fall or auto accident that quickly jars the spine. This can stretch muscles and ligaments, leading to spinal instability and early onset of arthritis and spinal degeneration. The second main cause of subluxations is also the most common, because it's the things we do every day, things that cause muscles to tighten and pull unevenly. These things include poor sitting posture (good sitting posture means having your back pressed back into a chair with a lumbar pillow), prolonged standing (which can cause your back to sway and misalign), improper lifting (you should always lift with legs bent and lower back straight), and improper sleeping position (sleeping on your side with one leg drawn up, or sleeping on your stomach, or sleeping on a non-supportive mattress and pillow.) These little things cause spinal misalignment, then spinal nerve pressure, then organ and gland dysfunction—often with little-to-no symptoms, perhaps some back or neck stiffness. *(See Causes of Spinal Subluxations chart)*

Look at the spinal nerve chart below and see if any of your spinal pains and stiffness might be related to your internal problems, and vice versa. A spinal problem does not have to hurt; it's just a misaligned spinal bone. It might cause stiffness in a particular joint, or you might feel nothing at all. If you have any internal problems, like stomach or intestine or respiratory tract problems, look at the chart to see how they can be improved by removing pressure from the corresponding spinal nerve. Nerve pressure works sort of like a dimmer switch; the lights work if you turn the dimmer down, but they don't work as they were meant to. Same with your organs and glands; the more nerve pressure, the less they function normally. As the spine continues to misalign, it squeezes the spinal nerve. If this is in the lower back it can press on the nerve that goes to the intestines, possibly resulting in constipation or colitis. Tissues need 100 percent of their nerve supply to function at their intended capacity. Subluxations cause decreased nerve supply to the organs, glands, tissues and cells. You need the electricity turned on for the glands and organs to work properly and not develop disease. Chiropractic physicians are highly trained spinal structural specialists who can detect and correct spinal subluxations and turn the electricity and power back on. *(See Effects of Spinal Misalignments chart)*

3) **Toxicity** damages cells by poking holes in membranes, causing premature death. Certain toxins are attracted to certain tissues; for example, neurotoxins primarily attack nervous tissue like the brain, spinal cord and spinal nerves and peripheral nerves. Toxins can be linked to tissue irritation and damage, along with cancer formation. Aspartame, the sweetening ingredient in the artificial sweetener Nutrasweet, may cause tumors in the

central nervous system, including the brain and spinal cord. Synthetic bovine growth hormone (SBGH), given to dairy cows to increase milk production, may be linked to breast cancer. Certain dyes are indicated in bladder cancers. So, to best protect your organs and glands, **get the good in** (the 90-plus essential nutrients, oxygen and simple carbohydrates from vegetable source and whole grain complex carbohydrates) and **get the bad out** (toxins, chemicals and drugs via detox programs.)

4) Organ/gland specific nutrition supplements the essential nutrients just mentioned. To help organ and gland function, God made specific plants to help specific organs and glands. These plants are rich in vitamins, minerals, trace mineral, phytochemicals and antioxidants. (Remember Ezekiel 47:12, which says "the fruit shall be their food and the leaf their medicine.") For instance, for a healthy heart, you could eat hawthorn berries. In a study on dogs in China, doctors clamped the major blood vessel to the heart, constricting it to cause a heart attack. They recorded the amount of constriction and the amount of permanent heart muscle damage. The next group of dogs was fed hawthorn berries and put through the same routine. Amazingly, dogs fed hawthorn berries took three times more constriction to cause a heart attack. When the dogs continued to eat hawthorn, their hearts repaired themselves with no permanent damage.[1] This is because God's pharmacy is perfectly balanced. But only when taken naturally. When man takes a chemical composition of hawthorn made in a lab as a drug, the results are not the same as they were for the dogs. Drugs and medications have side effects, because they're not perfectly balanced like plants from God are. Drugs not only yield side effects, but also cause a greater strain on the liver to detox all these unnatural medications and chemicals in your body. We don't want undue strain on our elimination organs (liver, kidneys, bowels), because they keep us as toxin-free as possible. This doesn't mean all medication is useless; some is necessary in emergency situations. But for the long haul of life, we should go to God's pharmacy of life-giving plants and herbs more than we go to man's pharmacy of drugs and chemicals.

What can I do for my organ/gland health?

1) Get the good in by ingesting essential nutrients.

2) Get the bad out by detoxifying regularly.

3) Exercise daily with rebounding cellular exercise or at least three times per week (30 minutes per day.)

Causes of Spinal Subluxations
STRESS
PHYSICAL

CHRONIC

1. Poor sitting posture
2. Poor standing posture
3. Poor lifting posture
4. Poor sleeping posture
5. Poor support mattress
6. Poor support pillow
7. Poor muscle tone
   - neck
   - upper back
   - middle back
   - lower back
   - pelvis/hip
8. Decreased muscle flexibility
   - neck
   - upper back
   - middle back
   - lower back
   - pelvis/hip
9. Overweight
10. Lack of movement
11. Repetitive stress
12. Above max work load capacity
13. Past accidents, falls, sudden stops, jars, hits or contact
14. Arthritis/Degeneration

ACUTE

1. Accidents
2. Falls
3. Hits
4. Jars
5. Contact
6. Sudden stops

THERMAL

1. Hypothermia
2. Hyperthermia
3. Weather
   - humidity
   - barometric pressure

MENTAL

1. Self induced
2. Personality
3. Problems with:
   - spouse
   - children
   - finances
   - relatives
   - friends
   - past memories
   - neighbors
   - job
   - health

GENERAL HEALTH

1. Illness past/present
2. Suboptimal
3. Poor fitness level
4. Lack of sleep
5. Genetic/Present organ gland weakness
6. Diet
   - food sensitivity
   - refined sugar
   - red meat
   - dairy
7. Malnutrition
8. Maldigestion
9. Malabsorption
10. Poor elimination
11. Toxicity

SPIRITUAL

1. Fear
2. Lonliness
3. Lack of love
4. Lack of joy
5. Lack of peace
6. Lack of relationship with God

CHART OF EFFECTS OF SPINAL MISALIGNMENTS

"The nervous system controls and coordinates all organs and structures of the human body." (*Gray's Anatomy*, 29th Ed., page 4). Misalignments of spinal vertebrae and discs may cause irritation to the nervous system and affect the structures, organs, and functions which may result in the conditions shown below

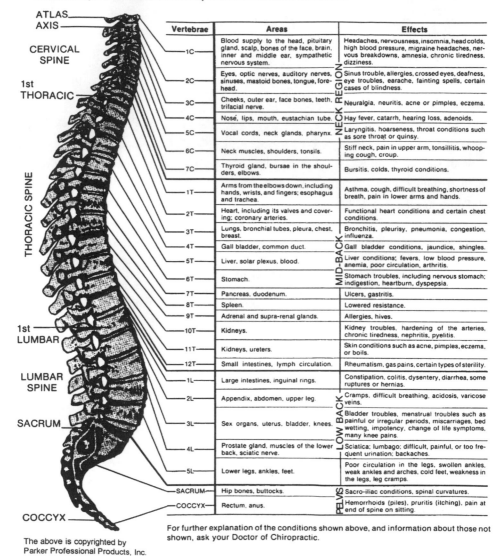

Vertebrae	Areas	Effects
1C	Blood supply to the head, pituitary gland, scalp, bones of the face, brain, inner and middle ear, sympathetic nervous system.	Headaches, nervousness, insomnia, head colds, high blood pressure, migraine headaches, nervous breakdowns, amnesia, chronic tiredness, dizziness.
2C	Eyes, optic nerves, auditory nerves, sinuses, mastoid bones, tongue, forehead.	Sinus trouble, allergies, crossed eyes, deafness, eye troubles, earache, fainting spells, certain cases of blindness.
3C	Cheeks, outer ear, face bones, teeth, trifacial nerve.	Neuralgia, neuritis, acne or pimples, eczema.
4C	Nose, lips, mouth, eustachian tube.	Hay fever, catarrh, hearing loss, adenoids.
5C	Vocal cords, neck glands, pharynx.	Laryngitis, hoarseness, throat conditions such as sore throat or quinsy.
6C	Neck muscles, shoulders, tonsils.	Stiff neck, pain in upper arm, tonsillitis, whooping cough, croup.
7C	Thyroid gland, bursae in the shoulders, elbows.	Bursitis, colds, thyroid conditions.
1T	Arms from the elbows down, including hands, wrists, and fingers; esophagus and trachea.	Asthma, cough, difficult breathing, shortness of breath, pain in lower arms and hands.
2T	Heart, including its valves and covering; coronary arteries.	Functional heart conditions and certain chest conditions.
3T	Lungs, bronchial tubes, pleura, chest, breast.	Bronchitis, pleurisy, pneumonia, congestion, influenza.
4T	Gall bladder, common duct.	Gall bladder conditions, jaundice, shingles.
5T	Liver, solar plexus, blood.	Liver conditions; fevers, low blood pressure, anemia, poor circulation, arthritis.
6T	Stomach.	Stomach troubles, including nervous stomach; indigestion, heartburn, dyspepsia.
7T	Pancreas, duodenum.	Ulcers, gastritis.
8T	Spleen.	Lowered resistance.
9T	Adrenal and supra-renal glands.	Allergies, hives.
10T	Kidneys.	Kidney troubles, hardening of the arteries, chronic tiredness, nephritis, pyelitis.
11T	Kidneys, ureters.	Skin conditions such as acne, pimples, eczema, or boils.
12T	Small intestines, lymph circulation.	Rheumatism, gas pains, certain types of sterility.
1L	Large intestines, inguinal rings.	Constipation, colitis, dysentery, diarrhea, some ruptures or hernias.
2L	Appendix, abdomen, upper leg.	Cramps, difficult breathing, acidosis, varicose veins.
3L	Sex organs, uterus, bladder, knees.	Bladder troubles, menstrual troubles such as painful or irregular periods, miscarriages, bed wetting, impotency, change of life symptoms, many knee pains.
4L	Prostate gland, muscles of the lower back, sciatic nerve.	Sciatica; lumbago; difficult, painful, or too frequent urination; backaches.
5L	Lower legs, ankles, feet.	Poor circulation in the legs, swollen ankles, weak ankles and arches, cold feet, weakness in the legs, leg cramps.
SACRUM	Hip bones, buttocks.	Sacro-iliac conditions, spinal curvatures.
COCCYX	Rectum, anus.	Hemorrhoids (piles), pruritis (itching), pain at end of spine on sitting.

For further explanation of the conditions shown above, and information about those not shown, ask your Doctor of Chiropractic.

The above is copyrighted by Parker Professional Products, Inc.

4) Have a chiropractic physician examine your spine for subluxations, which can cause nerve irritation and organ/gland dysfunction. Even if you're not experiencing any pain or problems, it's good to have your spine checked because many problems have no outward symptoms for years even though internally disease may have already begun.

5) Take the appropriate organ/gland specific herbs for areas you want to strengthen or maintain at optimal health. There is a specific herb or combination of herbs that will feed, regenerate, rejuvenate, and protect almost every organ and gland in your body. These herbs are great to take after you have done all other aspects of your *total health = wholeness* program.

The following list will help you choose the right herbs. Remember, choose organic first, and wildcrafted second. Herbs come in different forms for consumption: teas, tinctures, and capsule or powdered forms. To make herbal tea, put raw herbs in distilled water and let it sit a few hours or more. Simmer on low heat for 15 minutes, then strain and drink. Tinctures, made from herbs in concentrated liquid forms, can be stored for years without losing potency. (Teas and powdered herbs do lose potency over time.)

HERB	ORGAN/SYSTEM	USE
Ginko	Brain	Stimulates blood flow
Cayenne	Brain	Stimulates blood flow
Valerian	Nervous	Sedates/relaxes
Lobelia	Nervous	Antispasmodic/relaxes
St. Johns wort	Nervous	Nerve repair&healing, pain relief
Wild Yam	Nervous	Antispasmodic/relaxes
Wild Yam	Reproductive (female)	Hormone balancing/PMS/menopause
Angelica	Reproductive (female)	Hormone balancing/PMS/menopause
Damiana	Reproductive (female)	Female tonic
Licorice	Reproductive (female)	Hormone precursor
Ginseng	Reproductive (male)	Increases fertility/sexuality
Siberian Ginseng	Reproductive (male)	Hormone precursor
Saw Palmetto	Reproductive (male) Hormone precursor	Decreases prostate inflammation
Lobelia	Respiratory	Bronchial dialator/antispasmodic
Eucalyptus	Respiratory	Disinfectant, bronchial dialator
Peppermint	Respiratory	Disinfectant, bronchial dialator
Tea Tree	Respiratory	Anti-bacterial, fungal
Garlic	Respiratory	Expectorant/anti-bacterial,viral,fungal
Onion	Respiratory	Expectorant/anti-bacterial,viral,fungal
Hawthorn	Heart	Heart protector
Motherwort	Heart	Heart beat regulator
Ginger	Gastrointestinal	Digestive aid
Peppermint	Gastrointestinal	Digestive aid
Fennel	Gastrointestinal	Digestive aid
Licorice	Gastrointestinal	Aids in ulcer healing, stool softener, laxative
Slippery Elm	Gastrointestinal	Soothes GI tract
Aloe Vera	Gastrointestinal	Soothes GI tract, aids in tissue healing

	Anti-inflammatory	
Aloe Vera	Skin	Aids tissue repair, anti-inflammatory
JoJoba	Skin	Emollient, natural sun protective factor 16
Olive	Skin	Emollient
Tea Tree	Skin	Anti-fungal, bacterial
Eyebright	Eye	Promotes eye healing and health
Goldenseal	Eye	Eye disinfectant
Horseradish	Sinus/Nose	Decongests, stimulates
Onion	Sinus/Nose	Decongests, anti-bacterial
Eucalyptus	Sinus/Nose	Decongests, anti-bacterial
Mullein	Ear	Anti-Inflammatory, pain relief
St. Johns wort	Ear	Anti-inflammatory, pain relief
Clove	Teeth	Infection, pain relief
Oak bark	Teeth	Gum healing aid
Garlic	Teeth	Infection, abscess
Echinacea	Throat	Immune stimulant
Garlic	Throat	Anti-bacterial, viral, fungal
Cayenne	Throat	Circulates blood, pain relief
Peppermint	Throat	Soothes, disinfectant
Licorice	Throat	Soothes
Wintergreen	Muscular	Anti-inflammatory
Peppermint	Muscular	Increases blood flow to area
St. Johns wort	Muscular	Trauma repair
Marigold	Muscular	Trauma repair
Arnica	Muscular	Trauma repair

6) Support your major hormonal glands: pancreas, adrenals and thyroid. These glands are the movers and shakers of your entire body. Adrenal glands secrete adrenaline. (For a full discussion on adrenaline, see Chapter 17.) The thyroid is the hormonal gland of metabolism—a "thermostat" setting the temperature of your body's furnace. All bodily functions depend upon enzymes, and all enzymes depend upon proper body temperature. The pancreas secretes insulin and glucagon, regulating blood sugar so your body's cells have enough food for energy and in times of need. Problems arise when blood-sugar levels rise and fall too quickly, or remain at high or low levels. Symptoms of high blood-sugar include excessive thirst, hunger, urination and weight loss, while symptoms of low blood-sugar (hypoglycemia) are sudden mood swings, anxiety, weakness, headaches, hyperactivity, irritability, sweating, rapid heart rate, dizziness, memory problems, learning problems and digestive problems. Eating five smaller meals instead of three larger ones can control hypoglycemia. Also, refined sugars are to be strictly avoided. Time-released foods, like raw vegetables, are

ideal, especially mid-morning and mid-afternoon. Other things that affect blood-sugar levels include food sensitivity, allergy, stress levels and physical exercise.

Here's a list of natural foods and supplements to help keep your adrenals, thyroid and pancreas functioning properly.

Adrenal

DHEA	wild yam
B vitamins	SupremeFood, whole grains
Vitamin C	citrus, green and red peppers
Calcium and Magnesium	SupremeFood, plant based organic minerals in the form of sesame, pumpkin, sunflower seeds, dark green vegetables
Sedative, Antispasmodic Herbs	Valerian, hops, passion flower, sedative oil wild yam, black cohosh, blue cohosh

Thyroid

Iodine	kelp, dulse
Trace Minerals	SupremeFood, sesame, pumpkin, sunflower, and flax seeds
DHEA	wild yam
Radish juice	radish juice
(mixed with carrot juice)	

Pancreas

B vitamins	SupremeFood, whole grains
Chromium	SupremeFood, plant based organic minerals
Green bean juice	

CHAPTER 19

LIGHT AND ENERGY

In the book of Genesis, the first thing to be made was light, and without light no life would exist on the planet. Light energy can enter into our bodies in two ways:

1) Through sunlight
2) Through green food or plants that contain chlorophyll

SUNLIGHT

Sunlight is so vital to human health that one could write volumes to explain how intimately connected the two are. To keep it simple, one should know that there are eight basic ways to maintain proper health:

1. Pure air
2. Pure water
3. Pure food
4. Detoxification
5. Sunlight/energy balance
6. Exercise
7. Pure mind
8. Pure spirit

The sunlight-generated energy that our bodies are exposed to is extremely important to human health. I have summarized some of the many beneficial effects that sunlight has on our health.

Sunlight [1]
• Decreases blood pressure
• Decreases resting heart rate
• Decreases cholesterol
• Decreases blood sugar
• Increases energy, endurance and muscular strength
• Increases body's resistance to infection (increases white blood cell count, i.e.: lymphocytes and phagocytes)
• Increases tolerance to stress
• Increases sex hormones

Regular gradual exposure to sunlight has a very similar effect on the body as regular exercise and even has shown measurable increase in physical fitness.[2]

A cholesterol drop of 13 percent was recorded in a study of 30 patients after just one sunlight treatment.[3] One case study showed a female age 65 was given four successive days of sunlight treatment with no other changes in diet or lifestyle. Her cholesterol dropped from 333 to 221.[4]

Sunlight and skin cancer.

With the great rise of skin cancers and melanomas, how can the benefits of sunlight be received without causing increased cancer rates? The answer is found in our diet and lifestyle. Studies have shown that if ample amounts of natural occurring antioxidants are consumed in food, like vitamins A, C and E, these protective vitamins protect the skin from the damaging effects of sunlight.[5] If gradual exposure is practiced it can actually have the opposite effect and make the skin more flexible and youthful.

The other factor that affected the increase in skin cancer was increased amounts of fats and oils of all types. This also goes along with many studies that show all cancer rates increase as fat and oil consumption (even good fat and oil) increases.[6] So to get the health benefits from the sun, one must progressively increase their exposure from a few minutes up to approximately 30 minutes. This varies widely with the time of day. The sun is strongest from 10:00 a.m. to 2:00 p.m. each day. Seasons also affect exposure, as does skin type and color. You never want your skin to burn, redden or hurt.

Good sources to saturate tissues with the following vitamins are:

VITAMIN A
carrots
sweet potatoes
melons
corn
squash
apricots
peaches
bananas
dark green, leafy vegetables (kale, broccoli, collards)

VITAMIN E
whole grains
fresh vegetables
whole raw nuts and seeds

<u>VITAMIN C</u>

green peppers	red peppers
tomatoes	oranges
grapefruit	strawberries
dark green leafy vegetables	

<u>Sunlight</u>:
- Destroys bacteria [7]
- Increases lymphocyte production, which produces, increased interferon, which can dramatically help in reducing cancer and viral infections [8]
- Factory workers had 50 percent fewer colds in those that worked under ultraviolet light as opposed to standard light[9]
- Decreases CAMP (cyclic adenosine monophosphate.) CAMP is found in almost all cells in the body. If levels of CAMP build up in the body it causes depression of the immune system. What causes CAMP?
  - Stress and adrenaline production
  - Coffee, tea, chocolate
  - From polyunsaturated intake [10]

Any of these factors that cause increased CAMP decreases the immune system which greatly increases the chances of cancer formation or uncontrollable viral, bacteria, fungal or parasitic infections. So wonderful is that sunlight destroys CAMP and boosts the immune system by not only getting rid of the CAMP which suppresses the immune system but also by increasing the number of lymphocytes and increasing the ability of white blood cells to eat bacteria, viruses, fungi, parasites and cancer cells. Sunlight is a very powerful ally of the immune system.

Sunlight and ionization of air.

Sunlight causes air to be balanced at a ratio of 4:5 negative to positive ions.[11] This ratio is proper for good health. Positive ions increase various symptoms that can be felt as headaches, nasal obstruction, hoarseness, fatigue, dry throat and dizziness.[12] Negative ions cause more exhilaration and well being although they can have negative effects of longer periods if not in balance with positive ions.[13] Some other health effects of air from ions are:

Negative Ions
- Inhibit cancer growth [14]
- Lower blood pressure
- Decrease respiration rate
- Increase ease of breathing for hay fever and asthma patients
- Inhibit respiratory tract infections

Positive Ions
- Increase cancer growth
- Raise blood pressure
- Increase respiratory rate
- Depress adrenal gland function, which causes the body to be more susceptible to the negative effects of stress.[15]

Heating systems cause air to be positively charged[16] so it is very important to keep your windows open and keep the thermostat low. Also, a high quality air filtration system that both oxygenates and ionizes the air is highly recommended.

Sunlight and the Mind
Much has been written about Seasonal Affective Disorder (SAD) and how sunlight is important to our mind function. The lack of sunlight can cause a wide range of mental symptoms, the most prominent being depression. Lack of sunlight also causes an increase in CAMP, which causes people to become emotionally upset by putting the nervous system in a more hyperactive state.[17]

ENERGY
All living matter has energy that God gave it to maintain life. This energy is the basis of life and without this energy the organism ceases to exist. This energy field can even be seen with the advanced Kirlian Photography, which shows streams of energy emanating from growing plants or the body of a person.

What is this energy?
It is thought to be made up of bioelectrical charges. This bioelectricity is vital for functioning of the cells of your body, for them to rid themselves of toxins and bring into the cell the proper nutrients and oxygen. Cells start to die when their fluid becomes acidic and the energy drops too low to support the function of taking in nutrients and oxygen and

releasing toxins. When this bioelectricity of the cells drops it is the first step in the disease process and it occurs long before any laboratory test shows a problem. It also shows before symptoms develop.

How does living uncooked food help?

Dr. Hans Eppinger at the First Medical Clinic of the University of Vienna found that a living food diet increased the electrical potential between the tissue cells and the capillary cells. Dr. Eppinger also showed that the living food increased the absorption of nutrients and increased the release of toxins of the cells. Most important was that Dr. Eppinger found that living uncooked foods were the only kind of food that could restore the bioelectrical potential of the tissues once their electrical potential was weakened and cellular degeneration had begun.[18]

This could possibly be because living foods get their energy and bio-electrical charges from sunlight. In essence, the living food becomes a package or container of the sun's energy to enter our bodies and keep us healthy, or to restore to normal the lost electrical potential of abnormal or diseased cells, therefore restoring normal cellular function and affecting a healing in them. This is analogous to a car battery that has lost all of its charge and gone dead and once it is jump-started it regains its electrical charge and will operate correctly once again.

Dr. Valerie Hunt of the Bioenergy Fields Foundation in California has documented the bioelectricity of cells through Kirlian Photography. This ultraviolet film technique visually shows the bioelectricity of any life form. Dr. Hunt has shown how living food has a bioelectric field surrounding it whereas cooked food and junk foods lose their bioelectric energy field.[19]

The greatest bioelectrical charge is found in food that is still living (i.e. sprouts.) Once food has been cut, it starts to lose its bioelectricity. This is why the most health promoting foods are sprouted greens like wheat grass, barley grass, sunflower greens and buckwheat greens. Their bioelectricity is at the peak so as to "jump start" the weak or damaged cells, their enzyme content is greatest so as to give life, not take it away, their vitamin, mineral and phytochemical contents are also at their highest levels to add to the weakened cells.

To summarize, all living things have a bioelectric energy or field that emanates from them. This life force is seen in both animals and plants. Once the animal or plant dies, the bioelectric field is lost. When we eat cooked food it has no bioelectric charge to "jump start" our weakened or damaged cells. So although it supplies calories, minimal vitamins, minerals, phytochemicals and can sustain health, it can never regain health that is being lost. It supplies no bioelectrical charge, no enzymes, and no oxygen; the three most important components of maintaining life. So dead food eventually makes dead people whereas live food makes live people.

To summarize, God made light and we were meant to be in it. Our health is dependent upon it. The more we live in an artificial inside environment, the more negative the impact it will have on our *total health* = *wholeness*. The most current research on diet in the treatment of disease concludes that the most health promoting, most anti disease forming foods are green plants. Then God said...." everything that has breath of life in it—I give green plant for food." (Gen. 1:30)

CHAPTER 20

RECOMMENDATIONS FOR WHOLENESS

John 6:33 tells us that the Spirit gives life. The flow of life and health is from spirit to soul (mind, will and emotions) to body.

Here is how you should address your *total health = wholeness*:

1) Have a personal relationship with the Living God through His Son Jesus Christ—God incarnate, the perfect God-Man. This relationship requires only faith, one doesn't have to do anything to approach God. Jesus did it all when He died on the cross. He paid the price for our sins, erasing the Old Covenant and establishing the New—an unbreakable covenant between Himself, representing all mankind, and God the Father. This covenant means that all that is God's is also ours through His Holy Spirit, and all that is ours becomes His. We die to our old nature and become alive in Christ. This is the gospel, or "good news."

God loves us so much that He promises never to leave or forsake us. He promises to always comfort, guide, empower, teach and reveal all things to us. When we are in Christ, all the covenant blessings are ours because when Jesus died for us, His blood formed a new everlasting covenant. In Christianity, we don't get what we deserve. Jesus, the perfect God-man, didn't deserve to die for us. But in His death, He paid the price we deserved to pay, so that we would have eternal life, living forever with God in heaven and empowered on this earth. If we got what we deserved, we'd all be going to hell eternally separated from God, His Love, His joy and His peace. Through the disobedience of one man, Adam, we all became sinners. But through the obedience of one man, Jesus, all have become righteous in God's sight.

Communion with God is not a religion; it is a relationship with God through His Son Jesus Christ. God wants to talk to us and listen to us. He wants us to know He loves us and will do anything for us. When we ask Jesus Christ into our hearts, we become a new creation, and we begin to fall in love with the God who made us. We begin to serve and keep His commands not because we have to, but because we want to. When I got married, no one gave me a "book of marriage" that told me how to please my wife; that just came naturally because I loved her. It's the same with

God; as we pursue Him in love, He fills us with His love, joy and peace—the main ingredients in *total health = wholeness.*

Jesus said, "I am the way and the truth and the life. No one comes to the Father except through me." (John 14:6) The Apostle Paul, inspired by the Holy Spirit, told us how to have a personal relationship with God: "If you profess with your mouth that Jesus is Lord and believe in your heart that God raised Him from the dead, you will be saved" (Romans 10:9.)

If you haven't already, ask Jesus into your heart now and begin the most wonderful relationship you will ever experience. And it will last for eternity.

2) Live in love, joy and peace, which all come from our Father in heaven. Jesus promised to leave His Holy Spirit with us to live in our hearts—to always lead, guide, comfort, empower, help, and reveal all things to us. Galatians 5: 22-23 says, "The fruit of the spirit is love, joy, peace, patience, kindness, goodness, faithfulness, gentleness and self-control." If we know Jesus as Lord and Savior, this fruit will be evident in our lives once we understand how much God loves us and has poured His grace upon us. Grace means "unmerited favor." We don't deserve God's blessings; we can't earn salvation. They are a free gift received through our faith, our response to God's promises.

A life of love, joy and peace comes when you regularly meditate, commune and communicate with the Living God and listen to His voice spoken into your heart, letting the Holy Spirit bring it to life. So, fill your head and heart up with God's good promises to you, and pray that the Spirit makes them real and alive. This is how to know God's peace, which transcends all understanding. God's love, joy and peace don't depend on your circumstances; that's why Paul could praise Jesus in a Philippian jail after being beaten half to death. God's love, joy and peace depend upon your relationship with Him and your understanding of how much He loves you.

In a very small way, I experienced a type of this when I married the love of my life. Once I entered the covenant of marriage, I knew my wife loved me with all her heart, as I did her. This love gave me joy, knowing I will always be with the one God created for me, my Eve. This also gave me peace, knowing that my purpose in life was fulfilled; I had entered into a lifelong covenant with the one who made me complete. But the love, joy and peace I have with my wife is just a shadow of what we have when we enter into a covenant relationship with God through His Son Jesus Christ.

3) Give all your cares, worries and stress to God. It's vitally important to know how to minimize stress; doing so will increase the quantity and quality of your life. There's no other way to live life, except to give it to God and let Him handle it. Otherwise, you tend to take control, and that always fails. It's like dieting: You might lose weight on a diet plan. But eventually, you lose your self-discipline and go back to your old ways, gaining all the weight back. That's the difference between self-discipline, which comes from your own efforts, and self-control, which is a fruit of the Spirit and comes from God. How do you give it all to God? By understanding the new covenant promise, which says that all that God has, He gives to us through Jesus Christ. The evangelist Smith Wigglesworth once said, "God said it, I believe it, and that settles it."

Let's see what God has said through his Word:

a) "Cast all your cares upon Him because He cares for you" (1 Peter 5:7)

b) "My yoke is easy and my burden is light" (Matthew 11:30)

c) "I will never leave you nor forsake you" (Hebrews 13:5)

d) "You may ask me for anything in my name, and I will do it" (John 14:14)

e) "Do not be anxious about anything, but in everything, by prayer and petition, present your requests to God. And the peace of God, which transcends all understanding, will guard your heart and your minds in Christ Jesus" (Philippians 4:6-7)

f) If God knows the number of hairs on your head (Matthew 10:30), don't you think He knows what you need?

The Living God loves us so much that He died so that we may live. He always has our best interests in mind. He knows what we need, and He sees the whole picture. So by trusting Him, we put our lives in the best hands. We can stop worrying and cast our burdens on Him.

God will speak to us through His Holy Spirit. One day when my wife was getting dressed, the Holy Spirit spoke to her heart and said, "Don't put on your makeup." My wife thought it was just her own thoughts, but as soon as she put on the makeup, she had a reaction and her eyes swelled. If God helps us with the little things in life, He'll help us with the big things too. He loves us more than we can ever know, so give everything to Him and listen to His voice. He will guide you by speaking to your heart with love, joy and peace.

4) Seek God for your mission statement, the purpose for which He created you.

Everyone of us has a reason, a mission, a purpose for which God created them. This is God's will for our life. When and if we come to that place in life when we discover God's will for us we will soar higher than anyone else, because what ever specific task He has created us for no one else can do this quite like us. When we do it we actually do it effortlessly and with timelessness. Effortlessly because it is natural to us, it is what we were created for and when we are operating in the purpose we were designed for there is no effort, it just flows. Timelessness, because when we are performing the call for which we were made, it is pure joy, not work. When you are having fun time flies as if there was no time. When we are doing the exact thing God created us for, we also live and walk supernaturally in each moment. God releases supernatural gifts that enable you to perform your call like no one else in the world can. Things become naturally right when you are living your purpose, events just happen to move you forward in your purpose: doors open, contacts are made, timing is right, these are not coincidences, they are divine appointments.

Unfortunately many never find what their true purpose is, they never align their will with God's will for them. They do not seek Him and wait to be directed by Him. Instead they get a job or enter into a lifestyle that seems right to their mind. They settle because of what the world or their natural (without God) mind says when God has so much more for them. They end up living an ordinary life, missing out on the blessing of living a supernaturally extraordinary life. How do you find out what God's will is? Take time in meditation and prayer to listen every day. He speaks if you are listening, but He speaks to the heart and not to the head. Sometimes what is in your heart seems crazy in your mind. Continue to seek Him, if it is from Him the love, joy and peace will grow in your heart. This then will give you strength to overcome your mind and step out of your comfort zone to God's greater blessings. Living your purpose in life. Most all the great people in life that accomplished something to change the world, to further humanity in some way are those who DID discover their mission statement, their call, their purpose. It is then that the spirit, soul (mind, will and emotion) and body connect together in perfect balance and supernaturally the world is and can be changed like never before. God has placed this inside everyone of us, but so few of us take the quiet time in prayer and meditation to discover this gift God has given each one of us. Take the time and then begin to live the life you were created for.

5) Make your dreams become reality

God made us creative spirits because He is a creative Spirit and we were made in His image. Every invention, every innovation, everything that made this world what it is, started as a desire, a dream. How do dreams come true? It starts with knowing that God gives us the desires of our hearts. This is awesome. If we use the process below, our dreams can become reality. God made many laws both spiritual and physical that operate and govern the world. Spiritually, the law of sowing and reaping, the law of giving and receiving, the law of faith are a few. Physically, some of the laws include the law of gravity and the law of thermodynamics. What is a law? It means that if that an expected outcome is always produced when the principles are applied. If we jump off a building we will always fall down to the ground, when we plant corn, corn will always grow. When God says He will give you the desires of your heart, He will. His Word always is true and more constant than any law. Let us apply these principles to make your dreams become reality.

Desire

Desire comes from deep in your heart. It is what you want and how much you want it that determines your desire.

Envision

This is the process of painting the picture created with your desire on the canvass of your mind. This is seeing your desire already accomplished. Living as if it already was reality and enjoying it. Enjoying it means feeling the enjoyment in your heart as if it was already done. How would it feel if you really accomplished your dream? In this step you must see it, feel it and enjoy it no differently than if it truly had already occurred. This is the enjoyment of the journey.

Pray

In your quiet time before God you present your picture that you created before Him and seek His guidance to refine your picture, to show you the best path to complete the picture. This is crucial to the dream process because God knows all things and led by Him you will open the right doors along your journey. Without His guidance and input, the dream process becomes hard work instead of great joy.

Speak the Dream

Speak out the dream as if it were already reality because not only does it strengthen your faith in it, but it also strengthens the faith of those around you who start to see the picture of your dream. Your words give strength to your desire.

Know It

You live and believe as if your dream has already occurred so much so that when it really does occur your reaction is "no big deal" because you already lived it, experienced it and enjoyed it. The journey was the excitement, the destination is anticlimactic, it just leads you to new desires and the creative process begins again.

6) As much as possible, eat a living, raw, vegan, organic diet. Uncooked food is loaded with enzymes, vitamins, minerals, phytochemicals, oxygen, bioelectricity and antioxidants. Cooked food loses all enzymes, oxygen, bioelectrical charge and many vitamins. As you transition to this new lifestyle, don't compare yourself to anyone else; this can frustrate you. Instead, compare yourself to how you were a year ago: Are you growing in your *total health = wholeness*? If you don't like what you see, ask God to help you make some changes. (For more on this, see Chapter 11)

7) Eat the cleanest, purest food possible. When digested food enters your bloodstream, it can be classified in one of three ways: 1) vital nutrient, 2) chemical or toxin, or 3) additive/foreign particles/undigested food. Our goal is to be pure, to put as many vital nutrients and as few of the other two groups as possible. **Get the good in** and **get the bad out**. Stay away from the toxins and chemicals and other harmful debris. Buy organic (no added chemicals). Read labels; if it looks like chemistry, don't eat it. (For more information, see Chapter 11)

8) Eliminate these from your diet: refined sugar, hydrogenated fats and oils, animal fat and protein, salt, dairy products, excessive protein, refined flours/pastas, store bought juices and all perservatives. I have described the problems associated with all of these in great detail in earlier chapters. (For more information, see Chapters 6 and 11)

9) Check for food sensitivity/allergy, and eliminate the offenders. This is critical for living in *total health* = *wholeness* (For a review of this topic, see Chapter 13)

10) Make sure you are thoroughly digesting your food. Chew completely. Drink little fluid with meals. Eat smaller meals more frequently. Combine food properly. (To review this topic, see Chapter 12.)

11) Take vegetarian-based enzymes with all meals that are cooked. A simple rule and a life saver. Enzymes are the key to life and vitality (For more on digestive enzymes, see Chapter 11.)

12) Take SupremeFood every day. The next best thing to eating all the right food is taking Supremefood, which is loaded with vitamins and minerals from the best organic and wildcrafted sources. This is a God-made supplemental food which is totally absorbable into the body, unlike the extremely low absorption rates of man-made supplements. Clinically tested, I have found nothing better than Supremefood as an addition to whole organic food. (For more on Supremefood, see Chapter 11)

13) Take additional whole food supplements, like organic plant bound minerals in seed form, acidophilus/bifidus flora, antioxidants (found in Vitamins A, C, and E.) When possible, get these vitamin supplements from food sources (carrots and yams for Vitamin A, oranges, red and green pepper for C, whole grains, seeds and nuts for E.)

14) Detox your bowel two weeks every three months. With the proper herbs (see appendix), you can clean, purify, tone and increase blood flow to your bowel by removing toxins, bacteria, and other harmful residuals, including impacted fecal material. (For more information, see Chapter 14.)

15) Stay on bowel maintenance herbal formula daily to insure bowel health.

16) Detox your liver, kidneys and blood one week each, every three months. I recommend it every month for anyone who has been very sick in the past. The liver/kidney/blood detox program takes a total of three weeks (see appendix.) (For more information, see Chapter 14.)

17) Stay on liver maintenance herbal formula daily to insure liver protection and liver detoxification.

18) Drink at least one quart (32oz) of distilled water or reverse osmosis water per 50 lbs. of body weight per day. Drink as much as you can before noon and don't drink for 1 to 2 hours after a meal and no closer than ½ hour prior to a meal. (For more about water, see Chapter 7.)

19) Get 30 minutes of cardiovascular exercise per day. On a rebounder is ideal to decrease stress on joints and increase the strength of every cell. Have your family doctor examine you before you start any exercise program. (See Chapter 15)

20) Get 30 minutes of cellular lymphatic exercise per day by rebounding. This should be a combination of deep breathing and doing the health bounce on the rebounder. Also do deep breathing exercises through out the day whenever you have time like in the car to and from work. (See Chapter 15)

21) Boost your immune system. Do this by following the dietary recommendations in this book, and by staying as far away from sugar and stress as you can. (For a review of the best ways to help your immune system, see Chapter 16.)

22) Keep your diet high in natural antioxidants and phytochemicals. The best antioxidants are Vitamin A, Vitamin C, Vitamin E and selenium. (For more on antioxidants, see Chapter 17)

Phytochemicals are God-made, plant-bound chemicals with healing capabilities. I believe they're what God referred to in Ezekiel 47:12, "The fruit shall be their food and the leaf their medicine." Things like broccoli, cauliflower, brussel sprouts and cabbage are powerful anti-cancer foods, not only because of their vitamin/mineral/antioxidant/enzyme content, but because of their phytochemical content.

Here's a list of major phytochemical families and their food sources:

Phytochemical Family	**Food**
Allyl Sulfides	Garlic, onions, chives
Indoles	Broccoli, cabbage, kale, and cauliflower
Isoflavones	Soybeans (tofu, soy oils)
Phenolic acids	Tomatoes, citrus, carrots, whole grains, nuts
Polyphenols	Green tea, grapes
Saponine	Beans, legumes
Terpenes	Cherries, citrus fruit peel

23) Support your major hormonal glands: pancreas, adrenals and thyroid (see chapter 18.)

24) Support any other gland or organ weakness by consuming the right foods. Here's a list of God's pharmacy for specific weak areas and organs:

GI System	aloe, ginger, peppermint, licorice
Liver	milk thistle, chaparral
Immune	garlic, echinacea
Blood	red clover, garlic, chapparal, lobelia, cayenne
Urinary	juniper, parsley, uva ursi, cranberry
Cardiovascular	hawthorn berries, red clover, garlic
Brain	cayenne, ginkgo
Nervous System	valerian, lobelia, black cohosh, blue cohosh, wild yam
Female	wild yam, angelica, damiana, licorice
Male	ginseng, siberian ginseng, saw palmetto
Respiratory	lobelia, garlic,eucalyptus, peppermint, tea tree

25) Juice your own juice daily. Fresh, organic vegetable juices are blood transfusions. They are packed with enzymes, vitamins, minerals, antioxidants and phytochemicals, oxygen and bioelectricity that are easily absorbed, and cause no digestive overload. Juice is ideal for those who do not take the time to eat enough raw vegetables; the daily recommended amount is at least six servings of vegetables per day. (For a more detailed discussion on the benefits of juicing, see Chapter 11)

Green juices are the most health promoting, like wheat grass, sunflower sprouts, buckwheat sprouts, kale, collards, broccoli, dandelion and cucumber for water content. If you mix SupremeFood with your juice you greatly increase your health benefits.

A few pointers:

- Drink vegetable juice, not fruit juice. You do not want concentrated amounts of sugar in your blood even from fruit. This will weaken your immune system and throw your hormonal system out of balance.
- Drink fresh, preferably organic, juice within 15 minutes of making it.
- Start slow, diluting two ounces of juice with two ounces of water. Gradually build up so your digestive tract becomes accustomed to digesting juice. To help with the process, chew your juice so your saliva mixes with it, starting its digestion.

Always remember: Juicing is one of the best things you can do for your *total health = wholeness.*

26) Get the good in and get the bad out. Statistics show that we need to hear something seven times before it starts to sink in. And we've said this far more than seven times throughout this book. And I'm going to say it again: To live a healthy, vibrant life, you must get 90-plus nutrients into all your cells, along with oxygen and water and simple sugar from complex carbohydrate digestion. And because we live in a toxic world, we must regularly detoxify our bodies to keep our cells, tissues, glands and organs healthy and strong. If we don't, the oxidative damage from free-radical formation causes cellular damage and immune system suppression, which means we're on our way to getting sick.

27) Have the energy of your spirit, mind and body in balance. Spirit and mind were covered in chapters 9 and 10. Be examined by a wholistic chiropractic physician, the spinal structural specialist, who will find and remove any nerve pressure to glands or organs. Make sure your diet is filled with energy and oxygen rich green living sprouts and raw vegetables. Sunlight in moderation is tremendous for your *total health = wholeness* (see chapter 19.)

28) Address each point of the Total Health Checklist in the appendix daily.

The focus of my suggestions—of this entire book, for that matter—is mainly preventive health. We do these things to treat the cause of problems and to achieve *total health = wholeness*. We are moving away from taking medicine or even vitamin pills to treat the effects. We are achieving total health by addressing our diet, digestion, assimilation, detoxification, exercise, the nervous and energetic systems along with our mental and spiritual health.

Build your house on the strong foundation of these principles, and you will be well on your way to *total health = wholeness.*

APPENDIX I

TOTAL HEALTH CHECKLIST

1) Oxygen Intake
___Proper breathing technique
___High oxygen rich green plant food
___Cellular exercise-rebounding
___Cardiovascular exercise-rebounding

2) Water Intake
___Distilled or reverse osmosis filtered
___1 quart (32 oz.) per 50 lb. of body weight per day

3) Food Intake (Getting the Good In)
___Vegan (animal free) diet
___Living first, raw second, cooked last
___Low fat
___Low protein
___No dairy
___Low sugar (none refined)
___High vegetable
___Whole grains, sprouts, seeds, nuts, legumes and beans
___SupremeFood daily
___Seed "milk" daily

4) Digestion/Assimilation
___Chew every bite of food 25 times
___Don't drink with your meals (no more than 6 oz. of water)
___Eat in a non-rushed relaxed atmosphere
___Combine your food properly
___Eat only food that you are not sensitive or allergic to
___Take digestive enzymes with all cooked meals

5) Detoxify Your Body Daily and Seasonally (Getting the Bad Out)
___Proper breathing technique
___Proper water intake
___Proper diet (vegan and chemical free when possible)
___Bowel Cleanse Program every 3 months
___Bowel Maintenance every day

___Liver/Gall Bladder Program every 3 months
___Liver/Gall Bladder Maintenance daily
___Kidney/ Bladder Program every 6 months
___Blood Cleanse every 3 months

6) *Exercise*

___Lymphatic exercise (rebounding with breathing technique)
___Cellular exercise (rebounding) daily 2 minutes per hour
___Cardiovascular exercise (rebounding) daily for 30 minutes

7) *Structural/Nerve/ Organ/Gland Balance*

___Proper posture: sitting, standing, sleeping and lifting
___Proper nerve flow to every organ and gland: correct all spinal sub-
     luxations
___Proper spinal/postural exercise

8) *Energy Balance*

___Proper food (living or sprouted)
___Organ/Gland balance
___Decrease EMF exposure

9) *Light*

___Sunlight exposure at least 30 minutes per day

10) *Sleep*

___8 hours per night of non interrupted, deep sleep

11) *Emotion/Mind Balance*

___Your personal enjoyment time at least 30 minutes per day
___Organized   ___Time management
___Don't over commit   ___Have fun
___Laugh   ___Dream
___Check adrenals for breaking mind/body barrier
___Check the Spirit Emotion Mind Body connection (SEMB)
___SEMB remedies   ___Flower remedies

12) *Spiritual Balance*

___Quiet meditation time to be guided and empowered by God
___Prayer time: talking to God and listening to His answers
___Refining your dreams with wisdom from God
___Check the Spirit Emotion Mind Body Connection (SEMB)
___SEMB remedies

APPENDIX II

TOTAL HEALTH INSTITUTE'S PRODUCTS

1. SupremeFood
2. Enzymes
3. Bowel Move/Vac
4. Bowel Maintenance
5. Liver/Gall Bladder Program
6. Liver/Gall Bladder Maintenance
7. Kidney/Bladder Program
8. Blood Detox
9. Immune Program

1. SUPREMEFOOD

Nature's powerful organic whole foods supplement. It
- Increases energy & vitality.
- Provides complete nutrition.
- Builds a healthier body from the inside out.
- Establishes optimal weight.

Because of modern agricultural practices resulting in the depletion of the soil, nutritional supplementation is vital.

If you were limited to using only one product, it would have to be SupremeFood. This naturally balanced blend of whole foods is specifically formulated to supply you with natural food sources of vitamins, minerals, amino acids, enzymes, and essential trace nutrients. All of the ingredients are from the richest whole food sources on the planet. SupremeFood is rich in enzymes and is easily assimilated into your bloodstream. You'll definitely feel the difference.

Our bodies were designed to eat foods as they are found and designed by nature. Healthy bodies feel better and have abundant energy. What counts in building health is how much your body assimilates, absorbs, and utilizes, not the milligram dosages printed on a label.

Another benefit of SupremeFood is helping you reestablish your optimal weight. When your body gets the needed nutrients it becomes satisfied nutritionally (which means your appetite is satisfied.) Many find Supreme-

Food to be a great weight loss aid. An 8-oz. glass of water or juice and SupremeFood will give you organic, totally absorbable vitamins, minerals, trace minerals, enzymes and phytochemicals.

100% Organic Vegetarian and Natural Ingredients:

Spirulina blue green algae, chlorella-broken cell algae, alfalfa grass, barley grass, wheat grass, purple dulse seaweed, beet root, spinach leaf, rose hips, orange peel, astragalus, nettles and non-active nutritional yeast.

Recommended Use:

2 tablespoons of SupremeFood in 8 oz. of water or juice, shake up and drink. Or in a blender, mix 8 oz. of pure water with 1 banana and 2 heaping tablespoons of Supreme Food. (If not sugar sensitive)

2. ENZYMES

The life of food comes not only from the essential nutrients they contain, but even more importantly from the enzymes they have stored. It's not what you eat that counts but what you digest and assimilate into the cells of your body.

Enzymes are key to vibrant health and without them your health would steadily decline. God made all raw food to contain life, to contain enzymes. When we cook food we destroy its life, its enzymes. This can be seen when you plant sunflower seeds, one raw and one dry-roasted or cooked. Only the raw uncooked seed will grow. Every cellular reaction that takes place in your body is enzyme dependent and without them you would quickly die. So what is the answer to the vibrant health? Add enzymes to your meals! Four capsules per meal whenever you're eating a cooked meal.

Also, a lack of enzymes in your food causes a build-up of toxins via increased intestinal permeability (leaky gut syndrome) which is the primary cause of almost all disease. The most devastating fact is that without sufficient enzymes in your diet, your white blood cells have to eat your meal instead of eating bacteria, viruses, fungi, parasites and destroying cancer cells. You do not want your immune system depleted because this opens you up to cancer and all other types of disease. Our enzymes are vegetarian based. They are the type recommended by world renowned enzyme expert Dr. Howell, Author of "Enzyme Nutrition."

3. BOWEL CLEANSE PROGRAM

BOWEL MOVE

- Eliminate constipation
- Heal & strengthen the colon
- Anti-parasite
- Improve digestion
- Relieve gas and cramps

This stimulating formula is cleansing, healing and strengthening to the entire gastrointestinal system. Stimulating your peristaltic action (the muscular movement of the colon) and over time strengthens the muscles of the large intestines. This product disinfects, soothes and heals the mucous membrane lining of your entire digestive tract. This herbal formula also improves digestion, relieves gas and cramps, and increases the flow of bile which in turn cleanses the gall bladder and bile ducts, destroying candida albicans overgrowth, promotes a healthy intestinal flora, destroys and expels intestinal parasites, increases gastrointestinal circulation and is anti-bacterial, anti viral and antifungal.

This product, when combined with a nutritious, vegan (plant based) diet is a perfect aid to assist in the prevention of colon cancer, which is now the leading cancer among men and women within the U.S.

100% organic Vegetarian and Natural Ingredients:

Cape aloe leaf, senna leaves and/or pods, cascara sagrada aged bark, barberry root bark, ginger root, fennel seed, garlic bulb powder, cayenne pepper.

Recommended Use:

Begin with one capsule of this formula during or just after dinner. This formula works best when taken with food. The next morning you should notice an increase in your bowel action and in the amount of fecal matter that you eliminate. The consistency should be softer. If you do not notice any difference in your bowel behavior, increase your dosage by one capsule each night. A bowel movement corresponding with each meal per day (2 to 3 per day) is considered healthy. It has taken most of us years to create a sluggish bowel, so be patient and increase by only one capsule per day until you obtain the desired results. Continue with this daily dosage as long as needed to maintain optimal bowel function. As your diet improves, and your colon heals and strengthens, you will require less and less Bowel Move. *Be sure to drink lots of water, fresh vegetable juice and herb tea during the day.* This should be 32 oz of water per 50lbs. of body weight per day. Occasionally, some need no help at all having two to three normal bowel movements per day. In such cases begin with our Bowel Vac Formula, as it will sooth, detoxify and cleanse the bowel. *Not recommended if pregnant.*

BOWEL VAC

- Removes toxins
- Soothes Colon irritation
- Cleanses & heals lower bowel

This cleansing and soothing formula is to be used periodically in conjunction with the Bowel Move Formula. This formula is a strong purifier and intestinal vacuum, helping to draw out old fecal matter from the walls of your colon and out of any bowel pockets. Bowel Vac aids in the removal of poisons, toxins, parasites, heavy metals such as mercury and lead. This formula will also remove drug residues.

This product is designed to soften old hardened fecal matter for easy elimination. This is a soothing remedy for intestinal inflammation such as diverticulitis or irritable bowel syndrome.

Bowel Vac Formula can also be used as an antidote for food or other types of poisoning.

100% Organic Vegetarian and Natural Ingredients:

Flax seed, apple fruit pectin, pharmaceutical grade bentonite clay, psyllium seeds and husks, fennel seed, activated willow charcoal.

Recommended Use:

In a small jar, mix 1 heaping tablespoon of Bowel Vac Formula powder in 16 ounces of water, shake or blend and drink it all down. Take this formula three times each day beginning in the morning for seven consecutive days. One hour before your morning nutritional drink (SupremeFood) mix 1 heaping tablespoon of Bowel Vac Formula with 16 ounces of water. It mixes best if you blend or shake it in a small jar with a lid. Do the same 1 hour before lunch and between lunch and dinner. Make sure that you are consuming a total of 3 heaping tablespoons each day. Increase Bowel

Move Formula by one additional capsule, or more if necessary, to have sufficient bowel movements (2-3 per day.) It is helpful to drink additional liquid after each dose of Bowel Vac Formula, about 8 ounces. We also recommend that you do not take any other herbal formulas at the same time as this formula because the pectin, clay, and charcoal will absorb the nutrients taken with them. *Not recommended if pregnant.*

4. BOWEL MAINTENANCE

This is to be taken daily in-between the complete seasonal Bowel Move/Bowel Vac Program. This combines the Bowel Move and Bowel Vac into capsules to maintain bowel peristalsis, cleanse, strengthen and heal the entire gastrointestinal tract. Aids in the removal of poisons, toxins, parasites and heavy metals like mercury, lead and drug residues.
100% Organic Vegetarian and Natural Ingredients
Cascara Sagrada aged bark, Senna leaf, Psyllium seed, Turkey Rhubarb root Cape Aloe leaf, Barberry root bark, Slippery Elm bark, Cayenne pepper

Recommended Use:
Begin with 1 capsule during or following the evening meal. The following morning there should be an increase in bowel function. If no noticeable change occurs, increase dosage by one capsule each day until improved bowel function is achieved. *Not recommended if pregnant.*

5. LIVER/GALL BLADDER DETOX PROGRAM

LIVER DETOX TEA
- Increase energy
- Improve digestion
- Strengthen liver function
- Digest and assimilate food better
- Excellent coffee substitute

This tea has numerous health benefits. It will act as a stimulant to the entire digestive system. This tea also cleanses the blood, skin, liver and gallbladder. This is the tea to use with the liver/gallbladder flush program.

Liver Detox Tea flushes out the bile and fats from the liver. It is a diuretic and disinfectant to the kidneys and bladder causing you to urinate more within an hour after ingestion.

A proper- functioning liver will boost your energy, as the liver is the body's main source of glucose or stored energy.

This tea is also an excellent coffee replacement. It is a hot beverage, dark in color and tastes good.

100% Organic Vegetarian and Natural Ingredients:

Dandelion root, burdock root, pau d'arco, fennel seed, horsetail herb, orange peel, cardamon seed, cinnamon bark, licorice root, juniper berries, ginger root, black, peppercorns, uva ursi leaves, clove buds, dandelion leaf, sassafras root, parsley root or leaf.

Recommended Use:

Put 1 tablespoon (medium) or 2 tablespoons (strong) of this tea into 20 ounces of distilled or purified water. Be sure to use only stainless steel or glass cookware. Let the tea sit in the water overnight and in the morning heat up to a boil reduce heat and let simmer for 15 minutes. Strain out the herbs, do not discard them, let the tea cool a bit but drink it hot. Put the used herbs back into the pot, add 1 tablespoon of fresh herbs and 20 ounces of pure water. Let sit overnight and repeat the whole process again. Keep adding new herbs to the old ones with the addition of fresh distilled water until after the third day, then discard all herbs and start over. *Not recommended if pregnant.*

LIVER/GALLBLADDER FORMULA
- Increases energy
- Kills parasites
- Heals and protects liver function
- Stimulates liver detox function
- Stimulates digestion

The herbs in this formula are best known for their ability to stimulate, cleanse and protect the liver and gallbladder and rid the body of parasites.

This works best if used in conjunction with the Bowel Move. Use if parasites are suspected, or if there has been a history of bowel problems, constipation, eating of animal products, prolonged illness, serious disease or degeneration. Fatigue and lack of energy is often due to poor liver function, particularly if you are tired after a meal.

Milk Thistle contains chemicals that bind to and coat liver cells, which promote healing of previously damaged cells, protecting the liver from future damage. Oregon grape root bark, gentian root, wormwood leaves and dandelion root are all classic bitter tonic herbs. These herbs not only stimulate digestion but also stimulate the liver to excrete more bile, which in turn cleanses both the liver and the gallbladder. Black walnut hulls, wormwood and garlic are all strong anti-parasite herbs. Parasites are a fact of life. This formula will kill parasites as well as expel them from the bowel. Use this when returning from foreign travel.

100% Organic Vegetarian and Natural Ingredients:
Milk thistle seed, dandelion root, Oregon grape root, gentian root, wormwood leaf and flower, black walnut hulls, ginger root, garlic bulb, sweet fennel seed, fringe tree root bark. Extracted and preserved in U.S.P. Grade Grain Alcohol.

Recommended Use:
2 dropperfuls (70 drops) 4-5 times daily for one week. Most effective when used in conjunction with the Liver Detox Tea. *Not recommended if pregnant.*

6. LIVER/GALL BLADDER MAINTENANCE PROGRAM

This is to be taken daily in-between the Liver/Gall Bladder Program which should be done seasonally (every 3 months) This combines the Liver Detox Tea and Liver/Gall Bladder Formula into capsules to maintain healthy Liver/Gall Bladder function. The herbs in this formula stimulate, cleanse and protect the liver and gall bladder cells. This is a must for today's toxic environment. This keeps the Liver/Gall Bladder balanced, healthy and prevents toxins from damaging the liver and gall bladder.

100% Organic Vegetarian and Natural Ingredients:
Same as in the Liver Detox Tea and Liver/Gall Bladder Formula

7. KIDNEY/BLADDER PROGRAM

KIDNEY/BLADDER FORMULA
- Disinfects urinary tract
- Reduces edema (swelling)
- Strengthens the entire urinary tract

These formulas are both diuretic (increases flow of urine) and disinfectant. According to medical studies the herbs in this formula destroy the bacteria that cause kidney and bladder infections. Experience has shown this formula helps eliminate urinary tract infections, even after antibiotics had failed. This tonic works best if used along with the Kidney/Bladder Formula and Kidney/Bladder Tea.

Kidney/Bladder Formula:

100% Organic Vegetarian and natural Ingredients:
Juniper berries, uva ursi leaves, horsetail herb, pipsissewa leaf, burdock root, and goldenrod flower, dandelion root/leaf, hydranga root, gravel root, marshmallow root, and corn silk. Extracted and preserved in U.S.P. grade grain alcohol.

Recommended Use:
1 to 2 dropperfuls (35-70 drops) 3-4 times daily. Best results are obtained if used for 5 days consecutively and along with the Kidney / Bladder Tea. *Not recommended if pregnant.*

Kidney/Bladder Tea:

100% Organic Vegetarian and natural Ingredients:
Juniper berry, corn silk, uva ursi leaf, horsetail herb, parsley leaf/root, goldenrod flowers, dandelion leaf, orange peel, peppermint leaf, hydrangea root, gravel root, marshmallow root.

Recommended Use:
Pour 16 ounces of boiling distilled water over 1 rounded teaspoon of herbs and let steep. Drink two cups per day for seven days. For best results take Kidney/Bladder Formula along with the Kidney/Bladder Tea. *Not recommended if pregnant.*

8. BLOOD CLEANSING FORMULA

- Detoxifies blood and lymph
- Promotes quicker recovery from chronic illness

The formula is a very powerful blood and lymph cleansing formula and is based on the famous Hoxey formula; Dr. Christopher's Red Clover Tonic and many similar formulae from around the world. Make sure you consume a gallon of water each day of its use. The herbs in this formula are strong in taste, and very effective detoxifiers. Patients with a chronic illness or degenerative condition would benefit from this formula.

100% Organic Vegetarian and Natural Ingredients:

Red clover blossoms, chaparral herb, Oregon grape root, burdock root and seed, yellow dock root, wild indigo root, garlic juice, lobelia herb and seeds, habanero cayenne pepper. Extracted and preserved in U.S.P. Grade Grain Alcohol.

Recommended Use:

2 dropperfuls (70 drops) 4 to 6 times a day for a week. *Drink at least 96 to 128 ounces of water each day you use this formula.* A dropperful is one squeeze of the bulb. *Not recommended if pregnant.*

9. IMMUNE BOOST FORMULA

- Boost immune cell activity
- Increase natural resistance
- Recover from illness quickly

All of us are subject to illness and injury. Rather than taking drugs designed to suppress symptoms, take this herbal combination and boost your body's natural healing ability.

This formula works by boosting the number of your immune cells and amounts of natural chemicals that help to fight illness. Expect much shorter duration of colds, flu and sore throat. this formula also initiates and speeds up recovery from chronic and long term immune depression illnesses, diseases and degeneration.

Echinacea angustifolia is the primary herb in this formula. Squirt a dropperful of Immune Formula on your tongue. In a short time you will feel a tingling sensation. This is the signature of good Echinacea. If you don't experience this, you have a product of inferior quality. Echinacea is one of the strongest immune stimulators and enhancers known.

Siberian Ginseng helps to build stamina when under stress. Pau d'Arco is known to be antifungal, anti-candida and anti viral. Studies have shown Usnea to be effective in combating gram positive bacteria, such as those found in strep throat.

Garlic is a powerful broad-spectrum antibiotic, anti-viral, antifungal herb, as well as a great immune builder. We often recommend taking fresh garlic in addition to this formula. Three to five cloves per day. Cut into small pieces and swallow like you would a pill or capsule. It has to be fresh and is best if organically grown.

100% Organic Vegetarian and Natural Ingredients:

Echinacea Angustifolia, Siberian Ginseng root, Pau d'Arco, Usnea lichen, Cats Claw, fresh garlic. Extracted and preserved in U.S.P. Grade Grain Alcohol

Recommended Use:
For active or current illnesses: Take 2 dropperfuls (70 drops) 6 times per day for six to fourteen days. For general immune boost, take 1 dropperful (35 drops) 3 to 5 times per day for one to two weeks.

10. IMMUNE MAINTENANCE

This should be taken with Immune Boost at the start of any symptoms of cold, flu, fever or illness. This formula is very powerful yet does not over stimulate the immune system. This is why it is the ideal daily immune system strengthener.

100% Organic Vegetarian and Natural Ingredients:

Comfrey root, fresh garlic bulb, wormwood leaf, lobelia herb and seed, marshmallow root, white oak bark, black walnut hull, mullein leaf, skullcap herb, uva ursi leaf, hydranga root, gravel root, organic apple cider vinegar, preserved in pure vegetable glycerin.
Recommended Use:
As a general immune builder take 1-2 tablespoons 3 times per day. During illness 1 tablespoon every hour. If illness persists contact your healthcare professional. *Not recommended if pregnant.*

11. IMMUNE –VIRUS TEA

The third weapon in combating disease is Immune-Virus Tea. The tea is taken along with Immune Boost Formula and Immune Maintenance.

100% Organic Vegetarian and Natural Ingredients:
Organic red clover blossom, organic chaparral herb, organic echinacea angustifolia root, wildcrafted pau d' arco inner bark.
Recommended Use:
Add contents of one packet of dry herbal tea to 3 quarts of purified water. Bring to boil, reduce heat and let simmer for 15 minutes. Strain. Let tea cool and drink. Drink 3 to 6 cups per day. Refrigerate after each use.
Not recommended if pregnant.

For inquiries about products or services:
Total Health Institute
Wheaton, Illinois
630-871-0000

or visit us on-line at
www.totalhealthinstitute.com

**Dr. Keith Nemec is also available
for speaking engagements.**

Coming Soon!
FOODS FOR TOTAL HEALTH
by Laurie Nemec

NOTES

Chapter 2: Disease

1. Vital Statisitics of the United States, 1991, cited in the *Cancer Journal for Clinicians* 41:1 (February 1991):22.

2. Susan Stockton, *The Book of Health* (Mc Lean Publishing, Tampa, Fl 1990): p. 3.

3. John McDougall, *McDougall's Medicine: A Challanging Second Opinion* (Piscataway, NJ: New Century Publishers, 1985):101.

4. Dean Ornish M.D., *Dr. Dean Ornish's Program For Reversing Heart Disease* (Ballantine Books, New York, 1990), p. 11.

5. McDougall, p. 101.

6. Ibid, p. 65.

7. "Diet and Stress in Vascular Disease," JAMA June 3, 1961, p. 806

8. Ornish, pp. 133-4.

9. Patrick Quillin PhD, R.D., *Beating Cancer With Nutrition* (The Nutrition Times Press, Tulsa OK 1994), p. 27.

10. David & Anne Frahm, *Healthy Habits* (Pinon Press, Colorado Springs, CO 1993), p. 13.

11. Phil Gunby, "Battle Against Many Malignancies Lie Ahead as Federal War on Cancer Enters Third Decade," *JAMA* (April 8, 1992): 1891.

12. 1993 Statistical Abstract of U.S., US. National Cancer Center For Health Statistics

13. Charles B. Simone, M.D., "Cancer and Nutrition," (Avery Publishing Group Inc., New York, 1992.), p. 9.

14. Ibid, p. 10.

15. National Cancer Institute, "Cancer Rates and Risk," (Washington, D.C., 1985)

16. Frahm, p. 13

17. Frahm, p. 13.

18. National Academy of Sciences 1982. "Nutrition, Diet and Cancer"

19. Simone, p. 15.

20. Patrick Quillin, *Healing Nutrients*, (Contemporary Books, Chicago, 1987)

21. Cancer Rates and Risk

22. McDougall, p. 77

23. Armstrong B, Doll R., "Environmental factors and cancer incidence and mortality in different countries, with special reference to dietary practices," *Int J Cancer* 1975, !5: 617-31.

24. Rose DP, Boyar AP, Wynder El., "International comparison of mortality rates for cancer of the breast, ovary, prostate and colon, and per capita food consumption," *Cancer* 1986; 58: 2363-71.

25. Hirayama T., "Epidemiology of breast cancer with special reference to the role of diet," *Prev. Med* 1978, 7: 173-95.

26. U.S. Department of Health and Human Services. "Surgeon generals report on nutrition and health," *DHHS Publ No. 88-50210,* 1988.

27. Phillips RL, Garfinkel L, Kuzma JW, et al., "Mortality among California Seventh Day Adventists for selected cancer sites," *J. Natl Cancer Inst.* 1980; 65: 1097-1107.

28. Kinlen, L.J., "Meat and fat consumption and cancer mortality: a study of religious orders in Britian," *Lancet* 1982, 946-49.

29. Neal Barnard, M.D. Food For Life (Crown Publishers, Inc. New York, NY 1993) p. 63.

30. A Walker, Osteoporosis and Calcium Deficiency, Am J Clin Nutr 16(1965): 327

31. R Mazess, Bone Mineral Content of North Alaskan Eskimos, Am J Clin Nutr 27(1974): 916.

32. B. Brenner, "Dietary Protein Intake and the Progressive Nature of Kidney Disease: The Role of Hemodynamically Mediated Glomerular Injury in the Pathogenesis of Progressive Glomerular Sclerosis in Aging, Renal Ablation and Intrinsic Renal Disease," *N Engl J Med* 307 (1982): 652.

33. Pesticide Industry Usage and Sales: 1988 Market Estimates (EPA): 1989.

34. *Safe Food News* summer 1994, Food & Water, Inc. Marshfield, VT.

35. Jacobson, Lefferts, Garland, "Safe Food Eating Wisely in a Risky World" *Living Planet*, Venice Cal. 1991 p. 157.

36. Jacobson, Lefferts, Garland p. 155.

37. Ibid, p. 156.

38. Ibid, p. 164.

39. *Pediatrics* 83;27, 1989

40. Hoover, R., L. A. Gray, and B MacMahon 1976. "Menopausal estrogens and breast cancer," *NEJM* 295:401

41. Paffenberger, R.S., et al "Cancer risk as related to use of oral contraceptives during fertile years," *Cancer* 39: 1887.

42. Brinton, L.A., et al 1979 "Breast cancer risk factors among screening program participants," *J Natl Cancer Inst* 62:37.

43. Jacobson, Lefferts, Garland pp. 160-1

44. Simone, p. 106

45. Nan Kathryn Fuchs, *The Nutrition Detective* (Los Angeles: Jeremy P. Tarchers, 1985) p. 66.

46. Nathan Pritikin with Patrick M. McGrady Jr., *The Pritikin Program for Diet and Exercise* (New York: Grossett and Dunlap, 1974) p. 46.

47. Quillin, p. 113

48. Allan Luks and Joseph Barbato, *You Are What You Drink* (New York: Stonesong Press, 1989), p. 88

49. Frahm, p. 125.

50. Luks and Barbato, p. 59.

51. Fuchs, p. 66.

52. Annemarie Colbin, *Food and Healing* (New York: Ballantine Books, 1986), P. 162.

53. Maury M. Breecher and Shirley Linde, *Healthy Homes in a Toxic World* (New York: John Wiley and Sons, 1992), p. 34.

54. Mike Samuels and Nancy Samuels, *The Well Adult* (New York: Summit Books, 1988), p. 136.

55. Harper's Magazine, *The Complete Harper's Index* (New York: Henry Holt and Co., 1991), p. 149.

56. Joseph D. Weissman, *Choose to Live* (New York: Penguin Books, 1988), p. 31.

57. Frahm, p. 131

58. Harvey and Marilyn Diamond, *Living Health* (New York: Warner Books, 1987), pp. 69-70.

59. Frahm, p. 131.

60. Mary Kerney Levenstein, *Everyday Cancer Risks and How to Avoid Them* (Garden City Park, NY: Avery Publishing Group, 1992) p. 250.

61. Diamond, p. 75.

62. Levenstein, p. 250.

63. Weissman, p. 32.

64. Frahm, p. 134.

65. Karen Karvonen, "Toxic Tans: Why Healthy Tan Hurts," *Women's Sports and Fitness,* July-August 1992, p. 16.

66. Frances Munnings, "Sun Safety: Shedding Light on the Risks of Exposure," *The Physician and Sportmedicine,* July 1991, p. 100.

67. *Cancer Weekly,* 27 July 1992, p. 10.

68. Ibid, p. 10.

69. Sydney Hurwitz, as quoted by Alexandra Greely, "No Tan Is a Safe Tan:

Depletion of the Ozone Layer Impairs Protective Screen Against Cancer- causing Radiation," *Nutrition Health Review,* Summer 1991, p. 14.

70. Breecher, Linde, p. 13.

71. Ibid, p. 178.

72. Levenstein, p. 179.

73. Breecher, Linde, p. 179.

74. Levenstein, p. 180.

Chapter 3: My Health: Where Did I Lose It?

1. Dr. Eric Scott Kaplan, *Dr. Kaplan's Lifestyle of the Fit and Famous* (Lancaster, PA: Starburst Publishers, 1995), p. 259.

2. Kaplan, p. 258.

3. Mark and Patti Virkler, *Eden's Health Plan Go Natural!* (Shippensburg, PA: Destiny Image Publishers), 133.

4. Mark Bricklin and Maggie Spilner, *Walking for Health* (Emmaus, PA, 1992), 80.

5. Bricklin and Spilner, 5.

6. Ibid, 4.

7. Dean Ornish M.D., *Dr. Ornish's Program for Reversing Heart Disease,* (New York: Ballantine Books, 1990), 324.

8. Ibid, 325.

9. Albert E. Carter, The New Miracles of Rebound Exercise (A.L.M. Publishers, Fountain Hills, AZ, 1988), p. 50

10. Ibid, p. 38.

11. Ibid, p. 36.

12. Ibid, p.115.

13. Ibid, p. 40.

14. Ibid, pp., 31-2.

15. Ibid, p. 91.

Chapter 4: The Interrelation of Total Health

1. *Pediatrics* 83:27, 1989.

2. Emrika Padus, *The Complete Guide To Your Emotions And Your Health* (Rodale Press Inc., Emmaus, PA, 1992) pp. 99-100.

3. Ibid, p. 366.

Chapter 6: You Are What You Eat

1. J. Smith, "Hawaiian Milk Contamination Creates Alarm: A Sour Response by State Regulators," *Science* 217 (1982):137.

2. J. Ferrer, "Milk of Dairy Cows Frequently Contains Leukemogenic Virus," *Science* 213 (1981):1014.

3. Editorial, "Beware of the Cow," *Lancet* 2 (1974):30.

4. Harvey and Marilyn Diamond, *Living Health* (New York: Warner Books, 1987), p. 278.

5. Susan Stockton, *The Book of Health* (McLean Publishing, Tampa, FL, 1990), p. 140.

6. Ibid, pg 139-140.

7. Ibid, pg 140.

8. Ibid, pg 142.

9. Jacobson, Lefferts, Garland, "Safe Food: Eating Wisely in a Risky World" (Living Planet Press, Venice, CA, 1991), p. 83.

10. Jacobson, Lefferts, Garland, p. 79

11. Scott Fa, "Cow Milk and Insulin-Dependent Diabetes: Is There a Relationship?" *American Journal of Nutrition,* 1990; 51:489-91.

12. Frank A. Oski, M.D., *Don't Drink Your Milk!* (Teach Services, Brushton, NY, 1983), p. 56.

13. Oski, M.D., p. 55.

14. Ibid, p. 50.

15. John Robbins, Diet for a New America (Stillpoint Publishing, Walpole, NH, 1987), p. 195.

16. John A. McDougall, M.D., & Mary A. McDougall, The McDougall Plan (New Win Publishing, Inc., Clinton, NJ, 1983), p. 52.

17. S. Harris, "Statement of Stephanie G. Harris before the Subcommittee on Health and Scientific Research of the Senate Committee on Human Resources," 6-8-1977

18. B. Agranoff, "Diet and the Geographical Distribution of Multiple Sclerosis," *Lancet* 2 (1974):1061.

19. Oski, p. 22-24.

20. *Food & Water Journal* (Walden, VT, 1996), Volume 5, Number 1, p. 13.

21. Joseph D. Weissman, Choose to Live (New York: Penguin Books, 1988), p. 164.

22. Hulda Regehr Clark, The Cure for All Cancers (Promotion Publishing, San Diego, CA, 1993), p. 23.

23. Jacobson, Lifferts, Garland, p. 94.

24. James Michael Lennon *Health Science* (Tampa Fla, 1996) May/June, p. 38.

25. Biochem Biophys Res Commun 132(3): 1174-79, 1985

26. Agatha Thrash and Calvin Thrash Jr., "Nutrition for Vegetarians," (New Lifestyle Books, Seale, AL, 1982), p. 40.

27. Elson M. Haas, M.D., "Staying Healthy With Nutrition," (Celestial Arts Publishing, Berkeley, CA, 1992), p. 112.

28. Nancy Appleton, Ph.D., "Lick the Sugar Habit," (Avery Publishing Group Inc., Garden City Park, NY, 1988), p. 20.

29. Joel D. Wallach & Ma Lan, "Rare Earth's Forbidden Cures," (Double Happiness Publishing, Bonita, CA, 1996), p. 307.

30. Dr. Patrick Quillin, "Beating Cancer with Nutrition," (The Nutrition Times Press, Tulsa, OK, 1994), p. 62.

31. David Reuben, "Everything You Always Wanted to Know About Nutrition ," (New York: Simon and Schuster, 1978), p. 206.

Chapter 7: Water And Air

1. F. Batmanghelidj, M.D., "Your Body's Many Cries for Water," (Global Health Solutions, Falls Church, VA)

2. Jacobson, Lefferts, Garland, "Safe Food: Eating Wisely in a Risky World," (Living Planet Press, Venice, CA, 1981), p. 132.

3. Susan Stockton, *The Book of Health* (McLean Publishing, Tampa, FL, 1990), p. 116.

4. Ibid, p. 121.

5. Ibid, p. 124.

6. Ibid, p. 124.

7. Ibid, p. 125.

8. Ibid, p. 126.

9. Ibid, pp. 133-135.

10. Ibid, p. 135.

11. California Air Resources Staff Report (Sept. 1982)

12. Maury M. Breecher, Shirley Linde, Healthy Homes in a Toxic World (John Wiley & Sons, Inc., Toronto, 1992), pp 12-13.

Chapter 11: Nutritional Health

1. John Robbins, *Diet For A New America* (Stillpoint Publishing, Walpole, NH, 1987) p. 247.

2. Malter M., Schriever G., Eilber, U., "Natural Killer Cells, Vitamins and Other Blood Components of Vegetarian and Omnivorous Men." *Nutr Cancer,* (1989), 12:27, pp.1-78.

3. Patrick Quillin, Ph.D., R.D., Healing Nutrients (Random House Inc., New York, 1987) p. 127.

4. Foster, HD, *Int J Biosocial Res 10, 1, 17,* (1988).

5. Dean Ornish M.D., *Dr. Ornish's Program for Reversing Heart Disease* (New York: Ballantine Books, 1990), 324.

6. Edward Claflin, "Healing Yourself With Food" (Emmaus, PA: Rodale Press, Inc., 1995), 144.

7. John A. McDougall, M.D. & Mary A. McDougall, *The McDougall Plan* (New Win Publishing Inc., Clinton, NJ, 1983) p. 83.

8. Robbins, p. 270.

9. Ibid, p. 268.

10. Ibid, p. 195.

11. Dr. George H. Malkmus with Michael Dye, *God's Way To Ultimate Health* (Hallelujah Acres Publishing, Eidson, TN, 1995) p. 100.

12. T. Colin Campbell, Ph.D. and Christine Cox. "The China Project" (New Century Nutrition, Cornell Technology Park PO Box 4716 Ethaca, NY 14852, 1996)

13. Ihid, p. 27

14. Ibid, p. 29

15. Ibid, p. 29

16 Humbart Santillo, *Food Enzymes: The Missing Link to Radiant Health* (Prescott, AZ: Hohn Press, 1991) 26.

17. Dr. Edward Howell, *Enzyme Nutrition* (Wayne, NJ: Avery Publishing, 1985), 144.

18. Paavo, Airola, Ph.D, *How to Get Well* (Sherwood, OR: Health Plus, 1974), 210.

19. Paavo Airola, Ph.D, 210.

20. Ibid, p. 210.

21. Humbart Santillo, 16.

22. Ibid, p. 27.

23. Dr. Edward Howell, 27.

24. Jack Joseph Challem, *Spirulina: What It Is...The Health Benefits it Can Give You* (New Canaan, CT: Keats Publishing, Inc., 1981), 16.

25. Ibid, p. 16.

26. Robert Crayhon, *Total Health* (St. George, UT: Total Health Communicator, Inc., 1996), 27.

27. James F. Balch, M.D., Phyllis A. Balch, C.N.C., *Prescription for Nutritional Healing*, 2nd edition (Garden City Park, NY: Avery Publishing Group, 1997), 61.

28. Ibid, p. 61.

29. Ibid, p. 61.

30. John Heinerman, *Heinerman's Encyclopedia of Healing Juices* (West Nyack, NY: Packer Publishing Co., 1994), 37.

31. Dr. Edward Howel, p. 4.

32. Ibid

Chapter 12. Digestive Health

1. Humbart Santillo, *Food Enzymes: The Missing Link to Radiant Health* (Prescott, AZ: Hohn Press, 1991) 34-35.

2. Susan Stockton, *The Book of Health* (Tampa, FL: McLean Publishing, 1993), 140.

3. Santillo, 26.

4. Dr. Edward Howell, *Enzyme Nutrition* (Wayne, NJ: Avery Publishing, 1985), 144.

5. Santillo, 11.

6. Greg Anderson, *The 22 Non-Negotiable Laws of Wellness* (New York: Harper Collins Publishers, 1995), 45.

7. Stockton, 140.

8. Santillo, 12.

9. Ibid, 37.

10. Ibid, 37.

11. Howell, 116.

Chapter 13: Assimilative Health

1. *Lancet* 341; 49-:1993.

2. *Am. J. Physiol.* 258; 603: 1990.

3. *Annals Allergy*, 1990.

4. Elie Metchnikoff, *The Prolongation of Life* (New York & London: G.P. Putnam & Son's, The Knickerbocker Press, 1910).

5. Phylis Austin, Agatha Trash M.D., Calvin Thrash M.D., *Food Allergies Made Simple* (Sanfield, MI: Family Health Publications LLC, 1985), 5.

6. *Journal of Family Practice* 9 (2) 223-232, 1979.

7. Austin, Thrash M.D., Thrash M.D, 27.

8. Ibid, p. 27.

9. Ibid, p. 27.

Chapter 14: Eliminative Health

1. Hulda Regehr Clark, Ph.D., N.D. *The Cure For All Cancers* (San Diego, CA: ProMotion Publishing, 1993)

2. *Guyton and Hall Textbook of Medical Physiology*, 9th edition (Philadelphia, PA: WB Saunders Co., 1996), p. 503.

3. John A. McDougall, M.D. & Mary A. McDougall *The McDougall Plan* (Clinton, N.J.: New Win Publishing, 1983), p. 79

Chapter 15: Circulative Health

1. Susan Stockton, The Book of Health (MeLear Publishing, Tampa FL 1990) p.63

Chapter 16: Immune Health

1. *Biochem Biophys Res Commun* 132(3): 1174-79, 1985

2. Agatha Thrash and Calvin Thrash Jr., "Nutrition for Vegetarians," (New Lifestyle Books, Seale, AL, 1982) P. 40

3. Emricka Padus, *The Complete Guide to Your Emotions and Your Health* (Emmaus, PA: Rodale Press, 1992), 483

Chapter 17: Oxidative Health

1. Phylis Austin, Agatha Trash M.D., Calvin Thrash M.D., *Food Allergies Made Simple* (Sanfiled, MI: Family Health Publications LLC, 1985), 5

2. Majid Ali, M.D., *RDA Rats, Drugs and Assumptions* (Denville, N.J.: Life Span press, 1995), 198

3. Majid Ali, M.D., *The Butterfly and Life Span Nutrition* (Denville, J.J.: Institute of Preventative Medicine, 1992), 138

4. Majid Ali, M.D., *RDA*, 198

5. Ibid, p. 444

Chapter 18: Organ/Gland Health

1. *Journal of Traditional Chinese Medicine* 4 (4): pp. 283-288, 1984

Chapter 19 – Light And Energy

1. Kime, Z. *Sunlight* World Health Publications. Penryn CA, 1980. P. 31

2. Ibid, p. 47

3. Ibid, p. 53

4. Ibid, p. 53

5. Ibid, pp. 107-110

6. Ibid, p. 95

7. Ibid, p. 161

8. Ibid, p. 176

9. Ibid, p. 180

10. Ibid, p. 186

11. Ibid, p. 191

12. Ibid, pp. 191-192

13. Ibid, p. 192

14. Ibid, p. 192

15. Ibid, p. 193

16. Ibid, p. 193

17. Ibid, p. 207

18. Brian R. Clement with Theresa Foy DiGeronimo, *Living Foods for Optimum Health* (Prima Publishing, Rocklin, CA, 1996) p. 36

19. Ibid, pp. 36-37